Health Education

Health Education

Effectiveness and efficiency

KEITH TONES,
SYLVIA TILFORD
and
YVONNE KEELEY ROBINSON

London
CHAPMAN AND HALL

First published in 1990 by Chapman and Hall Ltd
11 New Fetter Lane, London EC4P 4EE

Published in the USA by Routledge, Chapman and Hall
29 West 35th Street, New York NY 10001

© 1990 Tones, Tilford and Robinson

Typeset in 10/12pt Plantin by EJS Chemical Composition, Bath, Avon
Printed in Great Britain by TJ Press Ltd,
Padstow, Cornwall

ISBN 0 412 32980 8

British Library Cataloguing in Publication Data

Tones, Keith
  Health Education.
  1. Health education
  I. Title   II. Tilford, Sylvia   III. Robinson, Yvonne Keeley
  613.07

  ISBN 0 412 32980 8

Library of Congress Cataloging in Publication Data available

CONTENTS

Contents

Contents

INTRODUCTION

It could be said with some justification that the task of education is to safe-guard people's right to learn about important aspects of human culture and experience. Since health and illness occupy a prominent place in our everyday experience, it might reasonably be argued that everyone is entitled to share whatever insights we possess into the state of being healthy and to benefit from what might be done to prevent and treat disease and discomfort. Health education's role in such an endeavour would be to create the necessary under-standing. No other justification would be needed.

In recent years, however, questions have been posed with increasing insistence and urgency about efficiency – both about education in general and health education in particular. We can be certain that such enquiries about effectiveness do not reflect a greater concern to know whether or not the population is better educated: they stem from more utilitarian motives.

It is apparent, even to the casual observer, that economic growth and productivity have become a central preoccupation in contemporary Britain. Economic success is seen as depending on the competitive urge which, among other things, should generate efficiency. It is, therefore, not surprising that health education should be required to prove itself – especially since both the education and health sectors have been subjected to critical scrutiny. In the first place, educational institutions are alleged to have failed to generate an entrepreneurial spirit; reforms have been urged which include setting attainment targets by which efficiency may be measured. Again, in the health service, alarm has been expressed at the seemingly insatiable demands for health care and ensuing galloping inflation. Economies have been required – again in the interests of efficiency; performance indicators have been developed to assess progress.

Unlike many traditional educational disciplines, health education has consistently sought not merely to provide understanding about its substantive subject matter but has concerned itself also with such goals as attitude change and lifestyle modification. Indicators of successful health education have, for this reason, defined much more than gains in knowledge and understanding. Moreover, since health education is regarded as an arm of preventive medicine (at any rate by health professionals), it has been subjected to the same economic imperative as other branches of the health service. Furthermore, since health education occasionally, and usually unwisely, claims that prevention can save money by reducing the need for expenditure on curative medicine, it is not at all surprising that the question 'Does health education work?' really means 'Is it successful in preventing unhealthy behaviours and reducing health service costs? Such a perspective is, of course, as limited as the narrowly-conceived view that economic growth and productivity is the most important recipe for human happiness. It is, nonetheless, important to recognize the impetus which economic philosophy provides in creating a demand that health education should prove itself.

This book is concerned with the effectiveness and efficiency of health education. The effectiveness question is important – for instance, we would like to know whether or not a 'self-empowerment model' of health education really can empower people – but the question of efficiency is usually more important. This is in part because we can, at a very general level, answer the question 'Does health education work?' with a simple affirmative: 'Yes, it does!' The reason for such a confident assertion derives from the fact that there have been major changes in health-related behaviours over the past decade and, in many instances, an associated decline in premature death and the incidence of disease. In the USA, Britain and many other developed nations, there has been a substantial reduction in smoking and other risk factors implicated in coronary heart disease. In many countries there has been a significant improvement in cardiovascular health. Since the factors influencing these changes – cultural, behavioural and, arguably, epidemiological – must have been mediated by various forms of information, communication, persuasion and other educational activities, it would be churlish not to credit health education with the achievement.

The important point to consider is, therefore, not so much **effectiveness** but rather **efficiency**. In other words we need to know not merely whether health education has been successful but rather how successful it has been. Efficiency is, thus, concerned with the extent to which health education has achieved a given outcome by comparison with some alternative intervention. In the economic context outlined above, the criterion might be one of relative cost. In another context the yardstick might be the extent to which dietary behaviour has changed and the explicit or implicit comparison might be between individually directed health education or the introduction of labelling or other controls on food production and distribution. It is much more difficult to respond to the question of how efficient a given programme has been in achieving some desirable goal than it is to examine the issue of effectiveness. The answer to such a question will almost inevitably be 'it depends'. It depends for instance on the nature of goals, the criteria of success, the way in which the education is delivered, the resources available. This is one of the issues which the book will seek to illuminate.

There are several reviews of published studies which report on the success achieved by various health education interventions. They all provide evidence of effectiveness (and ineffectiveness) but typically address the efficiency issue· either not at all or in an oblique way. For instance Gatherer *et al.* [1] ask 'Is health education effective?' He and his fellow authors then provide abstracts of research and an overview of evaluated studies. Bell *et al.* [2] provide an annotated bibliography of health education research in the UK which includes many studies of effectiveness. Green [3] has been assiduous over the years in producing comprehensive and detailed lists of evaluated work together with critiques of research design which make it possible to judge the reliability and validity of the studies. It is, however, difficult to draw conclusions of a general nature from this kind of work – except that many of the interventions they describe have been effective in the sense in which the term has been used above. Gatherer's review, for example, reported that 85% of 62 reported studies demonstrated an improvement in knowledge while 65% of 39 studies indicated that there had been a change of attitudes 'in the desired direction'. Of 123 studies which sought to produce behavioural change, 75% actually succeeded in doing so. However, apart from elementary questions about research design such as whether the claimed changes could really be attributed to the health education intervention, there are more fundamental issues to be addressed. Foremost among these is the question of practical as opposed to statistical significance. For instance, how big were the changes in knowledge, attitude and practice? Were they big enough to justify claims of success? How big should they have been before we could argue a programme had been effective? Do the studies which apparently showed no change demonstrate the inefficiency of health education – or was it merely the case that the methods used and the available resources were inappropriate to the task? Or was the task intrinsically unsuitable for treatment by health education? Certainly, the observations of Gatherer *et al.* [1] support the notion of ineffective delivery of the programme: 'The overall impression from much of the literature on health education is that too much of the health education practised is inappropriate for many, perhaps the majority, of the people for whom it is supposedly intended'.

It is, then, not possible to use reported research on effectiveness and efficiency – even when the research design has been impeccable – to reach conclusions about the success of health education. Before this is possible, we must be clear about the criteria by which a programme may be assessed and we must know a good deal about the circumstances associated with the design and delivery of the education. Two examples will serve to underline this assertion. The first of these describes a dietary intervention mounted in Spring, 1981, in a rural community in Finland [4].

Thirty Finnish couples were matched with 30 couples in southern Italy and an attempt was made to bring the Finns' dietary status more in line with the healthier status of the Italian group. They received intensive counselling and were provided with several '... strategic food items free of charge'. One dietitian visited six families frequently and also met them when they made a twice weekly visit to clinics for blood pressure measurement. The intervention was manifestly effective: by the end of the counselling the Finnish families' diets approximated to the healthier Mediterranean type of diet. The proportion of energy derived from fats declined from 39% to 24%; the ratio of polyunsaturated to saturated fats increased from less than 0.2 to more than 1.0 (as compared with a shift in the P/S ratio from 0.24 to 0.32 recommended by NACNE, [6]). The total serum cholesterol level also declined and there was a reduction in blood pressure in every subject. The intervention lasted six weeks and afterwards, subjects reverted to their normal (and presumably preferred) diets. The various physiological indicators followed suit along with their risk status.

The study appears to have been methodologically sound and the results genuine. Criteria of success were certainly consistent with a medical model – behaviour change associated with clinical improvement. Educational methods were appropriate and the choice of face-to-face counselling and behaviour modification techniques were consistent with learning theory. It was in most ways an efficient as well as an effective programme since it is hard to imagine how alternative educational strategies might have been used to achieve a better result. However, it is unlikely that such an approach would be widely used since the use of one dietitian per six families would almost certainly be considered too expensive. We cannot ignore the values underlying evaluation and the political factors which determine the priorities to be accorded to these. For instance it might well be the case that the alternative to the intervention described above would be to undertake the much more substantial costs involved in treating the disease which the intervention might well have prevented – probably because the necessary shift in resources from acute to preventive sectors would be politically unacceptable. The net result of the process of prioritization might well be a token mass media campaign which would be neither effective nor efficient.

The second example concerns the teaching of breast self-examination (BSE). This is a relatively inexpensive screening strategy designed to achieve early detection of potentially lethal abnormalities on the assumption that early intervention will result in a better chance of cure. A more expensive alternative device for detecting breast lumps in post-menopausal women is the technique of mammography. The study described here sought to compare the efficiency of BSE with mammography. Its starting point was that BSE is often ineffectively performed due to the use of inappropriate teaching techniques. Indeed, common sense, let alone learning theory, would suggest that the acquisition of the psychomotor skill involved in BSE will not be efficiently acquired by the use of, for instance, pamphlets or even filmed models. Pennypacker *et al.* [5] utilized learning theory to create the proper conditions for the acquisition of the skill: they provided an opportunity for skills practice and provided immediate knowledge of results of successful examination of breast tissues. They employed not only silicon models of the breast to provide practice but also supplied television and computer-assisted display of information when women transferred their learning from the silicon models to their own breasts. As a result women not only acquired efficient scanning techniques but also learned to exert the right degree of pressure and discriminate normal from abnormal tissue. According to the researchers, the sample studied was more efficient than a mammography unit at detecting small lumps (a 5.8% hit rate compared with 5.3%). However, rather like the first study cited above, although the relative effectiveness (i.e. the efficiency) of the method was superior to competing techniques, the costs involved in the high technology, staffing and training would render it inappropriate for general use.

Apart from illustrating the complexity of determining efficiency and the political problems associated with basing decisions purely on the evidence of the relative effectiveness of competing strategies, the two studies [4, 5] allow us to make an important generalization. Provided that a given teaching method is based on sound educational theory, it is usually possible to achieve desired objectives. A good understanding of the psycho–social factors underpinning decision-making and behaviour will help us design specific interventions which will be successful. However, the application of this understanding will often be severely curtailed by practical and political considerations. For instance there may be insufficient skilled personnel and resources to supply the conditions for efficient learning; the theoretically appropriate methods may be too time-consuming or even unethical. For these reasons this book will not make any further comment on the effectiveness and efficiency of particular methods – such as group discussion, role play and face-to-face counselling – it will confine its consideration of effectiveness and efficiency to the macro or strategic level. It will, in other words, relate the question of success to the broader strategies involved in delivering health education: mass media, schools, health service, workplace, community.

This book is concerned, then, with general questions of success. It will not provide a detailed compendium of exemplars of effectiveness, nor is it intended to be an evaluation primer – although in Chapter Two it does seek to remind readers of the major research approaches to evaluation. The first issue it addresses has to do with the meaning of success. Chapter One shows how the measurement of effectiveness and efficiency must ultimately depend on how success is defined. The definition of success will, in turn, be based on ideology and philosophy. Since there are wide divergences of view about the purpose of health education, indicators of performance should, logically, be derived from a statement of the values underpinning programme goals.

The second issue is more technical and concerns the design of evaluations. Research design, despite its image, is not a mechanically scientific process involving the choice of an off-the-peg formula. It requires careful thought about the nature of the successful outcome, the use to which results will be put and the degree of insight which these results will provide into programme efficiency. It will remind us that there are different kinds of evaluation all having different capabilities for application to practice; it will also remind us that, like health education itself, there are important ethical issues to be considered in the research process.

The third issue concerns the role of theory. Reference has already been made to the importance of learning theory in determining the choice of teaching method. The whole book, in fact, is based on the premise that sound theory is essential to the design of effective, efficient and practical programmes. This contention is illustrated by the particular case of the choice of indicators. There are a wide variety of markers which might be used as measures of performance, and selecting those which most readily reflect the nature and degree of success achieved by any given health education enterprise is no easy matter. Chapter Three attempts to show how theoretical considerations should influence choice of indicator. It illustrates the point by describing how the Health Action Model and Communication of Innovations Theory provide a basis for reasoned choice of measures of outcome and both indirect and intermediate indicators of programme efficiency.

The remainder of the book seeks to illuminate these and other evaluation issues in the general context of five main delivery strategies as indicated above: schools, health service, mass media, workplace and community. It is therefore appropriate at this point to make a second generalization about the potential efficiency of health education. In the first place, any given educational goals will be more efficiently achieved when the five strategies listed above operate as part of a coordinated community-wide programme. Secondly, there is a synergistic effect when health education is supported by policy: maximal efficiency will therefore occur when a coherent health education programme is supported by appropriate legal, fiscal, economic and environmental measures – and vice versa. Although this book does not directly address the effectiveness of social policy changes in enhancing health, the postulated synergism between education and social policy should always be borne in mind when considering the efficiency of either kind of intervention.

The education system has been widely seen as a major institution for the delivery of health education. Chapter Four will assess the contribution it makes at a number of levels – from individual outcomes within the classroom to national policies and activities which support school activities. Both hospital and primary care services have been urged to develop the educational component of their activities – not least because, as we have seen above, educational inputs have been viewed as means of contributing to cutting health care costs. Chapter Five will examine the philosophical approach adopted to education in a health care context, the success of education as exemplified by a small number of outcomes, and will conclude with a general discussion of factors which enhance educational activity in primary care and in hospitals.

Chapter Six seeks to provide a theoretical analysis of the use of mass media as a delivery strategy and identifies the features which distinguish this from all other strategies discussed here. In general it supports the view that the proper application of social marketing principles will increase the chances of success – while at the same time noting the fallacy of assuming that the process of marketing health is basically the same as that which is involved in selling commercial products. The chapter also reinforces the book's general contention about synergy and asserts that mass media are most effectively employed in the context of an integrated community programme. A larger and wider variety of specific evaluations have been included in this chapter compared with those chapters considering alternative delivery systems. This decision has been made because of the typically inflated aspirations entertained for mass media use. Attempts are therefore made to indicate the limitations of this particular strategy and also to show how different features of programme construction – the content of the messages, the target population and the intrinsic variations in the type of media used – can influence the chances of achieving success. It is hoped in this way to generate more realistic expectations of what mass media can achieve.

Chapter Seven examines health promotion in the workplace – a strategy which offers several interesting insights into the meaning of effectiveness and efficiency. The workplace provides excellent examples of the way in which different philosophies and models of health education give rise to widely divergent criteria of success. Moreover the worksite illustrates the potential synergy between health policy and education in the form of, for instance, alcohol policy development and employee assistance programmes. In addition, evaluation of health education in the workplace provides us with some of the hardest evidence of effectiveness and efficiency.

The final chapter can, in some way, be seen as integrative in that community initiatives on which it concentrates may incorporate each and every one of the strategies discussed in earlier chapters. However, this chapter's major value is probably the way in which it illustrates how substantial differences in philosophy can underpin superficially similar approaches and tactics – which may therefore require different evaluation designs and have to be judged by very different criteria. Chapter Eight also allows us to re-assert the primacy of theory in devising sensible evaluations and re-examining the relationship between quantitative and qualitative research tactics. When considering the most thoroughly documented, properly evaluated and comprehensively structured programmes, it is hard to escape the conclusion that health education can certainly be effective and even efficient when the interventions are theoretically sound and properly designed.

No attempt is made in this book to relate the contents specifically to the UK scene – nor to review the international literature systematically. Rather it selects eclectically whatever examples suit the purposes of any given chapter. We choose from whatever source seems most appropriate to provide evidence in support of our arguments and assertions. However, because our experience is primarily of UK situations and the available evidence of effectiveness and efficiency tends to have been generated in North America, most examples will be derived from Britain and USA.

REFERENCES

1. Gatherer, A., Parfit, J., Porter, E. and Vessey, M. (1979) *Is Health Education Effective?* Health Education Council, London.
2. Bell, J., Billington, D. R., Macdonald, M., Drummond, N. and Thompson, G. (1985) *Annotated Bibliography of Health Education Research completed in Britain from 1948–1978 and 1979–1983*, Scottish Health Education Group, Edinburgh.
3. Green, L. W. and Lewis, F. M. (1986) *Measurement and Evaluation in Health Education and Health Promotion*, Mayfield, Palo Alto, California.
4. Koskela Kaj (personal communication).
5. Pennypacker, H. S., Goldstein, M. K. and Stein, G. H. (1982) Efficient technology of training breast self-examination, in: *Public Education About Cancer* (ed. P. Hobbs), UICC Technical Report Series, UICC, Geneva.
6. NACNE (1983) A discussion paper on proposals for nutritional guidelines for health education in Britain, Health Education Council, London.

1

THE MEANING OF SUCCESS

The fundamental purpose of the evaluation process is to determine the value or worth of an activity. In passing judgement on this activity, the evaluator comments on its success or failure in respect of some valued goal. Evaluation is concerned with effectiveness, i.e. it says whether or not the valued goal has been achieved. It also makes statements about efficiency by providing an indication of the extent to which the measures designed to achieve the valued goal have been effective, by comparing them with alternative and competing measures.

The implicit assumption underlying health education is, of course, that it is a worthwhile activity and is in some way good for people. It would, however, be wrong to assume that health educators have a common value system. Health education is no mere technical operation: health educators have different philosophies of professional practice which reflect their own values and define what it is they believe to be worthwhile about their professional goals. Although this situation is not peculiar to health education, those who seek to educate about health are subject not only to the intrinsic controversies of education but have also to address the problem of defining the nebulous notion of health. The difficulties involved in clarifying professional values are compounded by health education's lack of professional status. Although many people have challenged the desirability of professionalizing health education, the absence of the unifying framework of theory and practice which this process normally provides will tend to generate disagreement about aims and values.

This whole rather confusing scenario is further clouded by the recent emergence of the **health promotion movement**. For some, health promotion is an activity synonymous with health education; for others it is a related but substantially different process having different goals and values. Since health education is not a unitary process having a universally accepted philosophy and clear goals, it therefore follows that it is not possible to provide an unequivocal definition of what constitutes success without first examining the values upon which different approaches to health education are based. And since there now appears to be some confusion between health education and health promotion it would seem appropriate to try to resolve this demarcation dispute prior to considering the nature of the different health education approaches. Accordingly this chapter will consider the ways in which health promotion relates to three different models of health education and will subsequently examine the implications of this analysis for the definition of success and failure which is central to the process of evaluation.

THE MEANING OF HEALTH PROMOTION

It is not the purpose of this chapter to provide a detailed analysis of health promotion; comprehensive reviews may be found elsewhere [1, 2]. The term health promotion has been associated with various undertakings [3]. For instance it has been used to distinguish attempts to foster positive health from those designed to prevent disease. It also figured prominently in the influential series of publications produced by the US Department of Health, Education and Welfare [4, 5, 6] where it was contrasted with 'Health Protection' and 'Preventive Health Services'. In that context it was characterized by the specification of a series of precise and specific 'Objectives for the Nation' which were concerned with primary prevention. In a third manifestation, health promotion has been the label attached to the marketing of health by means of the persuasive use of mass media and associated promotional tactics borrowed directly from commercial advertising practice. Others, however, have adopted what is semantically a more logical course and used the term to refer to any measure designed to promote health. In such a guise, health education will form an integral part of health promotion [7]. The World Health Organization [WHO] adopts this perspective [8], viewing health promotion as a '... unifying concept for those who recognize the need for change in the ways and conditions of living, in order to promote health.' Indeed the health promotion programme is considered to be the major strategy for achieving the global target of Health for All by the Year 2000 (HFA 2000). Health promotion in this sense is therefore concerned with all the factors which influence health. The most important of these are represented in Figure 1.1.

For present purposes, health is viewed as both a positive state of wellbeing and as absence of disease. Four major influences affect health status: (i) the health and medical services, (ii) genetic endowment, (iii) individual behaviours and (iv) the socio-economic and physical environment. How would health promotion conceived as a broad-based strategy seek to manipulate these four major influences?

First of all, it is clear that apart from genetic counselling little can be done to influence one of the most important inputs to health. It is perhaps unfortunate that the advice to choose one's parents carefully cannot be followed! It is however possible to influence individual behaviour and lifestyle and this has been the main goal of traditional health education. As for the health and medical services, an equally traditional goal has been to promote the proper use of such services. However, in addition to reasserting the hallowed principle that health is more than the absence of disease but rather a state of mental,

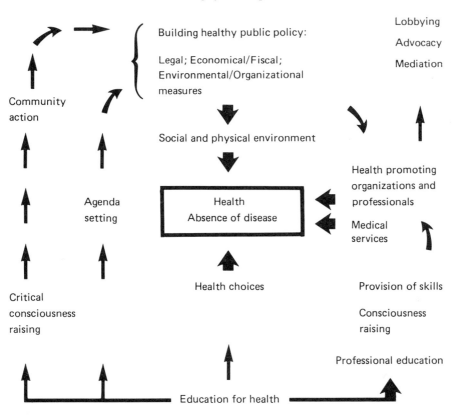

Figure 1.1 The contribution of education to health promotion. From Tones, B. K. (1987) *Promoting health: the contribution of education.* Paper presented at WHO Consultation on Co-ordinated Infrastructure for Health Education, Copenhagen.

physical and social wellbeing, the new health promotion programme of WHO differs from earlier concerns in the following important ways:

1. It acknowledges that health promotion is an intersectoral activity. Following the tenets of primary health care [9], health promotion is not considered to be the preserve of the medical services. As the Faculty of Community Medicine stated recently [10], '... the main responsibility for ensuring the prerequisites for health lies outside the health sector'; industry, trades unions and the professions must assume this responsibility.
2. The programme argues that health and medical services must be reoriented in order to meet consumer needs in a holistic and responsive way. This process of demedicalization should be paralleled by increasing lay involvement and community participation. People must be helped to gain control over their own health.

3

3. It asserts the supreme importance of the physical and socio-economic environment in determining health and illness. The World Health Organization seeks to achieve a new public health through political action [11]. In the words of the Ottawa Charter for Health Promotion [12], WHO is concerned to 'build healthy public policy' and 'create supportive environments'.

HEALTH EDUCATION AND HEALTH PROMOTION: A SYMBIOTIC RELATIONSHIP

The central feature of health promotion is its concern to build a system conducive to health through the development of policy at local and national levels. Health policies seek to achieve environmental change by implementing legal, fiscal and economic measures. They are also concerned to produce changes in organizations in the interests of the health of their members and their clients. The relative effectiveness of this social engineering approach has long been recognized. It has, for instance, been argued for many years that the best way to curb problem drinking is by means of regular increases in the taxation on alcohol. Again, it is generally accepted that the most efficient method of achieving the primary prevention of dental caries is through fluoridation of drinking water. At a more fundamental level, the association between health and socio-economic status has been unequivocally demonstrated [13] and, according to the Black Report [14], only a massive financial investment can radically alter the social class gradient in ill health and tackle the diseases of poverty. All such public policy measures have been said to improve health by 'making the healthy choice the easy choice' [15]. Health education has, self evidently, been concerned to influence health choices throughout its history, so what is its status in the context of the new health promotion movement? Is it now more or less important? Is it in danger of being marginalized, or has it moved closer to centre stage? In fact education for health (as it is now being called by WHO) is an essential prerequisite in all health promotion programmes. The relationship between health education and the process of building healthy public policy is symbiotic. Indeed it could be argued that health promotion consists of an amalgam of policy development and health education. Health promotion, therefore, consists of any combination of education and related legal, fiscal, economic, environmental and organizational interventions designed to facilitate the achievement of health and the prevention of disease.

The particular contributions made by education to health promotion may be seen in Figure 1.1. Its traditional function is to influence individual **health choices**; its more radical role is to influence the adoption of healthy public policies by raising public awareness of the issues in question. Two variations on this theme have been shown in Figure 1.1. One is that of **agenda setting** – a term which has been used to describe the process of generating public consciousness about a health problem prior to introducing some legislative measure. Since social engineering of this sort will normally involve some infringement of individual liberty, those whose liberty has been thus threatened may have to be softened up by precursor education before politicians – national or local – might be willing to take potentially unpopular actions. For example, although health education alone never succeeded in raising the level of front seat-belt wearing in UK by more than about 16% [16], it was manifestly successful in paving the way for subsequent legislation which has been effective in preventing injury and saving life lost in road traffic accidents.

The other variation on the awareness raising theme is more radical in intent and the term **critical consciousness raising** is reserved for this educational intervention. It is a translation of Freire's [17] notion of conscientizacion and, unlike agenda setting, is concerned not merely to have people think about issues but to examine critically their lives, their circumstances and the environment in which they live. They should then take action as a community and pressure politicians into implementing policies which they might find not only financially damaging but ideologically distasteful. For instance, whereas government might be willing to implement legislation to fluoridate public water supplies provided that it was convinced it would not suffer electoral disadvantage, it would in all probability baulk at the proposals of the Black Report [14] to deal with poverty. In August 1980, the then Secretary of State for Social Services pointed out that '... additional expenditure on the scale which could result from the report's recommendations – the amount involved could be upwards of £2 billion a year – is quite unrealistic ...' [18]. Presumably only concerted community action could result in a change of heart or a change of government.

It can also be seen from Figure 1.1 that another educational strand contributes to the overall health promotion process. This is labelled **professional education** and refers to attempts to influence health and other professionals. Its aim is twofold: first to persuade decision-makers to assume health promoting responsibilities and second to facilitate the delivery of health services which would meet real community needs. Professional education thus has a consciousness raising function and a second function which involves providing the skills which health personnel need in order to become effective health promoters and health educators.

It will be noted from Figure 1.1 that the related processes of lobbying, advocacy and mediation are an integral part of health promotion [12]. **Lobbying** refers to attempts to influence policy directly through the intervention of powerful individuals or pressure groups. **Advocacy** describes a similar activity but assumes that the lobbying is on behalf of a third party.

Mediation consists of a kind of arbitration which seeks to resolve the conflicting interests in society when these threaten health policy implementation. Although it is not easy to make any clear-cut distinctions, these three kinds of social encounter are not synonymous with health education – although clearly some education and teaching of individual decision-makers might be involved.

HEALTH EDUCATION: APPROACHES AND PHILOSOPHIES

Health education has thus far been defined in the context of health promotion in functional terms. However, if we are to base our discussion of evaluation on a firm foundation we need to give further thought to the values which govern interpretations of educational success. For instance we could say that health education has been successful if it raises awareness and leads to the implementation of policy: yet we have identified two varieties of awareness raising – agenda setting and critical consciousness raising – which differ not merely in their goals but in their underlying philosophy. Again, we might say that professional education has been effective if professionals have acquired certain skills. However, supposing that those skills helped the professional to coerce and manipulate patients into complying unthinkingly with medical advice – could we really say that the enterprise had been successful? While the learning might have been efficient, the education would have been a failure when judged by the WHO goal of HFA 2000 in that it would have disempowered patients rather than enhanced their participation. Furthermore, if we consider from Figure 1.1 the third contribution which health education may make to health promotion, it will be recalled that it has to do with influencing choices. What should be the direction of this influence? Should it, for example, be to change attitudes? Or should it be to facilitate decision-making? Clearly this will depend on the professional philosophy.

It is, of course, possible to describe the process of health education in a relatively neutral way. We could, for instance, define health education as any activity which promotes health-related learning, i.e. some relatively permanent change in an individual's competence or disposition. Effective health education may thus produce changes in understanding or ways of thinking; it may bring about some shift in belief or attitude; it may influence or clarify values; it may facilitate the acquisition of skills; it may even effect changes in behaviour or lifestyle. The task of evaluation for health education defined in this way would then be to determine to what extent health-related learning had taken place. More typically, however, health education is not defined in such a neutral manner. Indeed health education is frequently characterized by dialectical dispute and divisive debate and its rationale reflects the ideological differences of its practitioners. It is, therefore, hardly surprising that typologies of health education have been based on philosophy rather than function, on values rather than learning theory.

A review of contemporary models of health education is beyond the scope of this book. Suffice it to say that several interesting analyses have been produced in recent time [19, 20, 21, 22]. For the purpose of demonstrating the implications of adopting one or other approach for the practice of evaluation, a system derived from a paper by the author [23] will be discussed. This identifies three models for classifying health education.

THREE APPROACHES TO HEALTH EDUCATION

The Preventive Model

The first approach to be considered might be labelled a **Preventive Model**. While the term model is frequently misused, it is employed here because the meaning of Medical Model – from which the approach to health education currently under discussion is derived – is widely understood and accepted. The goal of the Preventive Model of Health Education is to persuade the individual to take responsible decisions, i.e. to adopt behaviours which will prevent disease at primary, secondary or tertiary levels (Table 1.1). This is the traditional and orthodox approach which also incorporates the sub-goal of proper utilization of health services (to prevent disease at primary, secondary and tertiary levels). Occasionally, in an attempt to refurbish a somewhat negative image, or as a deliberate marketing strategy, the Preventive Model may claim to be promoting positive health but its definition of success is unambiguous. It is concerned to produce behavioural outcomes. Health education will have been effective only to the extent that individuals or communities demonstrate that they have adopted a more healthy lifestyle. For instance, successful health education about heart disease would be able to show that there had been an increased level of exercise together with various medically approved dietary changes such as a reduction in the intake of saturated fats. People would also have stopped smoking. The individual designated at-risk would dutifully attend for screening and would comply with any anti-hypertensive medication prescribed by the GP. The ensuing measurable reduction in risk should ideally be supported by hard medical and epidemiological evidence of effectiveness. Decreases in blood pressure and serum lipid levels should be followed at a decent interval by an appropriate decline in coronary heart disease (CHD) morbidity and mortality.

The Preventive Model has been subjected to increasing criticism in recent years along with its parent Medical Model [24]. This critique considers the individual focus of the preventive approach to health education as both unethical and ineffective in that it ignores the real socio-political roots of ill health. This is classically illustrated by Zola's well known 'river analogy'

7

Table 1.1 Health education and the preventive model

Level of prevention	Function of health education
Primary	
Concerned to prevent onset of disease; reduce incidence	Persuade individuals to adopt behaviours believed to reduce the risk of disease; adopt healthy lifestyle. Persuade individuals to utilize preventive health services appropriately. NB Concerned with 'health behaviour', i.e. those activities undertaken by an individual who believes that (s)he is healthy in order to prevent future health problems or detect them at an asymptomatic stage.
Secondary	
Concerned to prevent development of existing disease, minimize its severity, reverse its progress; reduce prevalence	Persuade individuals to utilize screening services appropriately; learn appropriate self care; seek early diagnosis and treatment. Persuade individuals to comply with medical treatment and other recommendations.
Tertiary	
Concerned to prevent deterioration, relapse and complications; promote rehabilitation; help adjustment to terminal conditions	Persuade individuals to comply with medical treatment and adjust to limitations resulting from disease. Persuade patients to resume healthy state and abandon sick role. Provision of counselling for patients and caretakers.

of medical care (Zola [25] cited by McKinlay [26]). This parable describes a doctor's increasingly frenzied rescue efforts as he drags drowning men from the flood. The doctor says: 'You know I am so busy jumping in, pulling them to shore, applying artificial respiration, that I have no time to see who the hell is upstream pushing them all in'.

McKinlay would consider the individually oriented approach of preventive health education as an integral part of 'downsteam endeavours'. He points out the ultimate futility of this kind of strategy and argues that we should '... cease our preoccupation with this short-term problem-specific tinkering and begin focusing our attention upstream'.

If McKinlay's advice is followed and we refocus upstream, we find that the true origin of disease is not individual behaviour but a number of more fundamental social and economic influences. These comprise not only the manufacturers of unhealthy products but, according to some commentators, the very political fabric of society [27]. For instance the Politics for Health Group [28] argues that '... the major force responsible for the social production of an unhealthy diet is the drive of the food industry to accumulate profits ...'.

Crawford [29] and others have applied Ryan's seminal notion of **victim blaming** [30] to the Preventive Model of health education, claiming that it is not only inefficient but manifestly unethical to blame the victim for adopting an unhealthy lifestyle when society itself engenders and sustains the very unhealthy habits which health education seeks to eliminate. Indeed there are those who argue that the Preventive Model's acceptability to many western industrialized societies is due not only to the conviction that it may save money for hard-pressed health services, but also to its congruence with an ideology which emphasizes individual endeavour and competitiveness. Navarro [31] adopts this stance:

> ... rather then weakening, (health education) ... strengthens the basic tenets of bourgeois individualism ... far from being a threat to the power structure, this life-style politics complements and is easily co-optable by the controllers of the system.

This radical stance typically includes a critique of medicalization, i.e. the tendency of the medical profession to take over many of the normal aspects of living. It might be thought, therefore, that the holistic health movement, with its pursuit of positive health and high level wellness, would be considered an acceptable bedfellow for those arguing against a victim-blaming approach. On the contrary, the phalanx of narcissistic, non-smoking, diet-conscious joggers serves merely to distract attention from the true roots of ill health. Crawford [32], in an influential review of what he terms **healthism**, argues that a healthist ideology fosters a continued depoliticization and therefore an undermining of the social effort to improve health and wellbeing.

Radical–Political Model

So, those who reject the victim-blaming ideology of the Preventive Model might be said to advocate a **Radical–Political Model** of health education. Its goal is to get to the roots of the problem of ill health or, to change the metaphor, 'refocus upstream'. It is concerned to achieve social and environmental change by triggering political action. The critical consciousness raising aspect of the approach has already been described in the earlier discussion of health promotion. It should, however, be noted that while this strategy to promote health through the building of healthy public policy is by definition acceptable to the Radical–Political Model, the more limited agenda setting function is not. Indeed the agenda setting task of precursor health education described earlier is a logical extension of the Preventive Model in that it seeks to trigger change which is congruent with government policy and an ideology which, at the time of writing in the UK and USA, urges individuals to look after themselves as part of an emphasis on both self-reliance and economic productivity.

It is apparent that measures of success for a Radical–Political Model of health education would require very different evaluative measures than the narrower preventive approach. Health educators would need to demonstrate at the very least a heightened level of awareness or critical consciousness. Ideally a consciousness raising programme would also lead to measurable action. Freudenberg [33], arguing for an approach to health education which seeks to promote social rather than individual change, cites the following examples of effectiveness:

1. In the context of the women's health movement:
   (a) Writing papers individually or in groups and presenting these as a course for women on women and their bodies.
   (b) Forming a Committee Against Sterilization Abuse which led to a new law calling for mandatory counselling and a 30 day waiting period between the decision for sterilization and the surgery.
2. In the context of occupational safety and health:
   The formation of the Carolina Brown Lung Association which explains safety procedures to textile workers, teaches them how to monitor dust levels and how to take action when legal standards are violated.
3. In the context of the environmental movement:
   The case of a group of mothers in New Jersey who were alerted to a cluster of child cancer deaths in an industrial area and formed an organization which ultimately forced the State to begin an epidemiological investigation.

If we were to apply the Radical–Political Model to the prevention of CHD, its focus would not be on the individual but on the various social, economic and political factors promoting unhealthy products and practices. The tobacco manufacturers and the food and agriculture industries would be legitimate targets. Evaluation of such a health education programme would, therefore, include measures of public awareness of the ways in which certain commercial interests damaged health. More specifically, a local campaign might be judged a success if, after uniting a parent-teacher association and a school's governing body, it managed to influence the local education authority's school meals policy. In the last analysis effectiveness would consist of the establishment of a cafeteria system which did not promote the consumption of foods high in saturated fat content. Would it be a measure of even greater success if healthy food alone were on sale? Or should health education always provide for choice?

Self-Empowerment Model

The third model of health education to be considered is a **Self-Empowerment Model**. It derives from an Educational Model whose philosophy reflects the Society for Public Health Education of America's (SOPHE) goal of fostering informed choice. If there were such a thing as an official line on health education, then an educational model would have to receive such an accolade. In fact after a long and exhaustive debate – as part of an even longer process of professionalization – SOPHE has emphasized the principle of voluntariness as a *sine qua non* of professional practice. In its Code of Ethics [34], SOPHE asserts:

> Health Educators value privacy, dignity, and the worth of the individual, and use skills consistent with these values. Health educators observe the principle of informed consent with respect to individuals and groups served. Health Educators support change by choice, not by coercion.

After a little reflection on SOPHE's value position, it will be apparent that not only is the Preventive Model inconsistent with professional practice as thus defined but the Radical–Political Model – and even health promotion itself – would need careful reassessment. It is obvious that the goal of the Preventive Model is to change behaviour by fair means or foul – philosophically speaking. It would also appear on occasions that advocates of the Radical–Political Model are determined to massage the political consciousness of communities in order to bring about social changes dear to the heart of health educators rather than helping the community make its own decisions. Again, where the WHO stresses the principle of empowerment in health promotion, many of those who have enthusiastically adopted health promotion seem to be determined not merely to make the healthy choice the easy choice but rather to make the healthy choice the only choice! This model is consistent with the view of those philosophers who argue that education is a very different process from other attempts to influence people – such as propaganda, persuasion, instruction, training or any other non-rational methods which either rely on coercion in different degrees or give no thought to the moral nature of the outcome of the learning. At its simplest (and in some ways most naïve) form it would consist merely of providing knowledge. Success is not only easy to define but relatively easy to achieve in this model! A programme of education about contraception would need to demonstrate that the target group had understood and remembered the various facts, concepts and principles underlying the nature of contraception and contraceptive practice – together with related subordinate notions such as the physiology of reproduction. The naïvety of this model rests on the implication that knowledge is sufficient to facilitate informed decision-making. It may be necessary but it is certainly not sufficient. A more sophisticated version of this model would, therefore, argue that the cognitive input should be supplemented by non-traditional teaching methods which would ensure the clarification of values underlying decision-making and would also provide an opportunity to practice decision-making – albeit in a hypothetical context. This process is illustrated in Figure 1.2. These additions to a simple cognitive model will require additional evaluative criteria. The evaluator will now expect to find evidence that individuals have clarified their values and have acquired some new skill in making decisions in a situation simulating real life. Further consideration of this approach to fostering decision-making will, however, make it clear that the prospect of promoting genuine informed choice in this way is illusory.

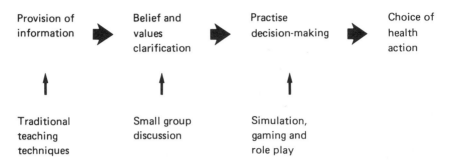

Figure 1.2 An educational model and associated methodology.

While the barriers of ignorance can be readily overcome, other barriers are less amenable to change. The nature of these obstacles to free and informed decision-making have been explored in depth elsewhere [35, 36]. For present purposes it is sufficient to comment that those who are already addicted to some substance have their freedom of choice curtailed. As McKeown [37] put it, '… with a drug of addiction the option is open only at the beginning'. Less obviously, decision-making may be restricted by an individual's primary socialization and previous life experiences. On the one hand it would be exceedingly difficult for a properly socialized Mormon or Seventh Day Adventist to choose not to be healthy while the socialization of children from a disadvantaged sector of society would militate against healthy decision-making. Of greater significance still are the environmental and social structural barriers frequently experienced by lower socio-economic groups – which are related to the adverse socialization mentioned above. It would, for example, be foolish, not to say callous, to claim that a middle-class man has the same options open to him as, say, a single woman having several children under 14 and living in deprived and impoverished circumstances and sub-standard housing. It is for these various reasons that advocates of an Educational Model would be accused of victim blaming by those who support radical–political action. However, the third model of health education considered here would seek to respond to this fully justifiable criticism of certain kinds of individually focused educational programmes by providing strategies for self-empowerment which are designed to remove at least some of the major barriers to genuine informed decision-making.

The Self-Empowerment Model, therefore, seeks to facilitate choice not merely by providing understanding, value clarification and practice in decision-making, but by attempting to empower the individual. It incorporates a fundamental tenet that in a democratic society social change can occur only by empowering individuals or groups of individuals to modify their environment. Self-empowerment will not, of course, occur as a mere by-product of critical consciousness raising. If it is to happen at all it will be as a result of training. There is a sound theoretical and practical basis for this work – for instance in Freire's work in developing countries [17] and in the various lifeskills strategies described by Hopson and Scally [38, 39, 40, 41]. At first glance, lifeskills training has some fairly specific health-related goals – such as stress management or ways of coping with unemployment. However, more important is the way in which the various specific lifeskills may contribute both directly and indirectly – and cumulatively – to changes in the way in which individuals view themselves. For instance, teaching people how to be assertive, to communicate effectively and to be positive about themselves, not only provides them with useful social skills to facilitate choice, but also promotes personal growth. More specifically, such personal growth would hopefully involve self-efficacy beliefs, i.e. a belief that it is possible to be in charge of one's life; it should include the capacity to resist social pressures and act proactively rather than merely reacting to the immediate demands of circumstances; it should result in enhanced self-esteem. Moreover, insofar as assertiveness and high self-esteem might be defined as mental and social health goals in their own right, a Self-Empowerment Model of health education could be said to promote health positively and directly as well as facilitating health choices of any and every kind. The process is outlined in Figure 1.3. It is worth

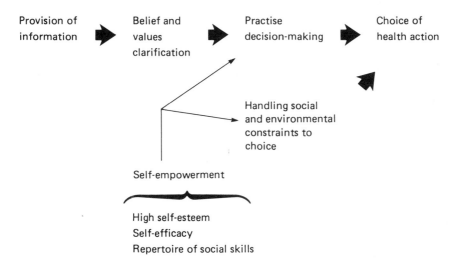

Figure 1.3 Major elements of a self-empowerment model.

observing here that the educational inputs which contribute to the kind of self-empowered choices referred to above may equally facilitate political activities congruent with the goals of the Radical–Political Model of health education, e.g. through the acquisition of skills enabling people to work in groups, organize and influence social and political systems [42]. It should also be clear from this analysis that an evaluation of the effectiveness of the Self-Empowerment Model (in addition to checking knowledge, beliefs, decision-making competences, etc.) would be concerned with measuring personal attributes such as self-esteem together with the variety of social and lifeskills described earlier.

CONCLUSION

So far an attempt has been made to describe the complementary processes of education and the development of social policy as synergistic components of the health promotion movement. The ways in which health education contributes to the overall process of health promotion have also been examined and three models of health education have been proposed to demonstrate how different values and philosophical issues can affect what, at first sight, might appear to be a relatively straightforward and unitary activity.

It would be wrong to exaggerate the degree of conflict existing between different approaches to health education. When faced with the mundane demands of occupational requirements, quite substantial ideological differences may be reconciled in practice! Again, at a theoretical level, the difference between a Radical–Political Model and the Self-Empowerment Model may be more imagined than real. However, there are fundamental dichotomies between, for example, the paternalistic and conservative values of those who subscribe to the Preventive Model, the tough-minded, radical philosophy of community activists and the more tender-minded radicalism which underpins the Self-Empowerment Model. Further discussion of this interesting issue is not a major concern for the present work. However, as has been stressed earlier, it is relevant for the measurement of effectiveness and efficiency. The nature of success depends on the values and philosophies inherent in the model which guides practice.

Although this book does not set out to provide a technical guide to evaluation, the next chapter will provide an overview of research design and perhaps alert readers to some of the different ways in which programme success may be assessed – and the difficulties inherent in doing so.

REFERENCES

1. Anderson, R. (1984) Health promotion: an overview, in: *European Monographs in Health Education Research, No. 6*, (ed. L. Baric) Scottish Health Education Group, Edinburgh, pp. 4–126.

References

2. Baric, L. (1985) The meaning of words: health promotion, *Journal of the Institute of Health Education*, **23**, 10–15.
3. Tones, B. K. (1985) Health promotion – a new panacea? *Journal of the Institute of Health Education*, **23**, 16–21.
4. US Department of Health, Education and Welfare (1978) *Disease Prevention and Health Promotion*, Washington, DC.
5. US Department of Health, Education and Welfare (1979) *Healthy People*, Washington, DC.
6. US Department of Health and Human Services (1980) *Promoting Health, Preventing Disease: Objectives for the Nation*, Washington, DC.
7. Dennis, J. *et al.* (1982) *Health Promotion in the Reorganised N.H.S.*, Report from a Study Group, Unit for the Study of Health Policy, 8 Newcomen Street, London SE1 1YR.
8. World Health Organization (1987) *Health Promotion: Concept and Principles in Action, a Policy Framework*, WHO Regional Office for Europe, Copenhagen.
9. World Health Organization (1978) *Report on the International Conference on Primary Health Care, Alma Ata, 6–12 September, 1978*, WHO, Geneva.
10. Faculty of Community Medicine (1986) *Health for all by the Year 2000: Charter for Action*, 4 St Andrew's Place, Regent's Park, London NW1 4LB.
11. Kickbusch, I. (1981) Involvement in health: a social concept of health education, *International Journal of Health Education*, Supplement to Vol. XXIV, No. 4.
12. World Health Organization (1986) *Ottawa Charter for Health Promotion, An International Conference on Health Promotion, November 17–21, 1986*, WHO Regional Office for Europe, Copenhagen.
13. Whitehead, M. (1987) *The Health Divide: Inequalities in Health in the 1980s*, Health Education Council, London.
14. Townsend, P. and Davidson, N. (1982) *Inequalities in Health*, Penguin, Harmondsworth.
15. Dennis *et al.* (1982) *Health Promotion in the Reorganised N.H.S.*, Report from a Study Group, Unit for the Study of Health Policy, 8 Newcomen Street, London, SE1 1YR.
16. Levens, G. E. and Rodnight, E. (1973) *The Application of Research in the Planning and Evaluation of Road Safety Publicity*, Proceedings of the European Society for Opinion in Marketing Conference, Budapest, pp. 197–227.
17. Freire, P. (1968) *Pedagogy of the Oppressed*, Seabury Press, New York.
18. Townsend, P. and Davidson, N. (1982) *Inequalities in Health*, Penguin, Harmondsworth.
19. Beattie, A. (1987) *Health Education in the Basic Nurse Curriculum* (unpublished paper presented at National Nursing Conference, King's College, London, 6th May, 1987).
20. Draper, P. *et al.* (1980) Three types of health education, *British Medical Journal*, **281**, 493–5.
21. Draper, P. (1983), Tackling the disease of ignorance, *Self Health*, Issue No. 1, November, 1983.
22. French, J. and Adams, L. (1986) From analysis to synthesis: theories of health education, *Health Education Journal*, **45**, 71–4.

23. Tones, B. K. (1981) Health education: prevention or subversion? *Royal Society of Health Journal*, **3**, 114–17.

24. Vuori, H. (1980) The medical model and the objectives of health education, *International Journal of Health Education*, **XXIII**, 1–8.

25. Zola, I. K. (1970) *Helping - Does it Matter? The Problems and Prospects of Mutual Aid Groups*, Address to United Ostomy Association.

26. McKinlay, J. B. (1979) A case for refocussing upstream: the political economy of illness, in: *Patients, Physicians and Illness*, (ed. E. G. Jaco), The Free Press, New York.

27. Draper, P., Best, G. and Dennis, J. (1977) Health and wealth, *Royal Society of Health Journal*, June.

28. The Politics of Health Group (1980), *Food and Profit*, Pamphlet No. 1, c/o British Society for Social Responsibility and Science, 25 Horsell Road, London, N1.

29. Crawford, R. (1977) You are dangerous to your health: the ideology and politics of victim blaming, *International Journal of Health Services*, **7**, 663–80.

30. Ryan, W. (1976) *Blaming the Victim*, Vintage Books, New York.

31. Navarro, V. (1976) The underdevelopment of health of working America: causes, consequences and possible solutions, *American Journal of Public Health*, **66**, 538–47.

32. Crawford, R. (1980) Healthism and the medicalization of everyday life, *International Journal of Health Services*, **10**, 365–88.

33. Freudenberg, N. (1981) Health education for social change: a strategy for public health in the US, *International Journal of Health Education*, **XXIV**, 1–8.

34. Society for Public Health Education (1976) *Code of Ethics*, October 15th, San Francisco, California.

35. Tones, B. K. (1987) Health education, PSE and the question of voluntarism, *Journal of the Institute of Health Education*, **25**, 41–52.

36. Tones, B. K. (1987) Health promotion, affective education and the personal-social development of young people, in: *Health Education in Schools*, (eds K. David and T. Williams), Harper and Row, London.

37. McKeown, T. (1976) The role of medicine: dream, mirage or nemesis? Nuffield Provincial Hospitals Trust, London.

38. Hopson, B. and Scally, M. (1981) *Lifeskills Teaching*, McGraw Hill, London.

39. Hopson, B. and Scally, M. (1980) *Lifeskills Teaching Programme No. 1*, Lifeskills Associates, Leeds.

40. Hopson, B. and Scally, M. (1983) *Lifeskills Teaching Programme No. 2*, Lifeskills Associates, Leeds.

41. Hopson, B. and Scally, M. (1986) *Lifeskills Teaching Programme No. 3*, Lifeskills Associates, Leeds.

42. Anderson, J. (1986) Health skills: the power to choose, *Health Education Journal*, **45**, 19–24.

2

RESEARCH DESIGN IN EVALUATION: CHOICES AND ISSUES

One of the purposes of this book is to stimulate reflection on the meaning of effectiveness and efficiency in health education. Moreover, although it is not concerned to offer detailed guidance on the measurement of success, it may well be worthwhile reminding readers of what is involved in evaluating programmes. Accordingly this chapter will provide a condensed account of the most common research designs used in **evaluation**. In so doing it will seek to underline some of the important issues involved in selecting an evaluation strategy and perhaps help potential evaluators make a pragmatic choice of method. It should also serve as a reminder that evaluation is not a mere technical activity: it incorporates philosophical issues and requires understanding of the purpose of research and the meaning of success. Above all, the reader should recall that there are often not inconsiderable difficulties involved in gaining unequivocal answers to the apparently simple question 'Has this health education programme been effective?'

More particularly this chapter will discuss experimental designs, will consider the meaning of surveys and formative evaluation and will compare all of these with ethnographic approaches. It will comment on the relative merits of qualitative and quantitative research techniques and emphasize the centrality of values in planning and implementing health education programmes by discussing the ethical dimension of evaluation.

We make the assumption in this chapter that evaluation is one of a range of research applications and not a separate area of enquiry. If research is taken to be the act of finding out about the world in a systematic way and making the process and product public, evaluation is clearly a research activity. It is, however, a research activity with particular characteristics which distinguish it from other forms of research. Jamieson [1] has suggested that evaluation differs from academic research in two important ways. The first concerns the choice of research questions. In evaluation, the researcher is usually employed by a sponsor to investigate the worth of a particular programme. Programmes are typically a form of social engineering and this tends to result in the investigation of variables which sponsors believe can be manipulated. Such enquiries may be at the expense of other factors which might have greater explanatory power in accounting for what happens but which are not amenable to change. Whereas academic research questions are theoretically constituted with reference to an academic community, evaluation questions are restricted to those with practical policy implications.

The second major difference between academic research and evaluation concerns the substance of the research report. In evaluation, the purpose of the final report is to inform and influence programme sponsors and other decision-makers. The publication of academic research, on the other hand, is directed at the scientific community to enhance understanding and knowledge irrespective of immediate application. While these are clearly real differences with undeniably practical significance, they suggest that evaluation is a form of research which differs from others in context and scope rather than underlying method. Once evaluation is accepted as one of a number of applications of research activity, it becomes clear that choice of appropriate method is as important for evaluators as for other social researchers. The following sections look at three research designs – experiments, surveys and ethnographic approaches – and seek to show how they can be used to answer different evaluation questions.

CHOOSING APPROPRIATE RESEARCH DESIGNS FOR EVALUATION

Research designs are the overall strategy for deciding what information is to be collected, from whom and when. Different designs have their advocates and critics but for most researchers decisions about design are determined by two major factors: the questions to be answered and the situational constraints. Choice of design is an important aspect of all research because it determines what can be legitimately and convincingly concluded from the data. Two aspects of research design which will affect the usefulness of results for evaluation studies are reliability and validity.

Reliability concerns consistency, that is the possibility, in principle at least, that the same results would be achieved on different occasions. Weighing scales which gave different readings for the same bag of flour would not be a very useful instrument. Similarly, research designs and methods which are unreliable yield results with limited application.

Validity has two aspects [2]. **Internal validity** refers to the appropriateness of a research method. How far does it measure what it is intended to measure and how certain can we be that what is claimed as a cause has actually produced the observed results in the piece of research? **External validity** is to do with how far the results of research are specific to a particular measure, group of people or setting. The more specific they are, the less results can be generalized. We shall see later in this chapter that different research designs differ in reliability and validity. Each is strong in some respects and weak in others.

In evaluation a distinction can usefully be drawn between questions about whether or not a programme has met its objectives or has had the intended effects and questions which concern the details of programme implementation and its effects on the various participants. Since the first set of questions is appropriately asked at the end of a programme, they form the basis of what is often called **summative evaluation**, whilst the investigation of the implementation of a programme is referred to as **formative** or **process evaluation**. Researchers carrying out summative evaluation will often be expected to remain rather detached from the programme and avoid, as far as possible, influencing the observed outcomes. By contrast, the role of the formative evaluator may well include feeding information back to programme participants to inform discussion about how a programme can best be developed or adapted to ensure effective implementation. Clearly summative and formative evaluations differ in terms of the kinds of question which are of primary interest, the time in the life of a programme when these questions can be answered and in the relationship between the evaluator and programme participants. These differences have implications for the choice of appropriate research design and in the following sections we shall consider some of the options.

EXPERIMENTAL DESIGN

Summative evaluation is very much concerned with the question of success. Have we achieved what we set out to do? Has this innovatory programme worked? Implicit in such questions is the notion of comparability. Would we achieve the same or better results by doing something different or even nothing at all? In order to be confident that the observed outcomes are attributable to a particular programme, the evaluator has to be able to rule out the possibility that outside influences – sometimes referred to as extraneous or confounding variables – have not also contributed to the results. The experimental method is the design which gives the researcher the greatest degree of control over outside influences. Its purpose is to create a standardized situation in which the researcher attempts to control all the main variables. The comparative question is resolved in experimental design by the use of (at least) two groups. In the simplest experimental design, one group, called the experimental or treatment group, receives the new programme which is being investigated (the term treatment is commonly used in experimental studies) while another does not. In order to ensure that there are no differences between the groups which could affect the outcome of the experiment, allocation to treatment and control group is done randomly. This does not mean that the two groups are identical in every respect, but it does reduce the risk of systematic bias that may arise if the groups are formed in some other way. Suppose, for example, that we wanted to evaluate the effectiveness of a school-based fitness and health project for young teenagers in increasing the uptake of exercise. If our treatment group consisted of schools which had volunteered to participate in the project and our control group was made up of schools which had shown no interest, we would have difficulty in interpreting our results. If it were demonstrated that the pupils in the treatment schools were taking more exercise a year after the project than those in the control schools, we could not unequivocally conclude that this difference must be due to the project. Sceptics could counter with the argument that the volunteer schools might well have been those which were already keen on promoting fitness and that this alone could account for the observed differences in the amount of exercise taken by pupils. By randomly allocating schools to the treatment and control groups, we can be more certain that any differences between pupils observed after the project are due to our intervention and not to other important school-related differences. The sequence of events in our experiment is illustrated in Table 2.1.

Table 2.1 Experimental design, post-test only, with schools allocated randomly to the two groups

Group	Experiment	Post-test
Treatment	New fitness and health programme	Amount of exercise taken
Control	Usual PE and sports lessons only	Amount of exercise taken

It is not always necessary for the control group to receive no treatment at all. Experimental design can also be used to test the merits of competing programmes. For example, we might already have evidence to suggest that fitness and health programmes in schools are successful in increasing the subsequent uptake of exercise but we might not be sure whether a programme which also included some written project work would produce better results than a programme which was entirely based on providing pupils with the opportunity to experience an extensive range of sport and exercise. To test this experimentally, schools, classes or pupils could be randomly allocated to two groups which would receive the different forms of the fitness and health programme.

In the example above, the evaluation design uses only **post-testing**, that is measurements are taken after the intervention has taken place. This is the form of experimental design frequently used in the biological and the physical sciences. In the social and behavioural sciences, however, we are often interested in finding out before an intervention takes place what people in the experimental and control groups already know or do. This is known as **pre-testing**. As well as providing a check on the comparability of the two groups, the use of pre-tests enables us to get a clearer and more sensitive picture of the specific effects of a programme. In the example of the fitness and health programme, the use of random allocation to an experimental and control group enables us to make inferences about the likely cause of differences in exercise levels which result from the programme using only a post-test. This is because it is assumed that exercise levels in the control group are what those of the experimental group would have been without the intervention. However, we might have been able to learn more about how the programme worked by looking at activity levels before as well as after the intervention. Pre-testing might have revealed, for instance, that the programme was particularly effective in increasing the amount of exercise taken by those pupils with initially low levels but made little impact on pupils already exercising at moderate to high levels. This information could be used to modify elements in the programme which could then be evaluated experimentally at a later date. The experimental procedure using both pre and post-testing is illustrated in Table 2.2.

Table 2.2 Experimental design, pre- and post-test, with schools allocated randomly to the two groups

Group	Pre-test	Experiment	Post-test
Treatment	Amount of exercise taken	New fitness and health programme	Amount of exercise taken
Control	Amount of exercise taken	Usual PE and sports lessons only	Amount of exercise taken

There are, however, some situations in which the use of pre-tests is not desirable or advantageous. If part of the fitness and health programme involved introducing pupils to a new sport, it would make little sense to pre-test levels of competence before the programme. There might also be situations in which the act of pre-testing could itself affect performance on a post-test. There is some evidence, for example, to suggest that the process of stating one's attitudes may itself bring about some modification in attitude. Where attitude change is to be measured as an outcome of a programme, there is the risk that this phenomenon may reduce the differences between experimental and control group, decreasing the apparent effectiveness of the programme. The basic experimental design can be modified to compensate for the effects of pre-testing attitudes. The Solomon Four Group Design (Table 2.3) combines pre and post-test and post-test only designs to determine the effects of pre-testing on outcome measures. Comparison of the post-test results of Groups 3 and 4 gives a measure of the main effects of the intervention. Comparison of the post-test results of Groups 2 and 4 provides a measure of the main effects of the pre-test.

Table 2.3 The Solomon Four Group Design, with subjects allocated randomly to the four groups

Group	Pre-test	Intervention	Post-test
1	√	√	√
2	√	×	√
3	×	√	√
4	×	×	√

FACTORIAL DESIGN

In social research there are often several variables of interest which are likely to interact to produce observed outcomes. As Fisher [3] states,

> We are usually ignorant which, out of innumerable possible factors, may prove ultimately to be the most important ... (and) we have usually no knowledge that any one factor will exert its effects independently of all others.

Factorial designs are variations of experimental design which allow us to examine the effects of the independent variables alone and also to look for their combined effects. A factorial design could be used to evaluate competing forms of a programme. Suppose we wanted to compare the effectiveness of two programmes intended to increase pupils' knowledge of the physiological effects of alcohol. One programme might consist of a video only, the other of a video with discussion guidelines. Four groups based on random allocation could be created, three receiving different interventions and the fourth, a control group, receiving nothing. This design is illustrated in Table 2.4. Let us

Table 2.4 An application of a factorial design, with subjects allocated randonly to the four groups

Group	Pre-test	Video	Guided discussion	Post-test
1	√	√	√	√
2	√	√	×	√
3	√	×	√	√
4	√	×	×	√

assume that the observed differences in knowledge-scores between pre- and post-test are as set out in Table 2.5.

In our hypothetical example, simply getting pupils to take and retake a test of knowledge about the physiological effects of alcohol (the control situation,

Table 2.5 An example of differences in pre- and post-test scores in a factorial design

	Video	*No video*
Guided discussion	(Group 1) 30	(Group 3) 15
No guided discussion	(Group 2) 25	Group 4) 20

Group 4) produced a gain of 20 points. Group 3, which received the guided discussion without the video, gained 15 points and actually scored worse in the post-test than the control group. Group 2, which saw the video but which had no guided discussion, improved by 25 points and so did better than the control group. Group 1, which received both video and guided discussion, made the greatest improvement in pre- and post-test scores. We can see from these results not only that the combined effects of the video and guided discussion are more effective than either on their own in raising levels of knowledge about alcohol but, more significantly, that this is an interactive effect: if it were simply additive, the gain of five points produced by the video alone would be cancelled out by the loss of five points in the guided discussion alone, giving an overall gain of only 20 points, thus equalling the score of the control group. The observed difference of ten points between Groups 1 and 4 indicates that the video and discussion notes in combination produced a greater effect than either alone.

Factorial designs have been used to assess quite complex interactions in teaching experiments which have compared combinations of different educational materials, teachers and teaching methods [4]. They offer the evaluator a useful method for assessing the effectiveness of different aspects of a programme.

QUASI-EXPERIMENTAL DESIGN

The experiment is the most powerful research design in terms of making causal connections between events. It is sometimes held up as the only research method, and one which the behavioural sciences should strive to emulate. As we shall see, however, experiments are not invariably the researcher's choice. Where the necessary degree of control over key variables can not be achieved, an approximation to the experiment, or a quasi-experiment may be preferable. It is usually impossible to match the rigour of the laboratory in the real world although, with flexibility, some difficulties can be overcome. In the example of the school fitness programme, for instance, it might be the case that a decision has been made to introduce it into all schools in the area. This does not mean that we need totally abandon the experimental design. Although it might not be possible to set up a control group which receives no intervention, it may be possible to arrange for the programme to be implemented in two phases. One group of pupils could act as a no-treatment control group until they entered the programme during its second phase. This design would allow for at least some aspects of the programme to be evaluated experimentally.

The very rigour which can be achieved in laboratory based experiments in the behavioural sciences can itself result in problems. The tendency of the subjects in contrived experimental situations to respond to this involvement has now become widely known as the 'Hawthorne effect' [5]. In an experimental investigation of the relationship between productivity and aspects of the working conditions in a factory, a number of systematic changes were made in the working conditions – such as varying the room temperature, lighting and length of rest breaks. Observation during the early months of the experiment showed that, almost irrespective of the changes made, productivity improved. This proved to be the case even where working conditions had been made worse. It was concluded that what was being observed was an experimental effect, sometimes called reactivity. The workers were responding to being involved in the experiment, had developed a strong group identity and were trying to please the experimenters. Partly as a result of this reactivity on the part of experimental subjects, many researchers have preferred to adapt the experimental method to more naturalistic settings, preferably in situations where those involved are unaware that an experiment is taking place. Such studies are often referred to as field experiments and make use of modified or **quasi-experimental design**. Quasi-experiments are an attempt to modify the basic experimental design to meet the demands of working within social contexts. They represent adaptations of the experimental method to research situations where randomization is not possible and where the researcher has little influence over when interventions are introduced. What is lost in control over subjects and manipulation of the variables being investigated is compensated for by gains in realism and reduced risk of reactivity. In their classic text, Campbell and Stanley [6] describe a number of quasi-experimental designs and assess their limitations. Four quasi-experimental designs are considered below.

Before and after Design with Comparison Group

Often the evaluator is not in a position to determine which groups will receive a programme and which will not, making it impossible to randomly allocate to intervention and control groups. A quasi-experimental design based on a comparison group can be used if a group can be found which resembles the one receiving the programme. This is illustrated in Table 2.6.

Caution is required in interpreting the results from this evaluation design. For example, there might be important factors which determine why one

Table 2.6 Before and after design with comparison group: subjects allocated non-randomly

Group	Pre-test	Receives programme	Post-test
1 Intervention	√	√	√
2 Comparison	√	×	√

group is recruited to the new programme in the first place. A group of enthusiastic teachers responsible for introducing a new health education programme into a school might encourage learning and attitude change in people whatever the resource material. This evaluation design cannot take account of such confounding variables and would not provide a conclusive test of the success of the programme. Nevertheless, it may reveal differences between people which require explanation. A logical argument would then be required to demonstrate that the activities in the health education programme were such that they would be expected to produce the observed outcomes.

Single Group Time Series

This is a design which uses a group involved in a programme as its own control. The same measurement is made at intervals before and after the intervention. The success or otherwise of the programme is assessed by whether or not it appears to change the observed trend. Suppose we wished to evaluate a campaign to promote safe handling of fireworks. We could compare the number of reported accidents from specific sources (e.g. local casualty departments) in the years before and after the campaign (Figure 2.1). We might conclude from this example that the campaign during 1985 was effective in reducing the number of reported accidents related to fireworks. Again, caution is necessary. There are other possible explanations for the findings. Perhaps the cost of fireworks had increased between 1985 and 1986 with the result that fewer people bought them. There may have been a general shift of public opinion in favour of organized firework displays so that fewer individuals were handling fireworks after 1985. It is clear that we cannot draw unambiguous conclusions about cause and effect from this quasi-experimental design.

Time Series Design with Comparison Group

The single group time series design can be strengthened by the addition of a comparison group. Trends in reported firework-related accidents in the

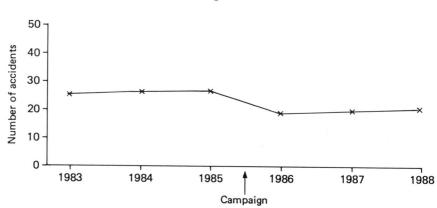

Figure 2.1 Number of recorded accidents by year in campaign area.

campaign area could be compared with those in a similar area matched in terms of important characteristics but which did not have a campaign (Figure 2.2).

This design allows us to compare trends in the intervention area with what are assumed to be more general trends reflected in the comparison area. The

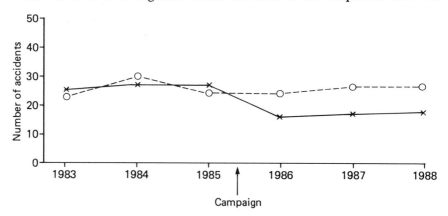

Figure 2.2 Number of recorded accidents by year in campaign and comparison areas: crosses – campaign area; open circles – comparison area (no campaign).

observation that there was no change in the number of firework-related accidents in an area with no campaign gives us greater confidence to suggest that it is the campaign which has led to the downturn in the trend in the intervention area. However, it should be remembered that matching cannot control for all of the relevant factors which may influence the results of the experiment. Indeed, it can often be difficult to decide exactly which attributes are the key ones for matching. As is always the case where there is no random allocation, groups which innovate may differ from others in a number of important ways likely to affect outcomes. Without randomization, it is always possible, in principle, that these differences account for the observed results.

Simple Before and After Design

Many evaluations, due to scarce resources, shortage of time for planning or lack of access to a comparison group, are based on pre and post-tests of a single group which is involved in a new programme (Figure 2.3).

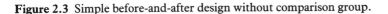

Non-random   ⟶   Intervention   ⟶   Pre-test   ⟶   Intervention   ⟶   Post-test
allocation   group

Figure 2.3 Simple before-and-after design without comparison group.

Clearly this is an extremely weak design for summative evaluation. It does not enable us to answer the essential comparative question, what would have happened without the programme? If this design is really the only evaluation option, the case for claiming that the intervention has been effective must be based on logic and theory rather than on the experimental result alone. This design can be strengthened by supplementing the results of pre and post-tests with a detailed description of the programme and how it has been implemented, supported by a well argued theoretical justification for the approaches used and how these might be expected to produce the observed results. As Cronbach [7] has suggested, interpretation of such evaluation

> is held in place by a chain (or cobwebs) of reasoning. Few links are formal and objective. Virtually any argument about the real event is rhetorical in the sense that ... the interpreter assembles information and assumptions to make a persuasive case.

THE STRENGTHS AND LIMITATIONS OF EXPERIMENTAL AND QUASI-EXPERIMENTAL DESIGN: A SUMMARY

The experiment offers the summative evaluator a research method for measuring outcomes of programmes. Experiments provide a powerful method for testing causal relationships, i.e. they have high internal validity. They provide a situation in which an independent variable can be carefully manipulated in order to observe very specific effects on dependent variables. Moreover, experimental procedures are typically easily replicated by others, ensuring high reliability. There are, however, a number of limitations associated with experimental design. Relatively few variables can be included for investigation in any one study. The degree of control necessary in experiments often results in unrealistic settings, making it difficult to generalize findings to other situations, i.e. there is low external validity. There may also be difficulties of reactivity and practical and ethical problems which arise in the allocation of people to treatment and control groups.

Quasi-experiments, on the other hand, by sacrificing experimental controls, lose internal validity and reliability but gain external validity, reduce reactivity and minimize practical and ethical problems.

SURVEY DESIGN

The survey offers another important research design which can be used in summative evaluation. It is a less powerful design than the experiment for making inferences about cause and effect but can be used to suggest relationships between variables and situations in which it is impossible to experiment. There are basically two kinds of survey: descriptive and explanatory. **Descriptive surveys** are used to provide a picture of what things are like. **Explanatory surveys** are concerned with attempts to explain observed states of affairs. Many of the most familiar surveys, such as public opinion polls, censuses and many of the surveys carried out on behalf of government, are descriptive. Investigations of this type have raised many important questions requiring explanation. A number of descriptive surveys have, for instance, linked indicators of social deprivation and poor health status. An explanatory survey, on the other hand, provides a research design which could be used to go beyond this observation to test hypothesized causal mechanisms linking these variables.

The survey is not synonymous with data based on self-reported behaviour or attitudes collected through interviews or questionnaires, although in practice most surveys are based on these research techniques. There is, however, no reason why surveys could not be based on data collected through observation. .Survey design is characterized not by specific research techniques but by two fundamental features of design [8]. Firstly, the survey is based on the standardized collection of information from a range of different cases (whether these be people, organizations or countries) about the same variables or characteristics to form a case-by-variable matrix (Table 2.7). Secondly, analysis proceeds by a systematic comparison of the different cases in order to look for relationships of co-variation between the variables. In a survey to look at the relationship between attitudes to health and the adoption of health promoting life-styles, for example, all respondents would be asked the same questions and the life-styles of those with favourable and unfavourable attitudes would be compared. This information might then be set out in a case matrix as in Table 2.7.

If it were found that those who thought that health was important were also the people taking exercise, eating a wholesome diet and so on, it would be

Table 2.7 A case matrix

Variables	Respondent 1	Respondent 2	Respondent 3	Respondent 4
Age (years)	40	31	58	20
Sex	M	F	F	M
Social class	Non-manual	Non-manual	Manual	Manual
Perceived importance of health	High	High	High	Low
Frequency of exercise	Regular	Regular	Infrequent	Infrequent

inferred that valuing one's health makes an individual more likely to adopt a healthy life-style.

This example highlights two important differences between experiments and surveys in the way in which inferences are drawn. The first concerns the presence or absence of direct intervention in the independent variable. Unlike the experimenter, survey researchers do not manipulate the independent variable in order to observe differences in an outcome or dependent variable. They observe and measure variations which already appear within the group being studied (in the previous example, attitudes towards health and aspects of life-style) and, by comparing cases, make inferences about cause and effect. The second difference relates to the use of random allocation to groups. In an experiment, the researcher randomly allocates subjects to an intervention or control group, thus eliminating any systematic bias. In surveys, the researcher may use random sampling, but this is only to select a range of cases for comparison and not to determine the composition of the groups. This absence of control means that the survey is potentially a less powerful tool than the experiment for inferring relationships of cause and effect. In this respect, surveys suffer from the same weakness as quasi-experiments. Despite observed co-variation of two variables, it is always possible, in principle, that some other factor is causing the variance in both. As we saw in the earlier examples of the health education fitness programme in schools, a positive attitude towards health might account for both the willingness of the school to adopt a health education programme and the tendency of pupils to take more exercise. Survey design in summative evaluation can give us what Marsh [8] has described as only 'a very indirect process of drawing inferences from already existing variance in the population'. Nevertheless, the explanatory power of surveys can be strengthened in two important ways: by careful choice of variables for measurement and the use of powerful statistical techniques in data analysis.

The choice of variables in surveys is crucial. We could not collect all the facts, even if we knew what these were. If we are restricted to collecting the relevant ones, we must have criteria by which to decide what these are. The choice of variables for measurement and the interpretation of subsequent observations are guided by some notion of how the variables might relate to each other, i.e. by theories or less formalized hunches about how the world works. As we have seen in earlier chapters, theories both define the criteria for success in evaluating health education intervention and suggest appropriate indicators for measurement. Theories about the importance of self efficacy beliefs in the adoption of specific health behaviours, for example, would lead the survey researcher to ask questions such as how far individuals feel that they rather than outside agents are in control of their lives. Differences in perceived locus of control could then be related to differences in the health behaviours of interest. Alternative explanations which stress social learning in the adoption of behaviours would suggest the collection of data about the health behaviours modelled by significant others. Both sets of questions could, of course, be included in one survey and their explanatory power in relation to reported health behaviour analysed and compared. The important point is to ensure at the outset of a survey that the important variables have been identified and all appropriate indicators included.

The process of analysing survey data also depends on a clear formulation of the hypothesized links between the variables and their indicators, although the process of analysis may itself suggest further questions or the reformulation of the original ones. A detailed account of the analysis of survey data is beyond the scope of this chapter, but the method of choice will depend in part on the number of variables being analysed. **Univariate techniques** are used to describe the characteristics of the sample in terms of one variable at a time, such as the distribution in the sample of age, social class or health behaviours. Bivariate techniques are used to compare two variables and multivariate methods to analyse relationships between three or more variables. **Bivariate techniques**, looking to see whether the values of one variable change as those of another are varied, are an important first step for the survey researcher in trying to explain the data. The purpose of the various bivariate analysis techniques is simply to see whether two variables are associated. Suppose we have evaluated an educational intervention for patients in a coronary care unit designed to increase their knowledge about self-care on discharge from hospital. Two instructional modes have been compared, a patient booklet and face-to-face teaching by a nurse. Learning is assessed using a questionnaire-based survey to test patients' knowledge of self-care strategies. Results appear to suggest that the booklet has been more successful than the face-to-face teaching in raising patients' levels of knowledge about self-care (Table 2.8).

For many, anticipating greater learning from a more active, participatory approach, this would be a surprising result. How could it be explained? Is some other important variable affecting the outcome? Other research suggests that the timing of health education for patients who have suffered a heart attack is crucial. If it is given too soon whilst the patient is in a state of shock or denial,

Table 2.8 Levels of knowledge by mode of patient education

Level of knowledge	Mode of instruction	
	Patients receiving booklet (%)	Patients receiving teaching (%)
High	55	45
Low	45	55

it appears to be less effective than if introduced at a later stage. Could the timing of the intervention explain the results? We could begin to elaborate the original bivariate analysis with the inclusion of this additional variable (Table 2.9).

Table 2.9 Levels of knowledge by mode and timing of patient education

Level of knowledge	Intervention early in patient's recovery		Intervention late in patient's recovery	
	Patients receiving booklet (%)	Patients receiving teaching (%)	Patients receiving booklet (%)	Patients receiving teaching (%)
High	5	25	50	20
Low	15	50	30	5

By elaborating our original analysis in this way, we can see that both the timing of the patient education and the mode of instruction are important. Learning is more effective if introduced later in the patient's recovery and based on a face-to-face teaching approach. This effect was masked by the fact that most face-to-face teaching was done during the early stages of recovery whilst the booklet was given out later on. This example highlights the importance of using theory as a basis for clarifying in advance the information to be included in a survey. Had the timing of the patient education not been recorded as part of the survey or available in some other form, such as patient records, its role in the outcome of the educational intervention would have been missed.

For evaluation in which there are more than two independent variables, **multivariate techniques** provide a powerful tool for assessing the impact of independent on dependent variables and for comparing the relative impact of a number of independent variables. A study of smoking in secondary school pupils [9], for instance, used multivariate analysis to compare the predictive power of a number of independent variables on pupils' smoking status. They found that beliefs about how enjoyable smoking is and whether their mother would mind if they smoked were stronger predictors of pupils' smoking status than beliefs about the associated health hazards. Such analysis can go beyond simple correlations to illuminate possible causal mechanisms between variables and may help in choosing between competing explanations or theories. It is important to remember, however, that statistically significant relationships between variables are not intrinsically of value to the researcher. The practice of 'data-dredging', i.e. of using multivariate techniques on a range of variables just to see if there are any statistically significant results, has sometimes brought surveys into disrepute. The ultimate significance of a relationship between variables lies in the theoretical reasoning that provides a model for understanding the meaning of that association.

SELECTING CASES:
THE USE OF SAMPLING IN SURVEYS

We have described the survey as a research design characterized by the creation of a case-by-variable matrix and have argued for the importance of theory and appropriately derived indicators in the choice of variables. We turn now to the selection of cases. Many statistical and research textbooks deal with the practicalities of sample size and the details of procedures for drawing samples, so we shall focus here on some general principles of sampling. Not all surveys use sampling to obtain cases. The term population is a technical one used to refer to all the people in a group being studied. Census surveys obtain information from everyone in a known population. This is obviously more practical where the population is a small one. Very often, however, it is neither feasible nor desirable to survey a whole population. In these situations information is sought from only some of the total group i.e. from a sample. Since survey design is based on interpretation of naturally occurring variance in the population, it is important that the sample is not too different from the population from which it is drawn. A sample obtained by standing in a shopping centre during the day would be likely to exclude, at the very least, people at work, the housebound and people unable to afford transport to the centre. Their exclusion could lead to serious errors in generalizing from the characteristics of the sample about the population in the locality.

There are a number of ways of selecting samples which can be broadly categorized into probability and non-probability sampling. A **probability sample** is one in which each person in a particular population has an equal chance of being included. Perhaps the best known method of drawing a probability sample is random selection. In order to do this a list, called a sampling frame, of all those units which make up the population must be available. A widely used sampling frame for individuals is the electoral roll. Names could be drawn out of a hat, but selection based on tables of random numbers is usually more practical. Other probability sampling methods include stratified sampling – a modification of simple random sampling – where the sampling frame is grouped according to a category considered important for the research, such as age or type of school, to ensure correct representation in the sample, and multi-stage cluster sampling where one sample is drawn from another, such as households from blocks which have been drawn from districts which, in turn, have been taken from cities. Samples are drawn to be representative of the population from which they have been carefully selected. If some of those selected do not respond or refuse to participate in the survey, the representativeness of the sample is diminished, reducing the certainty with which we can generalize from our observed responses to the population as a whole. This is because it is reasonable to assume that people who refuse to participate are different from those who do not refuse. Non-response is a particularly serious problem where we do not know the characteristics of non-respondents and cannot therefore estimate how their exclusion from the survey might bias the results. Any information about non-respondents which can be obtained is useful, even if it is only a description of where they live because it enables us to begin to identify specific biasing effects.

Probability sampling may not always be regarded as necessary. **Quota sampling** is a technique commonly used in market research. The interviewer is typically given set quotas of specified types of individual to interview. Where the distribution of the specified characteristics in the population is known, such as age, it can be reflected in the set quotas. The interviewer will look out for people to fill each quota. This is not a random method of selection as the interviewer can take anyone who fits the category. Quota sampling could be used to evaluate reactions to a series of health education articles in a local newspaper. An interviewer might be asked, for instance, to interview a predetermined number of people of whom half are to be men and half women and to ensure that a specified number of interviewees are within certain age groups.

Probability sampling relies on the availability of sampling frames. **Non-probability samples** do not have this basic requirement. Very often no sampling frame exists for groups of interest. If we wanted to evaluate the effectiveness of an AIDS campaign directed at intravenous drug users, no list exists of the target population. Registers of drug users are notoriously incomplete and do not provide an adequate sampling frame. In such cases, other sampling approaches would have to be used. Purposive sampling is a means of gathering a group or groups of respondents based on selection of individual cases because they typify people in a particular category. We could attempt, for example, to evaluate the effectiveness of an AIDS campaign by asking workers in agencies for drug users to suggest clients who might be willing to participate in the survey. We would be interested in finding individuals who might be considered typical by workers in a number of typical agencies. Drug users identified in this way could not be said to be representative of all intravenous drug users and this would, of course, limit the extent to which generalization about all drug users could be made on the basis of a survey of this kind. Other less systematic sampling procedures might include opportunistic sampling, i.e. surveying any drug user who can be found and who will agree to participate, and snowball sampling, where key individuals identified are asked to suggest other people who they think might be of interest to the researcher. Clearly, whilst these techniques may sometimes be the only option, samples formed on such a basis have little or no claim to representativeness.

THE STRENGTHS AND LIMITATIONS OF SURVEY DESIGN: A SUMMARY

There are many criticisms of surveys, ranging from their inherently deterministic nature to their role in the ideological manipulation of the public. Some of these could be said to refer to poorly conducted surveys rather than to the survey design itself and the reader is referred to Marsh [8] for a thorough exploration of the issues.

In summary then, the survey is a technique, which normally has high reliability and which can be used to collect data in sufficiently large numbers to make some generalizations beyond the research sample. It allows the researcher both to map existing variation within groups and to consider causal relationships between variables on the basis of naturally occurring differences. It provides a non-interventionist approach which can be used when experiments are impractical or considered unethical. There are three main limitations in survey design for summative evaluation. Firstly the survey researcher wishing to test causal relationships can only do so through measures of co-variance. It is always possible, in principle, that a variable not included in the survey accounts for all observed variance. Secondly, surveys typically rely on data collected in rather artificial settings, such as interviews, focusing on narrow aspects of respondents' lives. In this respect, survey design could be seen as low in external validity. Thirdly, in translating complex concepts such as health into indicators which can easily be quantified, important aspects of meaning may be lost, threatening the internal validity of some surveys.

DESIGNS FOR FORMATIVE EVALUATION

Formative evaluation is concerned with details of the implementation of programmes or initiatives. It looks inside the 'black box' which may be left unopened and unexplored by summative evaluation. No undertaking which asks people to do something different or to learn new procedures is likely to follow an entirely predictable course. Some aspects of a programme may be unworkable in practice, others will result in unanticipated consequences. These must be understood as the programme progresses so that changes can be made where appropriate and possible. Feuerstein [10] cites an analogy offered by a group of community development workers. Being involved in a new programme is seen as akin to taking a bus journey into unfamiliar territory:

> While they could see through the glass windows they were happy because they could see that they were making progress. Then rain forced them to put wooden shutters over the windows and they could no longer assess their progress. They knew they were moving forward but could not tell along which road, how fast, or even whether they were nearing their destination.

It is possible, of course, that the destination could be reached by a number of different routes. Formative evaluation can provide an account of the alternatives and compare them in terms of how acceptable they are to participants, how easy to implement, whether they are likely to be sustained and so on. It is clear that the canvas of the formative evaluator tends to be much broader than that of the summative evaluator. The purpose of evaluation has been described by Parlett and Hamilton [11] as illuminative and the task of the evaluator one of revealing the complex interplay of different aspects of a programme, describing what it is like to be involved and suggesting explanations for the programme effects. Whilst summative evaluators may be relatively detached from the day-to-day life of programmes whose outcome they measure, it is clear that formative evaluation requires much greater involvement and is, typically, an action research approach. Role ambiguity may be experienced by both researchers and programme participants, who may be suspicious of someone who, on the one hand helps them to monitor progress and improve programme implementation and, on the other, observes and comments on their performance.

THE ETHNOGRAPHIC APPROACH

Working on the broad canvas of a social context through involvement is a feature which typifies many ethnographic studies. Ethnography is perhaps not a research paradigm in the same sense as the experiment and the survey. Although it may be used for any evaluative purpose, it is a methodology with a characteristic approach which makes it especially useful for formative evaluation. Participant observation is a research technique particularly associated with ethnographic research. The ethnographic researcher participates, overtly or covertly, in people's daily lives for an extended period of time, watching what happens, listening to what is said and asking questions [12]. There is commitment to attempting to understand how people live and work within their own context. Ethnographic researchers are typically interested in revealing the concepts and perspectives of those they observe, which may be very different from those of the researcher, and in describing how they make sense of the world in which they live. Ethnography is a style of research which usually focuses on local communities, organizations or specific groups. Ethnographers are critical of research designs which disrupt the normal pattern of everyday life. Unlike experimental and survey researchers, they will usually begin an evaluation with a very broad perspective, making a conscious effort to avoid preconceived ideas about what to expect. As the researcher spends more time with programme participants, key issues and themes will become clearer. This process has been described as 'progressive focusing' [12].

The significance attached to issues during this process will be based on the researcher's judgement informed by a number of factors including theory, hunch, observation and the views of programme participants. In this way, analysis is woven into the fieldwork phase: it does not come as a distinct stage at the end of the data collection. This dialectic between theory and data is an important aspect of the ethnographic approach and one which makes it particularly useful in the evaluation of a 'moving target' such as programme implementation. Decisions about which aspects of a programme to observe, which events to record, who to interview and when, are clearly crucial. Some focus will be provided by the programme's goals. The objective of a community outreach project, for example, might specify target groups such as women living on an isolated housing estate, particular kinds of activity – such as setting up self-help groups – and might advocate the involvement of other key workers, such as community nurses. Part of the role of the formative evaluator would involve looking to see how far these objectives were being realized and describing the processes involved in their attainment.

Sampling of individuals, events and locations is as necessary in ethnographic evaluations as in surveys. The techniques of sampling are, however, very different. The ethnographic approach is based on what has been called **theoretical sampling** [13]. This is quite different from statistical sampling and rests not on randomness but on the deliberate selection of critical cases, i.e. individuals or situations which are thought to be of significance because they are typical or deviant or might in some other way be expected to shed light on explanations of what is happening. The potential significance of other facets of the research context will be suggested by previous research and relevant theories. These will be used not to formulate clear hypotheses but rather to suggest ideas, concepts or what have been termed 'foreshadowed problems' [14] which will guide the researcher's observations and questions. As we will see, the literature on the communication of innovations, for instance, would suggest the importance of local opinion leaders and a distinctive S-shaped curve of diffusion within the community in evaluating the progress of the outreach project in the previous example. The programme participants themselves will have views about the important aspects of what is going on which may also be used by the ethnographic evaluator as a framework for observation. Indeed, some evaluators have argued that programmes should be evaluated solely in the light of consumer-identified needs and concepts without reference to the goals of programme providers. Scriven [15], for example, goes further to suggest that knowledge about goals is prejudicial to unbiased evaluation. Most evaluators would probably not wish to limit their focus to any one of the multiple perspectives available, but it is important to remember that the views of the consumers may differ greatly from those of service planners and providers.

Ethnographic research relies heavily on the involvement of researchers themselves and on their skills of focused observation and interviewing. It also rests on the evaluator's ability to handle a mounting volume of field notes, documents and transcripts from taped interviews and to shape these into useful categories. Promising trains of thought and themes for analysis do not always come easily. Whereas in experiments and explanatory surveys the theoretical framework is clearly outlined before the stage of data collection, in ethnographic research links are developed as part of the continuing research process. Some are sceptical about the validity of data collected in this way. The logic of the ethnographic approach itself suggests that the activity and interpretations of the researcher must be regarded as social products in exactly the same way as those of the people whose lives they describe and seek to explain. If this is true, how can we assess what value to place on such interpretations? Ethnographers are aware of this problem and have described two processes to increase the validity of ethnographic accounts. The first is **reflexivity**, i.e. the process of taking into account the effects that researchers have on the social world they study. The second is **triangulation**, i.e. the practice of drawing on a number of different sources of information – which might include data sources, respondents or even different researchers – to check that they all lead to the same conclusion.

THE STRENGTHS AND LIMITATIONS OF THE ETHNOGRAPHIC APPROACH: A SUMMARY

The ethnographic style of research offers the evaluator an approach characterized by close involvement with the people being studied, an emphasis on the importance of multiple perspectives and the development of understanding and explanation closely linked to data drawn from a wide range of sources. Ethnographic research is typically carried out in naturalistic settings, giving it higher external validity than surveys and experiments. It allows for the inclusion of a wide range of variables and perspectives which can be progressively refined and tested for their explanatory power in the light of accumulating data. Finally, ethnographic research provides a means of illuminating the processes involved in implementation of programmes and innovations. There are, however, four important limitations to the ethnographic style of research. Firstly, it is typically done on a small scale, which limits the extent to which findings can be generalized to other contexts. Secondly, because the ethnographic approach relies heavily on the involvement of researchers, it can be difficult to ensure reliability. Thirdly, reliance on the researchers' interpretations of a large body of data results in unknown, and possibly low, internal validity. Finally, there may be ethical problems involving deception where researchers take the role of participant observers without disclosing their identity.

QUANTITATIVE AND QUALITATIVE APPROACHES

No discussion of the methodological choices available to the researcher would be complete without reference to a recurrent theme of recent years, namely the debate about the relative merits of quantitative and qualitative research. This centres not only on issues of methodology but also on differing views of the epistemology which underpins the research process itself. **Quantitative research** is typically identified with positivist philosophy, although in practice this is often a very over-simplified view of positivism. The natural sciences are taken to exemplify the positive research tradition. Here, the researcher strives to be an objective observer of the world, collecting data in order to discover general laws about how the world works. Facts are held to exist independently of the ways in which we understand them. The underlying logic of the positivist approach is deductive, i.e. the researcher starts with an hypothesis derived from theory and then puts it to the test empirically. **Qualitative research** is typically associated with the ethnographic or anthropological tradition. Qualitative techniques are generally taken to be those which are not statistically based and refer typically to participant observation, documentary analysis and unstructured in-depth interviews. Their philosophical foundation is one which holds that knowledge is a social construct based on learned, shared meanings. It follows from this that objectivity in research is unattainable. According to this view, human behaviour is not to be understood in causal terms based on laws governed by external forces but through revelation of the meanings that people attribute to their own lives and actions. The underlying logic of qualitative research is inductive: it is the process involved in moving from the particular to the general, from a detailed understanding of specific situations to the suggestion of more generalized explanations of events, i.e. to hypotheses.

More detailed consideration of the philosophical underpinnings of deductive and inductive research is not possible here, but the issues are fully discussed by many writers on the philosophy of science [16]. However, it is important to note that the apparently stark differences outlined in this simplified account of positivist and non-positivist views become blurred with the introduction of sophisticated arguments. As a result of studying the history of science, Kuhn [17] has suggested that the positivist view is not, after all, an accurate model for understanding how knowledge progresses even in the natural sciences. He argues that all scientists work within certain paradigms, or frameworks of assumptions about what the world is like, which guide the selection and interpretation of data. These paradigms change over time and are learned. That is, they are part of the social context. Thus a sharp distinction between quantitative and qualitative research can not be upheld philosophically. Neither can quantitative and qualitative research be clearly differentiated in terms of specific methodology. Particular research techniques, such as the interview and participant observation, can be used to generate quantitative or qualitative data. Both can be used as highly structured instruments providing the evaluator with a predetermined system for recording and quantifying data, or as unstructured exploratory techniques yielding descriptive information.

Choices in evaluation design, as we have seen earlier in this chapter, are not in practice dictated by adherence to particular philosophies but are attempts to find appropriate methods to shed light on different questions. In much research, a combination of approaches is used in order to maximize the extent to which important issues have been included and how far they can be generalized. Quasi-experimental design has features of both the experiment and the survey since naturally occurring variation is used to simulate treatment and control groups. Many quantitative surveys incorporate qualitative methods. A survey-based evaluation of a community health education programme, for example, would probably start with unstructured in-depth interviews to describe the range of evaluative criteria used by providers and consumers. These would then be developed into quantifiable indicators to answer such questions as how many people rated the programme as relevant to local concern. Other studies using surveys have supplemented quantitative data with qualitative information obtained from in-depth interviews with selected respondents. Similarly, experimental and ethnographic designs can be combined. Qualitative data obtained from in-depth interviews may provide the evaluator with insight into the outcomes of a particular experiment by revealing participants' understanding of what was taking place. Many researchers now argue that we should abandon the false dichotomy between qualitative and quantitative methods. McQueen [18] has advocated a pendular approach, where the researcher moves backwards and forwards between quantitative and qualitative strategies. As C. Wright Mills [19] has advised 'avoid the fetishism of method and technique. Urge the rehabilitation of the unpretentious intellectual craftsman and try to become such a craftsman yourself'.

ETHICAL CONSIDERATIONS IN EVALUATION DESIGN

Until this point, we have stressed the importance of matching methodology to problems in the choice of evaluation design. However, as an activity which involves social interaction, research is influenced by cultural mores governing social relationships. Ethical questions arise in research when we make choices between courses of action not on the basis of expediency but by reference to social standards of what is morally right or wrong. Ethical issues face the evaluator at every stage of the evaluation process. In the choice of problem, the question arises as to whose interests the evaluation serves. Sponsors, evaluators, programme employees and consumers may have different issues they consider important. Which of these will be addressed by the evaluation? Selection of research design also involves moral decisions about whether or not anyone will be hurt or harmed by the research, or deprived in some way of likely benefit. Choice of research techniques will raise questions about how far the subjects of the research are to be informed of its true purpose. In experiments and surveys, individuals are often deceived about researchers' intentions in order to minimize reactivity. Similarly, in ethnographic enquiry researchers may conceal their identity when joining a group in order to carry out their observations in a more naturalistic setting. In writing up and publishing evaluation reports, evaluators have to decide whose views are to be expressed, whether or not those who have been evaluated should be able to comment on what has been written and how differences in opinion are to be handled in published material. Similarly, decisions have to be made about how different views about what counts as success and failure are to be handled in writing up evaluation reports and making recommendations for future policy. Ethical questions also arise when action is taken on the basis of evaluation reports. How far, for example, should evaluators be held responsible for the uses to which their research might be put? What criteria should be used to assess how good or bad these uses are?

It is clear that these are not always easy questions to answer. The evaluator has few guidelines as to what a subject's rights might be in the research context. Some have asserted that ethnographic approaches to research are intrinsically more sensitive to ethical issues than others. It does appear to have been the case [20] that early social research in the positivist tradition produced little concern for ethical issues, probably because of the separation of facts from values and the search for external laws governing human behaviour. Science and ethics thus appeared to be logically distinct areas of concern. It is not the case, however, that ethnographic research is necessarily unproblematic ethically. Participant observational methods, for example, raise many problems to do with deception of subjects and denial of informed consent [21], while small-scale research may make confidentiality and anonymity impossible to guarantee. Indeed, it could be argued, as Fichter and Kolb [22] have suggested, that quantitative methods are preferable for social research, because, in presenting aggregated findings, they protect the identity of respondents.

The evaluator need not, of course, be alone in weighing up ethical considerations. Professional associations, such as the American Sociological Association [23] and groups of interested researchers, such as those working in the 'new paradigm' [24] have attempted to define the parameters for ethical research. However, very often these take the form of rather general statements. Rule 3 proposed by the American Sociological Association [23] states 'every person is entitled to the right of privacy and dignity of treatment', while Rule 5 proposes that 'confidential information provided by a research subject must be treated as such by the sociologist'. Such moral absolutes are difficult to apply in practice and it is clear that as a society we are not consistent in how we value them. For instance, we may well feel that confidential information and privacy should be sacrificed in cases where it might prevent individuals abusing positions of power. Galliher [25] has suggested alternatives for these rules to take account of the context within which an ethical decision is made. His revised Rule 3, for example, states that:

> Every person is entitled to equal privacy and treatment as a private citizen. However, equal protection may require unequal treatment of different types of subjects ... The sociologist must make the judgement regarding the amount of explanation required for adequate subject protection. When actors become involved in government and business or other organizations where they are accountable to the public, no right of privacy applies to conduct in such roles.

In practice, the evaluator must fall back on general ethical principles in making decisions about research design and methodology. Principles such as informed consent, freedom to withdraw that consent, confidentiality, concern for the welfare of subjects and the right to privacy apply as much to research activities as to general social conduct which demonstrates consideration for others. How these principles apply in any particular evaluative situation clearly creates choices for evaluators which will be informed by their own consciences and ethical judgements. Evaluators are, however, also part of a wider research community and their actions may have repercussions for others. Standards of colleagues and professional bodies should, perhaps, also be taken into account in exercising ethical judgement. In the end, however, individual evaluators must decide whose side they are on, for as Becker [26] has so forcefully argued

> We cannot avoid taking sides... Almost all the topics that sociologists study, at least those that have some relation to the real world around us, are seen by society as morality plays and we shall find ourselves, willy-nilly, taking part in those plays on one side or the other.

METHODOLOGICAL CHOICES FOR EVALUATION: A REVIEW

In this chapter we have looked at three research designs – experiments, surveys and ethnography – and considered how they can be used to answer different evaluation questions. We have distinguished between summative evaluation, i.e. questions concerned with measuring the outcomes and assessing the success of programmes, and formative evaluation in which the processes involved in programme implementation are the focus of interest. We have stressed that no one design is best in all research contexts and that different designs can be used in combination to complement the strengths and limitations of each. Similarly, we have argued for the imaginative combination of quantitative and qualitative research methods. Research is not an activity which should adhere rigidly to any particular approach. It is a means of enquiry in which appropriate methodology should be used to answer particular questions, drawing on the strengths and limitations of a range of approaches. Finally, we have recognized that methodological choices for research are not insulated from the wider ethical rules of conduct which govern social relations.

In the next chapter, we will give some detailed consideration to the criteria which may be used as indicators of success – and argue that the choice of such performance indicators should not be made mechanically but should, rather, be based on an understanding of theories which attempt to explain the various factors which influence the outcomes which the strategies described in this chapter might be used to evaluate.

REFERENCES

1. Jamieson, I. (1984) Evaluation: a case of research in chains? in: *The Politics and Ethics of Evaluation*, (ed. C. Adelman), Croom Helm, London.
2. Campbell, D. T. (1969) Reforms as experiments. *American Psychologist*, **24**, 409–29.
3. Fisher, R. A. (1935) *The Design of Experiments*, Oliver and Boyd, London.
4. Shacklock Evans, E. G. (1962) The design of teaching experiments in education, *Educational Research*, 5, 37–52.
5. Roethlisberger, F. J. and Dickson, W. J. (1939) *Management and the Worker*, Harvard University Press, Cambridge.

References

6. Campbell, D. T. and Stanley, J.C. (1963) *Experimental and Quasi-Experimental Designs for Research*, Rand University, Chicago.
7. Cronbach, L. (1983) *Designing Evaluation of Educational and Social Programmes*, Jossey Bass, San Francisco.
8. Marsh, C. (1982) *The Survey Method: The Contribution of Surveys to Sociological Explanation*, George Allen and Unwin, London.
9. Nelson, S. C., Budd, R. J. and Eiser, J. R. (1985) The Avon prevalence study: a survey of cigarette smoking in secondary school children, *Health Education Journal*, **44**, 12–14.
10. Feuerstein, M. T. (1986) *Partners in Evaluation. Evaluating Development and Community Programmes with Participants*. Macmillan, London.
11. Parlett, M. and Hamilton, D. (1972) *Evaluation as Illumination*, Centre for Research in Educational Sciences, University of Edinburgh.
12. Hammersley, M. and Atkinson, P. (1983) *Ethnography Principles in Practice*, Tavistock, London.
13. Glaser, B. and Strauss, A. (1967) *The Discovery of Grounded Theory*, Aldine, Chicago.
14. Malinowski, B. (1922) *Argonauts of the Western Pacific*, Routledge and Kegan Paul, London.
15. Scriven, M. (1973) Goal-free evaluation, in: *School Evaluation: The Politics and Process* (ed. E. R. House), McCutchan, California.
16. Chalmers, A. F. (1982) *What is This Thing Called Science?* (2nd edn) Open University Press, Milton Keynes.
17. Kuhn, T. S. (1970) *The Structure of Scientific Revolutions*, University of Chicago Press, Chicago.
18. McQueen, D. V. (1986) Health education research: the problem of linkages, *Health Education Research*, **1**, 289–94.
19. Wright Mills, C. (1970) Appendix: on intellectual craftsmanship, in: *The Sociological Imagination*, Penguin, London.
20. Barnes, J. A. (1979) *Who Should Know What?* Penguin, London.
21. Bulmer, M. (Ed) (1982) *Social Research Ethics*, Macmillan, London.
22. Fichter, J. H. and Kolb, W. L. (1953) Ethical limitations in sociological reporting, *American Sociological Review*, **18**, 544–50.
23. American Sociological Association (1968) Towards a code of ethics for sociologists, *American Sociologists*, **3**, 316–8.
24. Reason, P. and Rowan, J. (1981) *Human Inquiry. A Sourcebook of New Paradigm Research*, Wiley, London.
25. Galliher, J. (1973) The protection of human subjects: a re-examination of the professional code of ethics, *American Sociologist*, **8**, 93–100.
26. Becker, H. (1967) Whose side are we on? *Social Problems*, **14**, 239–47.

3

INDICATORS OF SUCCESS AND MEASURES OF PERFORMANCE: THE IMPORTANCE OF THEORY

In Chapter One we argued that the meaning of success in health education is dependent on the values and philosophies of practitioners. The measures used to indicate a successful outcome will in turn depend on the model of health education which is guiding practice. Indicators of effectiveness for a Preventive Model would consist of the adoption of appropriate behaviours and, possibly, the medical or epidemiological outcomes assumed to result from such behaviours. A Radical–Political Model would look for outcomes which would indicate community action and possibly a change in public policy. Again, in the absence of a global measure of self-empowerment, appropriate outcome measures for a Self-Empowerment Model might indicate enhanced self-esteem, increased internality and the acquisition of certain key social skills.

However, irrespective of the model of health education adopted, the use of **outcome indicators** will often be inappropriate. Indeed most programmes require a range of **intermediate indicators** of success. Moreover, in many instances even intermediate indicators may not provide the best way of evaluating a particular programme and an **indirect indicator** may be needed. Accordingly, this chapter will consider what it means to gauge the success of a health education venture by using 'distal' as well as 'proximal' indicators. More importantly, however, it will emphasize the need for programme planners and evaluators to base their activities on sound theory. Without a sound theoretical model, the selection of intermediate and indirect indicators from what at first sight would appear to be a bewildering variety of alternatives would be a difficult and even arbitrary operation. For this reason, two theoretical models will be described. The first of these, the **Health Action Model**, will be discussed in some detail in order to show how theoretical understanding can assist with making a rational rather than a less informed choice of intermediate indicator. Similarly, **Communication of Innovations Theory** will be cited as a basis for selecting indirect indicators. Both theories will also assist with the process of generating a list of indicators for use in pre-testing target groups and programmes.

The chapter will also draw the reader's attention to the importance of indicators of subjective dimensions of health and will comment on the recent interest in so-called **performance indicators**. The importance of objectives in programme evaluation will also be raised and their relevance for standards of performance – including cost-effectiveness – will be discussed.

THE IMPORTANCE OF INTERMEDIATE INDICATORS

At first glance it would seem sensible to determine the effectiveness and efficiency of health education programmes in terms of the ultimate desired outcomes. For various reasons this is rarely possible and sometimes not desirable. The three most important situations in which intermediate indicators are needed are described below.

The first and most obvious instance of the inappropriateness of an outcome measure is where the link between an epidemiological or medical outcome and some precursor event may be in some way dubious. For example, the assumed causal link between a human attribute or behaviour and a disease process may be unproven. The association between Type A Behaviour and coronary heart disease (CHD) [1] would fall into this category and it would, therefore, be unwise to judge the effectiveness of a health education programme designed to produce a shift towards Type B characteristics in terms of a reduced incidence of acute myocardial infarction.

Again, the link between a given behaviour and a medical outcome might have been epidemiologically established to the satisfaction of a majority of experts but the specific behaviour in question might operate only in the presence of other factors – or at any rate be potentiated by them. The classic instance of such synergism is provided by the aetiology of CHD. It would clearly be foolish to expect a programme which was confined only to increasing levels of exercise to have a measurable effect on the incidence of CHD within the target population. Similarly it would be wrong to judge the effectiveness of a practice nurse's 'broad spectrum' risk factor counselling in terms of an individual's subsequent experience of CHD since she clearly cannot influence the patient's genetic predisposition or previous history. Furthermore, a health education programme might have been singularly successful in influencing exercise patterns but, because the exercise regime had not been tailored to the particular physiological needs of each individual, it might well have been insufficient to strengthen the cardiovascular system significantly. It could not, therefore, be expected to affect the natural history of the population's coronary disease in any way. The failure would have been one of epidemiological and physiological diagnosis: in other words, the educational operation had been successful but the patients died.

And so, in the context of a Preventive Model, health educators would be rash to allow themselves to be assessed by epidemiological or medical indicators. The endpoint indicator for the Preventive Model would thus be the adoption of a healthy behaviour or lifestyle and/or changes in existing unhealthy practices. This kind of behavioural outcome would thus be an intermediate indicator within the context of a broader community health promotion programme seeking to improve health and prevent disease.

The second situation in which health education must look for an intermediate indicator is analogous with the one just discussed in that it relates to the kind of all-embracing approach to health promotion discussed in Chapter One. It will be recalled that the ultimate health outcome (achievement of health and/or prevention of disease) depends on a kind of synergy between educational input and changes in policy. For instance, anti-smoking legislation and related educational/publicity initiatives may, arguably, have a much greater combined impact than either one operating singly (note Warner's [2] claim that the joint effect of cigarette price increases and associated publicity in the USA was to 'decrease consumption by 41.5% below what it otherwise would have been'.) It would thus be fatuous to expect health education to achieve substantial social change in the absence of supportive public policy which makes the healthy choice the easy choice. It would equally be unrealistic to expect major policy changes to happen in the absence of a health education programme which seeks to raise consciousness about the need for such changes.

In both of the situations described thus far we must, therefore, assess separately a variety of sub-programmes which are individually necessary but not sufficient to achieve an ultimate health promotion outcome. Even so, within each of these sub-programmes we will often be unable to use outcome measures because of an inevitable time lag between educational input and the attainment of the desired goal. This is the third of the three situations referred to earlier and will now be considered.

One of the more common difficulties faced by evaluators is that posed by the gap between the completion of a given educational programme and the desired outcome. An obvious instance is the delay which would inevitably be expected between changes in behaviour, consequent reduction in risks and the final epidemiological outcome. This phenomenon was illustrated by an earlier example which described the links between exercise and the incidence of CHD. It has been argued, however, that health education should not be evaluated according to such criteria and so the following example is of greater interest. This considers the time gap between the delivery of health education and the opportunity to put what has been learned into practice.

Consider the case of a school-based programme of cancer education. Let us assume that the prevailing model of health education is preventive and the goal is secondary prevention. The purpose of the teaching is to contribute to the achievement of early diagnosis and thus to persuade individuals to seek early medical advice whenever one of the classic early warning signs and symptoms of cancer present (cough or hoarseness, change in appearance of wart or mole, etc.). Clearly such symptoms are unlikely to occur and require attention for perhaps 20 or 30 years or more after the teaching has taken place. Any meaningful evaluative study of the effectiveness of the educational input would thus require a cohort study if the causal chain between education and behavioural outcome were to be established. Such a study would be too costly to contemplate – even if all the extraneous inputs of information and influences occurring over 20 years or more could be controlled. Intermediate indicators of the acquisition of knowledge, beliefs and attitude would have to suffice.

The kind of time lag examined above, is, of course, apparent to anyone who cares to think about the situation for more than a couple of moments. Less obvious is the time lag imposed by the dictates of sound educational theory and practice. For instance, recognition of the ways in which the various processes of socialization contribute to the development of a health career – the development over an individual's lifespan of health-related behaviours and the psycho-social factors underpinning these – should lead educational planners to devise a 'spiral curriculum'. This seeks to provide appropriate teaching at significant points on the health career such that a topic is not merely taught at only one point in time but is rather re-visited and handled in a manner appropriate to the developmental requirements of the student. The adoption of a health career approach should thus ensure that a planned and cumulative series of educational inputs have been provided prior to the moment when an individual is expected to make a given health choice. The concept of a smoking career exemplifies this process since research on the natural history of smoking has made it clear that a single lesson or even a series of lessons on smoking will neither prevent recruitment nor facilitate genuine decision-making about whether to smoke or not. A programme must be started long before early secondary school age and the time when experimentation starts in earnest. Such a programme will require not only differential provision of biological and social knowledge related to the children's developmental age but also expert teaching which will equip young people with social interaction skills so that they might be 'inoculated' against various pressures to smoke. Each element in the 'smoking career' is necessary and intermediate indicators are needed *en route* to check that each stage of the programme has been effective. (This should, ideally, be part of the process of formative evaluation – to which reference was made in the previous chapter.)

A sound programme of health education will thus require not only coordination of inputs throughout the health career but also coordination across the range of inputs provided at any one time. In other words both longitudinal and cross-sectional integration are a prerequisite for most complex programmes since the influences on health-related behaviours are many and varied and are brought to bear in a cumulative way over time. This complex of psycho–social and environmental influences is illustrated in Figure 3.1 and describes the multifactorial nature of drug misuse.

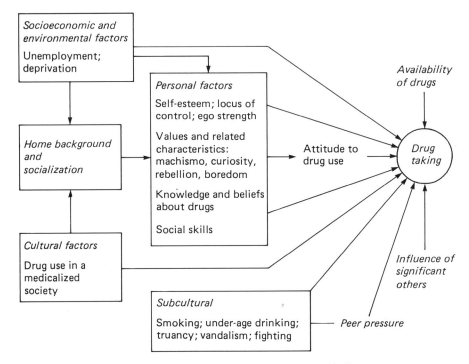

Figure 3.1 Misuse of drugs: psycho-social and environmental influences.

A detailed discussion of the nature of these causal factors and their interplay is beyond the scope of this book [3, 4] but two things should be apparent from Figure 3.1 in addition to the complexity of the factors contributing to drug use and misuse. Firstly, the multifactorial nature of many health problems requires a multifactorial educational programme if success is to be a real possibility. Secondly, each sub-programme will generate intermediate indicators. In the context of Figure 3.1 these will include: knowledge of the nature and effect of drugs; the acquisition of skills to resist social pressures; the acquisition of alternative forms of gratification; the modification of beliefs about drug misusers; enhancement of self-esteem, and so on. Figure 3.1 also serves to demonstrate the need for a theoretical framework which will help the health educator in the task of selecting intermediate indicators judiciously – and also help him or her devise a sound health education programme to evaluate!

CRITERIA FOR SELECTING A THEORETICAL MODEL

A sound theoretical framework will provide a substantial basis for practice. It should explain how individuals make health-related decisions. It will attempt to define the ways in which social and environmental factors influence these decisions and will provide insight into the nature of both inter- and intrapersonal dynamics governing behaviours. If we have some understanding of the constellation of factors influencing human behaviour in health and illness, we will be in a better position to devise strategies and formulate methods which will achieve our health education goals – no matter what our philosophy or what model we choose to follow. Again, if we understand the existing relationships between, for example, knowledge, beliefs, skills, attitudes, social pressures and environmental constraints, we should have some insight into the likely effects of a given educational programme and might, thus, select our indicators of success in a more rational and meaningful way. For instance, we might on the basis of theoretical understanding expect a conventionally taught and essentially didactic lesson on drugs to produce an increase in knowledge but little else. We would not expect it to affect attitudes or any of the other factors which Figure 3.1 suggests will influence drug misuse. We would, therefore, have a limited expectation of what the lesson might achieve and what it might contribute to a more comprehensive drug education programme. We would also know that the only appropriate indicator to use would be one which measured recall of information.

General principle: the North Karelia example

As Green has recently pointed out [5], there are many theoretical models at our disposal. A good model will present a comprehensive analysis of the factors which influence behaviours in a real life situation. A better model would be able to define and perhaps even quantify the relationships between the various elements of which the whole system is composed. Some models offer no more than a useful but limited formula which may provide a rough guide to practice and the evaluation of practice. For instance, consider the '... framework of general goals and theoretical principles for health promotion ...' which was used in the successful North Karelia health promotion programme established to reduce the high rate of cardiovascular disease in that Finnish county. The framework required the provision of six programme elements (McAlister *et al.* [6]):

1. Improved preventive services;
2. Information ('to educate people about their health...');
3. Persuasion ('to motivate people...');
4. Training ('to increase skills of self-control, environmental management, and social action...');
5. Community organization ('to create social support...');
6. Environmental change.

This scheme is clearly a much improved version of the simplistic KAP (i.e. the suggestion that Knowledge, supported by Attitude change, will routinely lead to a change in Practice) formula referred to in Chapter One. It provides a guide for programme planning and offers clear indicators for evaluation: they include performance indicators, such as provision of services to detect and control hypertension, and various intermediate indicators – such as knowledge of CHD risk, positive attitudes to reducing risk and the acquisition of culinary skills for a healthy diet. It also offers examples of indicators which may be used as measures of social and environmental change – such as the establishment of networks of lay leaders and the development of healthy nutritional policy which among other innovations gave rise to the Karelian low-fat mushroom sausage!

The Health Belief Model

Rather more refined theoretical models provide a narrower and sharper focus. Probably the best known of these is the **Health Belief Model** (HBM) [7]. Although the HBM has undergone revisions [8], its main contribution to programme planning has been the way it has highlighted the role of certain beliefs in stimulating preventive health actions. The HBM asserts that an individual must believe, (i) that (s)he is susceptible to a given disease, (ii) that the disease or disorder is serious, (iii) that the proposed preventive action will be beneficial – i.e. will effectively protect the individual from the threatening disease, and (iv) that these benefits will outweigh any costs or disadvantages that (s)he believes will be incurred as a result of the recommended preventive health action. In addition the likelihood of action will be enhanced if the individual has a generally positive attitude to health (typically measured by totting up the number of preventive measures adopted by the individual in addition to the preventive action currently under consideration) and if some cue or trigger is provided. The most important indicators of success which are highlighted by the HBM are the four key beliefs (how many of these does the individual hold and how strongly are they held?), the number of preventive actions undertaken and the successful delivery of appropriate 'cues to action'.

The Theory of Reasoned Action

A second model merits comment in this context since it has frequently been used to good effect in the health field. This is Fishbein's **Theory of Reasoned Action** [9, 10]. Fishbein and Ajzen complement and improve on aspects of an HBM analysis of health decision-making by separating belief from attitude and emphasizing the paramount importance of the influence of 'significant others' on an individual's 'intention to act'. The often substantial gap between intention and practice is acknowledged and the relationship between beliefs, attitudes, normative factors, intention and practice are expressed in mathematical terms. The Fishbein model would typically generate the following indicators: (i) an often long list of different beliefs about a given specific health action, (ii) the attitude which is created by these beliefs, (iii) a series of beliefs about the likely reaction of various significant others to the proposed behaviour, (iv) the individual's degree of motivation to comply with the perceived wishes of the significant others, (v) the strength of the resulting behavioural intention, and (vi) the actual behavioural outcome itself. One final model, the Health Action Model, will receive more detailed consideration below.

THE HEALTH ACTION MODEL

The **Health Action Model** (HAM) is a mapping model which seeks to provide a comprehensive framework within which the major variables influencing health choices and actions, and their interrelationships, are described and categorized. This model is capable of incorporating conceptually both the Health Belief Model and Fishbein's Theory of Reasoned Action. Various other health-related theories, such as Baric's Social Intervention Model [11], Freidson's Lay Referral System [12], and the important work on Health Locus of Control [13] are also congruent with HAM. The Health Action Model has been described elsewhere in the context of school health education [14] and drug misuse [15]: its main purpose here is to serve as a basis for enumerating indicators of success and to provide understanding of the ways in which these indicators relate to each other. Figure 3.2 provides a general overview of HAM's main components.

HAM and Behavioural Outcomes

Three categories of health action may usefully be identified. These are Routines, Quasi-routines and Discrete Single Time Choices. **Routines** are those behaviours which have become habitualized – often as a result of previous socialization. For instance brushing teeth, washing hands and similar hygienic practices are typically established during primary socialization under parental influence. Clearly the acquisition of routine behaviours is not only limited to influences of this sort; adults may learn a wide variety of psychomotor skills, for instance, at any stage in their lives. However, routine practices of any kind are not under direct conscious control and do not, therefore, require a conscious decision – except perhaps when they are becoming established, when they are disrupted or when attempts are made to change them. For example, drivers need to make a deliberate choice once they have formed an intention to wear seat-belts; however, once the choice has become routine, it will recur automatically. It is obvious that one of the main goals of health education is to ensure that many health practices do in fact become automatic.

The Health Action Model, however, is primarily concerned with deliberate **Discrete Single Time Choices**. It attempts to define the factors leading to an individual deciding to perform a specific act – such as visiting a GP for a

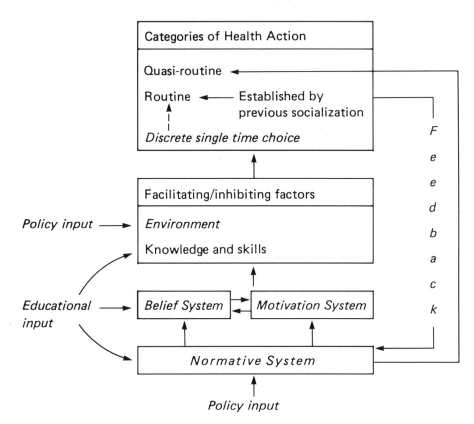

Figure 3.2 The health action model: an overview.

cytology appointment or writing to a local MP to complain about infringements of advertising regulations by tobacco manufacturers and their agencies. As indicated above, the choice may also be the first step towards changing a lifelong habit – for instance not adding salt to food. It may similarly be the first step in establishing a completely new practice such as adopting regular patterns of exercise.

Whatever the nature of the choice, three major systems influence it. These are the Belief System, the Motivation System and the Normative System. This latter is directly responsible for the third category of behavioural outcome shown in Figure 3.2 – **quasi routines**. The Normative System, as we shall see, comprises the whole range of norms and interpersonal pressures which may be so important in affecting individual decision-making. Indeed normative pressure may be so great that it effectively precludes choice. For instance a particular practice may be so unusual in a given community and/or so reprehensible that only the most reckless of deviants would ever contemplate such a course of action. In a case of this kind, the 'normal' alternative is described as a quasi-routine. This phenomenon is related to the process of inferior decision-making which Janis and Mann [16] described as Quasi-Satisficing.

The feedback loops in Figure 3.2 serve to remind us that experience is one of the most powerful influences on beliefs and attitudes. At any point in time a decision may be reversed as a result of experience. Similarly, even routinized behaviours may be abandoned as a result of experience.

The HAM analysis so far identifies three behavioural indicators: routines, quasi-routines and discrete single time choices. A variety of major intermediate indicators may be identified by considering the Belief System.

HAM and the Belief System

Some indication of the importance of health beliefs has already been provided in the earlier discussion of the Health Belief Model (HBM). A full and detailed discussion of the significance of beliefs is not possible in the present context; it should however be noted that they are defined in HAM as cognitive variables following Fishbein [17]:

> A belief is a probability judgement that links some object or concept to some attribute. (The term 'object' and 'attribute' are used in a generic sense and both terms may refer to any discriminable aspect of an individual's world. For example, I may believe that PILL (an object) is a DEPRESSANT (an attribute). The content of the belief is defined by the person's subjective probability that the object–attribute relationship exists (or is true).

Again, although the HBM's set of beliefs will often be important indicators of success, they are by no means the only ones and many subordinate beliefs will contribute to beliefs about costs and benefits, effectiveness, susceptibility and seriousness. Consider, for instance, the often cited pessimism about the curability of cancer. In HBM terms this represents a serious omission: people should believe in the effectiveness of treatment and detection services if they are to accept that seeking early medical advice about what they suspect might be a potentially cancerous sore is worth doing. The origin of this hypothetical situation might be found in two contributing beliefs: (i) a belief that treatment is generally ineffective and (ii) a belief about the nature of cancer. The latter belief will probably be derived from certain beliefs about cause, e.g. that cancer is inherited or is due to fate or retribution for real or imagined misdeeds, and a belief about the fundamental nature of the disease. According to audience research by the BBC [18], many people apparently consider that cancer is one single undifferentiated disease. This belief about its intrinsic nature will in turn affect a higher order belief that cancer may not be curable (after all, if people know that in many cases treatment fails and they believe that all cancer is the same, they may reasonably suspect that all treatment is ineffective). This relationship is illustrated in Figure 3.3. Each of the beliefs shown in Figure 3.3 represents both an objective of a cancer education programme and a measure of its effectiveness.

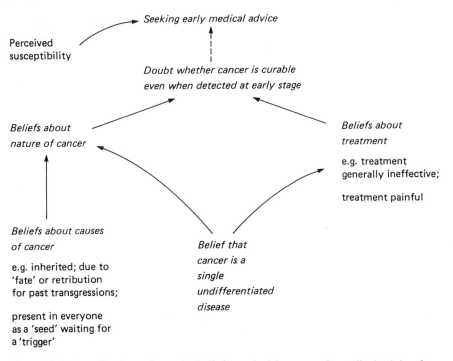

Figure 3.3 Contribution of certain beliefs to decision to seek medical advice for a persistent sore.

Two of Fishbein's notions about beliefs should be noted in passing. First, he argues that beliefs may be salient or latent. Salient beliefs are conscious and arguably more likely to influence health actions. However, latent beliefs may well make a significant impact if made salient by, for example a process of 'values clarification'. Secondly, belief strength will vary and is quantifiable. Clearly a high level of conviction will be more likely to contribute to a decision than a state of doubt and uncertainty. And so, indicators of belief should provide not only a measure of whether they are subordinate or superordinate but also should indicate the strength with which they are held and whether or not they are salient or latent.

Perhaps the most important category of belief is that set of beliefs which an individual holds about self. The sum total of such beliefs is usually known as **self-concept**. This includes the HBM variable of **perceived susceptibility**: its potential importance can be illustrated by referring again to Figure 3.3.

Perception of susceptibility should, other things being equal, facilitate action. An avid blond sun-worshipper who has dutifully absorbed the health education message about skin cancer and exposure to ultra-violet rays would in theory be more likely to suspect the potential malignancy of a persistent sore than someone believing that (s)he is less at risk.

More importantly, if individuals perceive themselves as 'copers'; if they believe that they are in control of their lives and have the capacity to act logically and decisively, then their chance of adopting a given health action which they believe to be sensible is that much greater than those having a different self-concept. On the other hand, action is less likely where someone's Perceived Locus of Control (to use Rotter's term [13]) is external. In other words a person who believes that life's choices are governed by the vagaries of fate or determined by a conspiracy of powerful others and faceless organizations will be less likely to mobilize the personal resources needed to face a potentially threatening situation. The importance of beliefs about self-efficacy and internality has already been considered in Chapter One in discussion of the Self-Empowerment Model. A further major indicator was that of self-esteem which, in HAM, is a key component within the Motivation System – which will now be described.

HAM: the Motivation System

The **Motivation System** describes a complex of affective elements which ultimately determines the individual's attitude to the specific action and his or her intention of adopting it. Part of this complex is the individual's value system. Values are acquired through socialization; they are affectively charged sets of beliefs referring to particular aspects of experience (see Rokeach [19] for more detailed discussion). Religious and moral issues relate to all-embracing values; the feelings one has for a career or in relation to family or spouse may be important in underpinning many health-related actions.

Attitudes, on the other hand, are more specific than values. They describe feelings towards particular issues. Fishbein and Ajzen [20] provide a definition which is both congruent with the HAM perspective and which shows how attitudes relate to beliefs:

> ... an attitude (refers) solely to a person's location on a bipolar evaluative or affective dimension with respect to some object, action, or event. An attitude represents a person's general feeling of favourableness or unfavourableness towards some stimulus object ...

> Each belief links the object to some attribute; the person's attitude toward the object is a function of his evaluations of these attributes.

Each value will thus produce a large number of attitudes. For instance, the value associated with sex and gender roles will give rise to a series of attitudes towards, say, the employment of women, the nature of the marriage contract, the role of women in trade unions, the adequacy of medical care for female maladies, and so on. The acquisition of new beliefs will, in turn, generate new attitudes energized by the value systems. For example, a belief that breastfeeding would militate against full sharing of the parental role might lead to a negative attitude to breastfeeding derived originally from the gender value mentioned above.

Obviously several values may conspire to produce one single attitude and this situation is illustrated in Figure 3.4. It is apparent from this analysis –

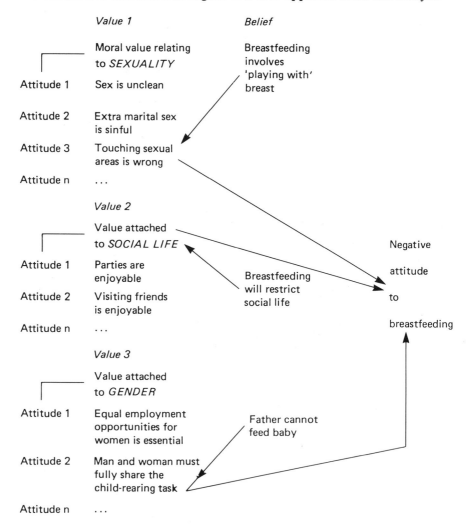

Figure 3.4 The contribution of values to attitude to breastfeeding.

indeed it is a truism – that it will be much more difficult to change an attitude which derives its motivational force from several values – especially where such values are deep-seated and salient. Almost by definition, one of the most powerful and influential values is that of self-esteem – just as the associated set of beliefs, the self-concept, plays a nuclear role in decision-making and behaviour. Self-esteem refers to the extent to which the individual values the attributes which make up the self-concept. Just as we formulate attitudes to any aspect of our world in accordance with our value system, we develop attitudes to ourselves. The sum of these attitudes defines our self-esteem or self-sentiment. The centrality of this notion to the Self-Empowerment Model has already been mentioned and needs no further comment here.

In addition to values and attitudes, the Motivation System incorporates 'drives'. The Health Action Model differs from some of the approaches already mentioned in that it recognizes the fact that certain basic and powerful influences may override socially acquired values and attitudes. The term **drive** is therefore used to describe largely inherited, species-specific motivational factors such as hunger, sex and pain. It is also used here to refer to those acquired motivators having drive-like qualities – such as addictions to drugs. The importance of drives is obvious at the commonsense level of explanation. For instance, a teenager might believe in the benefits of contraception and have acquired the appropriate techniques in using them; he or she may also have a well developed moral sense – but congruent beliefs, values and attitudes may yield to the pressures of sexual passion! Similarly, the alcoholic may well know the damage he is causing to his or her family life and may value children and spouse highly – but it is the drive-like influence of the addiction which may determine behaviour.

Frequently, however, there may be no obvious drive influencing intention to act. Nonetheless the presence of certain emotional states may signify the existence of motivational factors derived from drives. For instance guilt and anxiety may usefully be considered a fractionated or watered down version of pain or fear. Again at a commonsense level it is apparent that nagging feelings of anxiety at the prospect of a spouse's disapproval may prevent a person undertaking some otherwise valued healthy action.

It is thus possible to derive a further set of indicators from the Motivation System. In addition to the traditional measurement of attitudes (about which numerous volumes have been written) we might wish to gain some indication of individual values, drives (including acquired and derived) and self-esteem.

As we have seen, the Motivation System is a composite of different drives, values and attitudes having different emotional charges and giving rise to a particular level of arousal – or 'push' to take action. The Normative System contributes to this level of arousal in the form of an individual's motivation to conform to pressures from other people or, conversely, to resist interpersonal influence and/or deviant status.

HAM: the Normative System

The term 'norm' describes cultural, subcultural and group behaviours together with the various values, beliefs and routines associated with such behaviours. The actual observable behaviours may be termed statistical norms while the beliefs held by the relevant population about such behaviours may be called social norms. Current figures on the prevalence of smoking in, for example, the UK and USA would indicate that the smoker is a deviant in higher social class groups. The notion of deviance underlines the importance of the coercive power of norms and their influence on behavioural intentions and decision-making. The effect of the social norm is clearly most important here, for although it would often be correlated with the statistical norm, it is an individual's belief about other people's activities which is influential rather than the extent of the activities themselves.

Norms do not only operate within relatively large cultural units. The influence of norms within a small group on its individual members may be very powerful indeed and has been widely documented; the effect does of course depend on the extent to which the group member values membership of the group in question. Again the norms of a reference group, i.e. a group to which an individual does not belong but for which (s)he has membership aspirations, may also be influential in determining attitudes and behaviours. As indicated earlier, where norms exert a very high degree of coercive pressure, decisions may be reduced to the status of quasi-routines.

The Health Action Model describes the **Normative System** from an individual and therefore psychological perspective (for a sociological point of view of normative influences, see Baric [21]). This individual perspective includes not only a person's belief about normal practices in the local or national community but also beliefs about the likely reaction of significant others – as described earlier in the discussion of Fishbein's model. It is, however, obvious – again as Fishbein indicated – that such beliefs will only influence behaviour where the individual is motivated to comply with the wishes of significant others or to conform to what (s)he perceives as acceptable norms.

It is apparent that the Normative System generates further variables which might be used as diagnostic measures and indicators of success. These will include a description of the actual normative status quo (statistical norms), e.g. the prevalence of a particular practice in a given community; the 'norm-sending' aspects of the environment – such as the advertising of unhealthy products or the availability of smoke-free places; the nature of the 'lay referral system' [12]; the nature of social support networks; group behaviours; the actions and attitudes of significant others. The catalogue of normative indicators would also incorporate individual perceptions and beliefs about all of the aforementioned measures – such as people's interpretations of the significance of the presence or absence of healthy foods in works canteens; their awareness of prevalent lay constructions of illness; their beliefs about the level of peer smoking and the likely reaction of their friends to their proposed membership of a health and fitness club. Incidentally, these indicators might be used in an evaluation of a health promotion programme having as its goal either a change in the normative status quo, or a change in people's beliefs about the normative situation.

HAM and Health Promotion

It will be noted from Figure 3.2 that the various elements of which HAM is composed may be influenced by two kinds of input. These are the mutually interdependent processes of education and public policy-making which were described in Chapter One. Policy-making involves various legal, fiscal, economic and environmental strategies and these have an essential part to play if an individual's 'intention to act' is to materialize. Their function is to facilitate the translation of intention into practice and/or remove various environmental or social barriers – thus helping make the 'healthy choice the easy choice'.

The complementary processes of health education will in their turn – through consciousness raising – increase the likelihood that these policy decisions will be made. Health education will also facilitate intention to act by providing necessary knowledge and skills. It is worth emphasizing the difference between those health education programmes which are designed to facilitate a pre-existing behavioural intention and those which seek to create such an intention – for example by seeking to influence beliefs and attitudes. The latter kind of programme is typically more problematical.

INDIRECT INDICATORS

At the beginning of this chapter we identified three major kinds of indicator: indicators of outcome, intermediate indicators and indirect indicators. As discussed earlier, intermediate indicators are frequently more appropriate or practicable measures of success than outcome indicators. However, even intermediate indicators may prove to be impracticable in certain instances and planners must resort to indirect measures of success.

As we have seen from Figure 3.2, educational inputs are designed to influence one or more of the various psycho–social or environmental factors affecting health-related decision-making. If the measurement of these factors should prove problematical – perhaps because of lack of time or resources – or if it should be considered unnecessary because the effectiveness of a given educational input had already been demonstrated, then an evaluation may be concerned only with verifying that the educational programme in question had been properly delivered.

For instance, let us consider an educational programme in which family doctors routinely provide their patients with advice about smoking cessation as part of opportunistic health promotion during the consultation. As Russell *et al.* [22] have demonstrated, the provision of such advice can produce a smoking cessation rate of 5.1% after one year when supportive leaflets are given to patients. This compares with a rate of 0.3% in a control group. If all 20 000 general practitioners were to adopt this approach as a matter of course, then the researchers argued there would be half a million fewer smokers in the first year. This level of success could only be matched by increasing the number of special smoking cessation clinics to 10 000! Having demonstrated this cost-effective result – and in the absence of unlimited resources – it would make sense to assume that a programme of this sort would be at least as effective in future and would continue to reduce smoking in a practice population. An indirect measure of effectiveness might then legitimately be used to monitor the extent to which doctors delivered the service – for instance by recording the number of practitioners who requested dispensers of leaflets designed to be used as a support for the interpersonal advice on smoking cessation.

Other examples of commonly used indirect indicators of anticipated success would include the following: (i) adoption by schools of a new curriculum package, (ii) teacher attendance at courses designed to familiarize them with the package and, most indirect of all, (iii) the pre-testing of the package during construction to determine reading ease and consumer acceptability. In other words, it is often possible to describe a chain of indicators starting with an indirect measure and leading on through other indirect measures via various intermediate indicators until finally some indication of a successful outcome is reached. A record of the successful completion of the early links in the chain may be all that is needed or all that is possible in the case of many evaluation enterprises. This chain of possible indicators is illustrated in Figure 3.5.

McGuire's discussion [23] of this chain of indicators might usefully be noted at this point. He refers to the 'distal measure fallacy' involved in evaluating a campaign solely on the basis of the early indicators and describes also an 'attenuated effects fallacy' where the evaluator fails to take account of the 12 or so links in the chain and recognize that the probability of achieving all of them is a function of the probability of achieving step one multiplied by the probability of achieving step two and so on until step 12 is reached. In other words the chances of success are relatively small!

COMMUNICATION OF INNOVATIONS THEORY

The discussion of indirect indicators has referred to the importance of client groups adopting innovations. These groups would include both the population whose health will hopefully be enhanced by the educational programme and

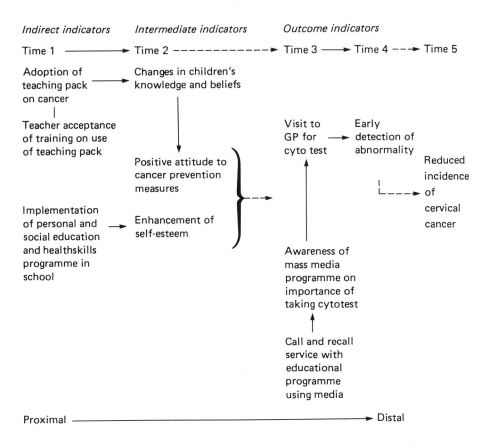

Figure 3.5 Temporal relationship between indicators.

the professionals who have to be persuaded to utilize the means to influence the population at risk. In the cases discussed in the previous section, the consumers would include the patients receiving the advice on smoking and the pupils who would benefit from the curriculum package; the health or education professionals in question would be the doctors and the teachers.

Again, as with the choice of intermediate indicators, it is not possible to influence the adoption of innovations effectively and measure the programme's impact without the guidance of theory – and theories defining the parameters governing the adoption of innovations are quite well developed. Discussion of these is not appropriate here but one example will be provided which will serve to illustrate the relevance of theory for interpreting the success of programmes which aim to stimulate the adoption of new ideas or practices (whether these involve outcome, intermediate or indirect indicators).

Communication of Innovations Theory allows us to make several generalizations – for example an innovation is more likely to be adopted if it is relatively simple and can be assimilated readily into existing practices or norms. This will also be more likely to happen if it can be tried out and the results of the trial observed quickly and if it offers some significant advantage compared with previous practices. A further and particularly important generalization has to do with the rate of adoption of an innovation. As Rogers and Shoemaker [24] have pointed out, this is invariably S-shaped (although the precise form of the S may vary). The shape is determined by the differential rate of adoption of the innovation by the target population. Those who adopt first of all are labelled innovators; these are closely followed by early adopters who are, in turn, succeeded by the early majority. Bringing up the rear are the late majority and, last of all, the laggards. This phenomenon is described in Figure 3.6.

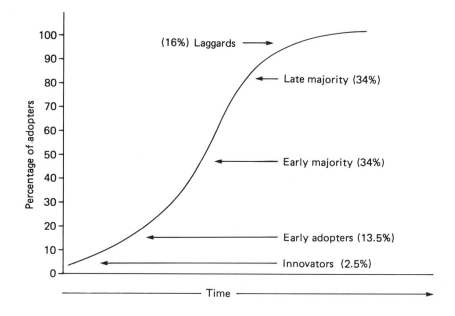

Figure 3.6 The S-shaped diffusion curve and adopter categories (after [23]).

Now since it is clearly increasingly difficult to influence later adopters and practically impossible to shift a residual hard core within the broader category of laggards, a law of diminishing returns will operate in health education programmes seeking to influence large groups of people. Evaluators should, therefore, build some form of compensation into their calculations. Green has recently argued [25] that this ceiling effect, originally noted by Hovland *et al.*

[26] in the field of mass communications, may be countered by means of an effectiveness index derived from the following formula:

$$EI = \frac{(P_2 - P_1)}{(100 - P_1)}$$

Where EI = Effectiveness Index; P_1 is the percentage of the population adopting the innovation prior to the educational intervention and P_2 is the percentage adopting at a given time after the programme.

Apart from arguing, as Green has done here, that a relatively small change in the hard core of resisting laggards might be a cause for self-congratulation while the same degree of change in an unexposed population might well demand a change of programme and personnel, we should also ask more general questions about standards of success. For example, how should we decide whether a particular percentage increase in a desired outcome ought to be considered a success or a failure? How should we determine standards of success? What levels of achievement have we, or our managers, a right to expect before we can claim that our interventions have been effective and efficient? These questions are best addressed by considering the ways in which programme goals are established and, in particular, by examining the role of objectives.

AIMS AND OBJECTIVES

There is some degree of terminological confusion between various statements of educational intent. Reference is made to aims, goals, targets and objectives almost interchangeably and indiscriminately. While there may be no universal agreement about the meaning of all of the above terms, there is general agreement about the difference between two of them: aims and objectives. An **aim** would normally describe a general statement of intent; it would usually provide an indication of the value underpinning a given health education programme – but little else. For instance, an aim for a nutrition education programme might be to improve the nutritional status of the nation. The implicit assumption is that this is worth doing, but because of the generality of the aim and the value position embodied within it, it is difficult to challenge its appropriateness (as opposed, say, to its practicability). On the other hand, **objectives** are much more specific and precise. Any one aim might generate a large number of objectives. The nutritional aim referred to above might be translated into dozens of objectives including, for example, that a target group should reduce '... average saturated fatty acids (SFA) intake from 59 g (18% of total energy) to 50 g (15% of total); i.e. a 15% reduction.' (NACNE Report, [27]).

Two observations may be made about the term objective: firstly, an objective is likely to generate more controversy than an aim – because it provides specific details of what is intended – and secondly, it is considerably easier to measure (for the same reason). Objectives have an especially important part to play in evaluation. On the one hand it has been argued that evaluation designs derived from objectives may well corrupt the educational programme while, on the other hand, it has been stated with equal vigour that the attainment of properly constructed objectives provides the best of all possible indicators of programme success. For the present, however, we will merely consider the objective as an indicator of performance. Before doing so, we need to give some further thought to the question of specificity.

It is possible to envisage a spectrum of specificity ranging from the delightfully vague to the almost pedantically precise. The aim would be located at the general end of this spectrum while the other pole would be occupied by a particularly specific variety of goal statement generally known as a behavioural objective. This highly refined statement describes the behaviours which a learner (as opposed to a teacher, educator or instructor) will produce in order to demonstrate that the desired terminal outcome has been achieved. The behavioural objective will, moreover, specify the conditions under which the learned outcome will emerge and criteria (or standards of acceptable performance) which will be used to signal success. Figure 3.7 illustrates this specificity spectrum as a goal continuum. In accordance with standard practice, an aim is positioned at the general end of the continuum while a behavioural objective is located at the other end in acknowledgement of its

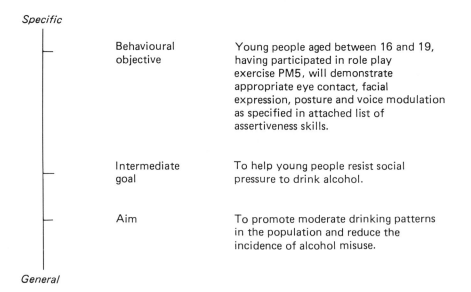

Specific

Behavioural objective	Young people aged between 16 and 19, having participated in role play exercise PM5, will demonstrate appropriate eye contact, facial expression, posture and voice modulation as specified in attached list of assertiveness skills.
Intermediate goal	To help young people resist social pressure to drink alcohol.
Aim	To promote moderate drinking patterns in the population and reduce the incidence of alcohol misuse.

General

Figure 3.7 A goal continuum: An example from alcohol education.

high degree of specificity. While a properly constructed behavioural objective could hardly be rendered more specific – being, as it were at a pinnacle of precision – other educational goals could be placed at virtually any point on the continuum. Their location would depend entirely on how general or specific they were. The example of alcohol education has been used to illustrate the potential variation in specificity and it can immediately be seen that the general aim of promoting moderate drinking could be translated into literally hundreds of more specific goals. The intermediate goal of helping young people to resist social pressure represents one of these and, in turn, could be translated into a much more limited number of more detailed, precise objectives.

It is not the purpose of this book to explore the merits and demerits of using behavioural objectives – although earlier discussion of quantitative and qualitative research methods has an important bearing on this. However, the interested reader should consult an amusing article by Popham [28] in which he describes the rise and fall of the 'behavioural objectives movement'. The zenith of this quest for precision and specificity in his own personal position is symbolized by a 1962 bumper sticker which read 'Help stamp out non behavioural objectives' and which indicates the degree of emotional involvement which curriculum design can inspire in its devotees. Since that highpoint, there has been a move away from what Parlett and Hamilton [29] have called the 'agricultural-botany paradigm' of educational evaluation and this has been accompanied by a demise in the popularity of the behavioral objective – certainly among educationalists (Popham modified his position to the point at which his bumper sticker read 'Help stamp out *some* non-behavioural objectives!).

However, whatever the fashion, the advantages of the behavioural objective are very real. Once the objective has been constructed, the success of the related educational programme can be determined in an objective, reliable and observable way by merely noting whether or not the objective has been attained – in other words by means of a simple yes/no decision. It is worth adding here the observation made by a doyen of the behavioural objective movement, R.F. Mager [30]: '... if you give each learner a copy of your objectives, you may not have to do much else'. This somewhat cryptic statement makes the entirely justifiable assertion that in many instances the specificity and clarity of the goal statement embodied in behavioural objectives is sufficient to generate learning. Unfortunately, one of the main difficulties in constructing this kind of goal statement stems from the fact that many educators are insufficiently clear about their goals! Without such clarity a behavioural objective cannot be produced.

It would, at first glance, appear that a behavioural objective might be inappropriate for programmes which measure their effectiveness by means of intermediate indicators of success. This would, however, be a misconception since the behaviour in question may refer not only to an 'action' outcome – such as attending a clinic for immunization – but may equally well apply to such cognitive or affective indicators as the acquisition of knowledge or attitude change. Behaviour therefore refers to any observable act: for instance a behavioural indication of successful learning about the involvement of fats in coronary heart disease might include producing a list (verbally or in writing) of various cooking oils and fats which correctly indicated which of these were saturated and which were polyunsaturated.

Apart from the advantages of specificity, behavioural objectives have two further benefits to offer evaluators. These derive from their emphasis on the importance of including the conditions under which a given learned outcome is to be demonstrated and the standards which have to be met if the learning is to be adjudged successful. The former requirement serves as a useful reminder that a given learning outcome will only be achieved if the conditions necessary for any learning situation are fulfilled (for instance the acquisition of social interaction skill requires repeated practice and feedback – perhaps using a role-play technique; attitude change on the other hand might require the use of 'group discussion–decision' [31] or some other appropriate methodological tactic). The matter of standards merits rather more detailed consideration since it has an important bearing on the politics of evaluation.

Standards

Green and Lewis [32] identify four kinds of standard which might be used to determine the relative success of any given intervention. The results of a health education programme might simply be compared with the degree of success achieved in previous ventures of a similar kind (historical standards) or, alternatively, a comparison might be made with the level of performance produced by other workers in programmes of a similar nature designed for similar target groups (normative standards). A third kind of yardstick is provided by 'theoretical standards' in which the criteria of success are derived from a knowledge of relevant theory – which indicates what one might reasonably expect on the basis of a conceptual analysis which is ultimately derived from all previous research in a given area. Green and Lewis contrast these with a fourth level of expectation based on 'absolute standards' – which demand nothing less than perfection, i.e. 100% success!

The reference to absolute standards should remind us of the important political dimension to evaluation – a dimension which we ignore at our peril. While our political paymasters may not really be so naïve as to expect complete success, they frequently appear to have entirely unrealistic expectations of what health education might achieve – both in general and in relation to particular programmes. It is an interesting paradox that these same politicians – whose whole experience in politics will typically have lead them to redefine the ambitious and idealistic goals of their youth so that their expectations have come to be more consistent with the 'art of the possible' – may expect health education to achieve substantial switches in public opinion and the deep-seated values which frequently underpin these attitudes. For instance a mass media campaign might be expected to significantly shift life-styles in a way which is largely inconsistent with existing social norms. If such a change were to happen in the political arena, it would be akin to achieving a dramatic reversal of political allegiance in large sectors of the population as a result of a series of party political broadcasts. It would rightly be viewed as little short of miraculous!

More commonly perhaps, political goals for a programme may differ – consciously or unconsciously – from overt health education goals. On the surface an hypothetical media-based drug education programme might be seeking to harden attitudes against heroin use or even to reduce the proportion of the population misusing that substance. However, the hidden agenda may well be to demonstrate governmental concern to an irrationally anxious public and to placate vocal and influential party supporters who have been outraged at what they perceive to be a major social and moral problem. In such cases it is essential that this hidden agenda be explored with the paymasters so that false expectations are not established and the subsequent and often inevitable failure of the programme is not used as evidence of the ineffectual nature of health education. Logically, the purpose of evaluation in these circumstances should be to provide a kind of performance indicator which will record activity, energy and perhaps enthusiasm! It should not seek to measure changes in the stated target population, i.e. drug abusers or those at high risk of misusing drugs; only minimal change would be set as a theoretical standard in a programme of this sort.

While it may not be possible to precisely specify standards of success, a sound understanding of existing theory in health education should allow us to establish criteria for programme evaluation and to indicate what we might expect from any given intervention. Clearly, past experience and specific *ad hoc* research will sharpen our predictions but even where such prior knowledge is limited, our understanding of health-related behaviour and educational theory should enable us to make realistic estimations of likely success. For example, we should be able to comment on the very best standard we could hope to achieve (a theory-based 'absolute standard'). The so-called 90/90 rule, which was used as a rough guide in developing linear teaching programmes in the heyday of programmed learning, would attempt to achieve a success rate of 90% in 90% of a relatively homogeneous target group. This is sometimes expressed as a 90/90/90 criterion [33], i.e. 90% of students will achieve 90% of the objectives 90% of the time. Further attempts at refining programmes would be subject to a law of diminishing returns and not be cost-effective. One might therefore say that a properly structured and essentially cognitive programme which has been pretested on a homogeneous target group might hope to achieve a comparable 90% success rate – but no more.

Let us consider a second hypothetical example – this time in the affective area. Let us assume that a vaccine has been developed to immunize against AIDS. The vaccine can be administered in a one shot, once for all form on a lump of sugar at any doctor's surgery, out-patient department, health centre or chemist. There are no side-effects and effectiveness has been proven. Little knowledge of attitude change theory is required to predict the success rate of a properly pre-tested mass media based programme which utilizes all appropriate channels to deliver the message and which provides specific information about where to obtain the vaccine – and, of course, uses minimal fear appeal! The 90/90/90 criterion mentioned above might even be surpassed in certain high risk groups!

SOME REFLECTIONS ON COST-EFFECTIVENESS

Before closing the discussion on standards of success, it is important to give some consideration to the measurement of effectiveness in economic terms. In other words we must confront some of the thorny issues raised by cost-effectiveness and cost-benefit analysis. In a very real sense economics is the ultimate arbiter of programme implementation even if, on occasions, it is not the primary concern. All programmes must take account of cost since all programmes consume resources and resources are finite. The most obvious situation where economic analysis is viewed as an essential part of programme planning and evaluation is where health education's *raison d'être* is considered to be one of saving on expensive health care costs so that money may be spent on other and presumably better things. However, even where the health education model of choice is, say, to create a sense of wonder at the marvellous workings of the human body, resources are necessary. Even where society values knowledge for its own sake (currently a somewhat eccentric view), it is manifestly better to create such knowledge efficiently, i.e. with minimal rather than profligate use of resources.

We can therefore argue that whatever the precision of the objectives set or the sophistication of the criteria of success adopted by a programme, some measure of efficiency should be considered. The term **effectiveness** is commonly used to denote the extent to which programme objectives have been achieved. The term **efficiency** normally refers to relative effectiveness, i.e. how well a programme has done by comparison with actual or potential competing programmes and strategies – or specific methods within programmes. Behavioural objectives have, of course, an inbuilt measure of efficiency in the form of conditions and standards. Health economics seeks to quantify efficiency by expressing it in monetary terms.

Three common analytical tools are employed in health economics:

1. Cost analysis – which merely indicates the financial cost of competing programmes or other initiatives.
2. Cost-effectiveness analysis – which compares the efficiency of competing interventions in achieving a given goal by stating the relative financial costs involved.
3. Cost-benefit analysis – which, unlike cost-effectiveness analysis (CEA), not only states the costs in monetary terms but also seeks to fix a price tag on the benefits accruing from the programme. A calculation of the cost per given benefit is then possible (typically expressed as a cost-benefit ratio).

It is important to note the difference between cost-benefit analysis (CBA) and CEA. Cost-effectiveness analysis seeks only to state the cost involved in, say, using smoking cessation clinics compared with family doctors providing routine advice on giving up smoking (as illustrated earlier in this chapter). On the basis of the quoted study, GP involvement is clearly more cost-effective.

Cost-benefit analysis, on the other hand, would not necessarily assume that smoking cessation was a worthwhile goal under any circumstances and would compare the financial costs of delivering the programme with the financial costs of the benefits resulting from smoking cessation. It is therefore controversial insofar as many people will fundamentally question the morality of attaching a financial label to human life and health; others will merely question the feasibility of doing so. The arguments used here are somewhat similar to those involved in the debate about behavioural objectives. The objection on grounds of ethical principle suggests that cherished human values are somehow demeaned by the process of subjecting them to critical analysis. The second category of objection is manifestly different: its criticism is based on accusations of incompleteness or naïvety.

The fact is, however, that just as behavioural objectives clarify goals through their precision and specificity, CBA and CEA may provide useful information to help decision-making under conditions of resource limitation. They may also be politically useful for health educators who, in the face of criticism of the costs of proposed programmes and demands for proof of efficiency, may be able to point out the relative cost of routinely accepted medical practices and non-educational preventive procedures. It is clear that the amount of money spent on different life-saving interventions varies enormously in relation to the pay-off in terms of lives saved – as may be seen in Table 3.1.

An important health economics concept is that of opportunity cost. Any service expenditure involves not only the cost of delivering that service but also the loss of some other facility which might have been financed by the money spent on that service provision. Thus while it might be argued that the money spent on prevention and health education could have been spent on curative services, it would seem equally reasonable to stand the argument on its head

Table 3.1 Cost per life saved for various preventive measure

Preventive measure	*Cost per life saved (£)*
Screening for stillbirth	50
Childproof containers	1 000
Department of Environment (road saftey)	39 300
Screening for cancer of the cervix	10 000–
	41 700
Trawler saftey	1 000 000
Alterations to high rise flats after Ronan Point disaster	20 000 000

Derived from Mooney, G.H. [33]

and assert that the resources used in high technology acute medicine might be better spent on health education and preventive services. Cochrane's classic 'random reflections on the health service' [35] showed how many routinely practised medical procedures had never been evaluated. Townsend [36], in discussing cost-effectiveness, cites Bodmer [37] who commented on the escalating cost of chemotherapies in the treatment of cancers and asserted that despite '... very serious side effects ...' these had '... no more than a marginal effect at the present time on increased survival'. Again, if we were to take account of evaluations of coronary care units [38, 39] we would conclude that the prospect of surviving an acute myocardial infarction would be enhanced by being nursed at home or in a general hospital ward rather than in a coronary care unit.

It is certainly not the intention of this book to even begin to explore the intricacies of CEA and CBA – and interested readers are referred to authoritative discussions [40, 41]. Two points are worth making however. First there is evidence that health education has been both effective and efficient – even when judged by the rigorous criteria of CBA. Second, despite such evidence of success, we would be very careful before allowing ourselves to be seduced into making such analyses routinely. Prevention in general and health education in particular may prove to be eminently worthwhile but intrinsically expensive!

Let us, nonetheless, consider an example where on the basis of existing theory a health education intervention could be expected to be cost effective. Townsend [36] considered how a hypothetical mass media anti-smoking campaign costing £250 000 might be judged in a cost-effectiveness analysis. Assuming that 1000 people gave up smoking permanently, 10 000 gave up temporarily, 2000 cut down temporarily and 15 000 seriously considered giving up, then 2 991 life years would be saved at a cost of £84 per life. The cost would appear to be reasonable by comparison with Table 3.1. The reader will be better able to judge whether, on the basis of historical, normative and theoretical standards, such a campaign could be expected to deliver these results after referring to Chapter six which discusses the effectiveness and efficiency of mass media.

Terris [42] has enthusiastically argued the cost-effectiveness case for prevention, estimating that a moderately effective programme in the USA might save each year at least 400 000 lives, six million person-years of life and five billion dollars' worth of medical costs. Green has provided several much more closely argued examples of favourable cost-benefit ratios for specific health education programmes [43]. One of these demonstrates a saving of $7.81 per dollar invested in a hypertension screening and education programme; the other, which analysed the impact of using group discussion techniques to modify unnecessary use of emergency rooms for asthma patients, notched up a cost-benefit ratio of 1:5.

A recent British study by the Policy Studies Institute [44] on the benefits and costs of family planning identified conservative benefit to cost ratios of 1.3:1 for the typical prevented unplanned pregnancy; a ratio of 4.5:1 for prevented pregnancies among mothers of three or more children; and a 5.3:1 ratio for unplanned, premarital conceptions. In other words, '... for every £100 spent on family planning services, the public sector can expect a benefit of £130, £450 and £530 respectively'. Although this illustration does not refer to a health education programme *per se*, it is clear that family planning, like other health promotion initiatives, cannot be achieved without an educational component.

There is, then, clear evidence that health education may not only be effective but its benefits can outweigh programme costs. However, as indicated above, we must strike a cautionary note. Just as health education should resist attempts to cajole it into using medical or epidemiological indicators of success, it should also be wary of adopting CBA too enthusiastically. While a favourable cost-benefit ratio is possible, there will be many instances where health education may in the long run prove expensive. For example the cost of successful alcohol and smoking programmes in terms of lost employment in those industries and lost govenment revenues is well known and although many if not all of these costs can be offset by savings on health service treatment costs, the balance sheet is still complex. The longer people live, the more demands they make on the welfare state. As Smith [45] elegantly reminds us, 'Various kinds of false optimism are invoked by many doctors ... First, they argue that preventive and curative medicine may one day be as successful with diseases that are currently chronic and incurable as it has been in the past with those acute diseases that relatively speaking no longer trouble us. But unless we succeed in abolishing death we shall always have to treat the dying. The optimists sometimes seem to look forward to a time when most people will make their exit from this world without causing inconvenience to doctors. The evidence provides little ground for any such hope. In general, the older we are when we die the longer the period of alleviative care we require before death. Since it seems reasonable to suppose that the older we are when we die the more likely it is that we have died of old age, it follows that when most people die of old age rather than intercurrent disease, the demands they make on medical care are greater. When we all die of old age, after a life-time of health, the main task of the health service will be with the alleviative care of terminal illness. If we should succeed in abolishing death the main preoccupation of the health service will be with contraception.'

Although health economists may offset some of the costs of future health care by the process of 'discounting' – so that future costs are rated as less important than current costs – or by resorting to the somewhat casuistic notion of 'merit good' [46] which appears to acknowledge that some social benefits are so intrinsically meritorious that financial costs are deemed irrelevant, nonetheless and in the last analysis, we have to be prepared to pay for health.

If the entire focus of our evaluation is, however, to be on achieving favourable cost-benefit ratios, presumably the ideal intervention is one which ensures that individuals achieve a level of health which is just sufficient to enable them to carry out an approved social role while indulging themselves in unhealthy activities to the extent that they avoid sickness absence, are productive but manage to damage their constitution to the extent that they die quickly on the day after they achieve pensionable age. In reality though, Draper's observations are nearer the mark: health promotion, he argues, is inherently inconsistent with the goal of economic productivity. In which case we are more likely to have to choose health or wealth [47].

INDICATORS OF WELL-BEING

Before reviewing this chapter's discussion of indicators of success, it is important to give some consideration to measures which might be used to indicate well-being. Reference was made in Chapter One to the concern felt by some people involved in health promotion that there should be a greater emphasis on promoting positive health in order to counterbalance the predominant orientation towards cure and prevention of disease – a viewpoint which is, of course, entirely consistent with the WHO's seminal concept of 'well-being'.

As Hunt and McEwen [48, 49] point out in their rationale for the development of the Nottingham Health Profile, the philosophical shift from logical positivism and empiricism combined with the changing nature of disease and disability in contemporary society, has lead to a concern to devise more subjective measures of well-being and quality of life. In the context of this book, such indicators are the positive analogues of the traditional medical outcome measures such as mortality, morbidity or individual clinical measures such as level of serum cholesterol or number of decayed, missing and filled teeth. A brief comment will, therefore, be made about the kinds of subjective indicator which have been used and are available to the evaluator.

Briscoe, writing from a social work perspective [50], comments that '... subjective measures of well-being are therefore needed in order adequately to assess – and hence treat – a wide spectrum of psychosocial dysfunction.' The reference to 'dysfunction' and to 'psychosocial' should incidentally remind us that it is difficult to completely distance oneself from negative aspects of health. Hall [51] underlines this point in his observation that two of the best buys in subjective indicators are the Housing Nuisance Index and the Health Symptom Index!

Hall describes the development of a variety of subjective measures of quality of life in Britain between 1971 and 1975. Clearly the most problematical aspect of measuring quality of life is defining it. Hall cites Tom Harrisson, the founder of Mass Observation, who said, 'You cannot, yet, take a census of love in Liverpool, or random sample the effect that fear of the future has on the total pattern of contemporary life in Leeds.' Nonetheless, Hall describes the result of the Social Science Research Council's 1975 survey in which respondents were asked to define 'quality of life'. The results are particularly revealing – not only for the construction of subjective indicators but also for the way they provide an insight into perceptions of health and well-being. For instance 23% of the sample of 932 people of all social groups referred to 'family, home-life, marriage' while 19% made rather more vague references to being contented or happy. A further 17% and 18% valued decent living conditions and money respectively. Health was relegated to a 10% response rate while more abstract and altruistic aspects of quality of life, such as equality and justice, were mentioned by only 2% of the sample. These findings confirm the view that many people's notions of positive health or well-being derive from whatever happens to be their salient value system and/or from a meaning of health which is consistent with the medical model perspective – lack of disease or social impairment.

Measures of quality of life, therefore, included people's level of satisfaction with the various 'life domains' mentioned above: more particularly, housing, health, standard of living, etc. In addition, more global measures of well-being were used. These sought to measure personal competence and trust in others and positive and negative affect (using for example Bradburn's Affect Balance Scale [52]).

By contrast, the Nottingham Health Profile (Hunt and McEwen, [47, 48]) adopted an approach which focused more on personal than social well-being. The Profile consists of six sections referring to: emotional life; experience of pain; energy levels; social integration; physical mobility; and sleep patterns.

While this brief glimpse of indicators of quality of life reveals the richness and variety of possible measures by comparison with traditional epidemiological indicators, we should still remember the cautionary note about using certain classes of outcome indicator as measures of health education success. Although positive health indicators will probably be more appealing to health educators than illness-related measures, they may prove to be equally, if not more, problematic. Like mortality and morbidity, quality of life will be affected by a wide variety of social and environmental influences beyond the control of even the most thorough programme. It would, therefore, be just as unwise to use well-being as an indicator of success as it would be to employ 'medical' indicators.

PERFORMANCE INDICATORS

Recent years have seen the development of indicators to monitor performance within the NHS. Government commitment to a free market economy and efforts to curb or reduce public expenditure on welfare services have given a new urgency to the debate about the costs of health care delivery. The question of relating public expenditure on health care to performance has become a central theme and the creation of systems of performance assessment a major initiative within the NHS. The original **performance indicators** (PIs) are based on statistical data already routinely collected in the NHS. What is new is the attempt to present this information clearly and systematically and in a form which will permit comparison between districts and over time.

Most PIs consist of simple ratios, such as costs per case, length of stay of patients in hospital, numbers of nursing staff per occupied bed, deaths and discharges per available bed. At present, the majority of PIs are indirect indicators exclusively concerned with inputs, such as cost per patient, and processes or activities, such as numbers of patients treated or the frequency of use of particular treatments or procedures. Their usefulness is based on the assumption that, given the appropriate resources and medical procedures, satisfactory health care will result.

Indicators, as we have already seen, are not to be equated with measures of outcome. Performance indicators alone, therefore, can not provide health service managers with direct information about the effectiveness of their activities. They are intended to highlight areas of performance which are believed to be related to outcome, for scrutiny and comparison. In other words, PIs are to be used to 'help illuminate local activity and use of resources, which will enable people to spotlight aspects of their services which warrant investigation ... PIs will not give them answers, but they will certainly help them to pose questions' [53].

There are, however, a number of difficulties associated with even this specifically limited use of PIs. It may not always be clear, for example, exactly what a set of PIs does illuminate. Suppose that comparison of PIs relating to neonatal mortality revealed large differences between two district health authorities. What questions should this information pose for health service managers? Little can be said about the quality of care in the two districts because just as indirect indicators are related to intermediate and outcome indicators in a complicated way, neonatal mortality reflects a complex relationship between medical care and health status. Birth weight is known to be an important factor in neonatal deaths, but is itself linked to a range of social factors. In the absence of information relating to these wider aspects of health status, it is difficult to interpret observed differences in indicator values between districts.

Routine statistics based on NHS activity will inevitably provide incomplete information about the effectiveness of services, making comparison between districts difficult. Data relating to the population served by a district and information about the provision and use of other services such as those provided by local authorities are essential if the impact of health care is to be seen in perspective. This difficulty underlines a general problem associated with PIs, even relatively simple ones. Many PI data sets are almost overwhelming in terms of the volume of data presented. Yet in any one area they often lack sufficiently detailed information to illuminate interpretation and comparison.

There may also be doubt about what the value of a specific PI should be. Where a policy statement explicitly quantifies its objective, it is clear that any indicator which falls short of this value is undesirable. The policy objective that there should be a health education co-ordinator in every secondary school, for instance, could be relatively easily monitored and although different rates of achievement of this objective between schools would require explanation, it would be clear that education authorities without a co-ordinator in every secondary school would not be achieving the goal. For most PIs, probably because so little is known in most cases about the relationship of inputs to outcomes, there is no 'right value', nor is it clear whether a change in the value of the indicator is a good or bad thing.

It has been suggested [54] that one effect of this ambiguity is the likelihood that health service managers will attempt to fall in line with average PI values. Yet, as Klein [55] points out, health service resources can be used in many different combinations and the use of average PI values may make the unwarranted assumption that a particular pattern of inputs and activities will necessarily produce the best results in all circumstances. Average PI values may also fail to take into account important differences between districts, such as patient mix and availability of other services. In a district with weak community support services, for example, it might be more efficient to keep some patients in hospital than would be the case where aftercare is easily obtainable. An atypical PI value for length of stay in hospital, although deviant, would reflect efficient use of resources in this case.

Performance Indicators and Outcomes

Performance indicators are useful to the extent that they relate to outcomes. Unless we know how PIs relate to a healthier (however defined) or more empowered or more satisfied population, it will not be clear what implications PIs, or changes in PI values, have for action. It is not, however, just a question of improving the validity of indicators. The outcomes against which they are to be validated may themselves be problematic. Even at a simple level, there may be confusion about what counts as an outcome. If a health education unit has run a course to improve the group work skills of health visitors, for instance, should increased group work activity by health visitors be seen as an outcome or as an input? At a more profound level, as we have seen in Chapter One, there may be disagreements surrounding the objectives and thus the appropriate outcomes of health service activity. The aims of the NHS have always been somewhat vague but most would probably agree that important goals are the reduction of death, disease, disability and distress. Mortality statistics, which are currently used as outcome measures in some sets of PIs, cover only the first of these. They indicate little about caring for the ill and nothing about the relief of disability and distress. Others, and most health educators would probably be included among these, would argue that it is also an objective of the NHS to promote health, yet the current sets of PIs do not relate to measures of health.

Even in cases where there is consensus about desired outcomes, there may be disagreement about how these are to be measured. Some outcomes are not readily translated into statistical indicators. This is not just a problem for health education. Similar difficulties exist in the area of psychiatry, for example. Key objectives of psychiatric services include not only improvements in symptoms, but also less tangible outcomes such as the social and occupational adjustment of patients and the impact of the illness on their families. The inherent difficulty of operationalizing significant but complex objectives such as these is well known in much social research. It may be a reflection of these difficulties that performance in psychiatry is assessed by on-site visits as well as by statistical indicators. Kushlik [56] has described areas of work which are difficult, if not impossible, to quantify, as 'fuzzies'. Many goals of health education fall into this category. Concepts such as personal growth, feelings of efficacy and self-empowerment are likely to defy reduction to a set of simple statistical indicators. We may in such cases choose to agree with Patton that it is preferable to devise 'soft or rough measures of important goals rather than have precise and quantitative measures of goals that no-one really cares about' [57].

Performance Indicators and Quality of Services

The DHSS has acknowledged [58] that is has proved difficult to devise PIs which relate to quality or acceptability of services. Statistics which are taken to indicate quality, such as staffing ratios and drug costs per patient, fall very far short of the aspects of health care which might be taken to contribute to its acceptability. Moreover, the notion of quality is itself not straightforward. Professional standards for assessing the acceptability of a service may conflict with those of its consumers. Hospital delivery may be preferred to home confinement by doctors but the reverse is the case for many women. The difficulty here lies not so much in the technicalities of developing PIs but in recognizing and taking account of conflicting views about the acceptability of particular aspects of health care. The Griffiths Inquiry [59] recommended the use of techniques such as market research to assess customer satisfaction with health services. Community health councils and voluntary groups might also be involved in developing indicators of acceptability and it is likely that this will be a more successful development at the local rather than the national level. The development of such indicators is, of course, as relevant to health education as to any other health service.

Performance Indicators and Health Education

If PIs developed from specialty-specific data have posed problems of selection and interpretation, it is not difficult to see why no national PIs have been developed for health education. Health educators in the NHS work with a variety of client groups, may be involved in a number of different programme areas and draw on a range of approaches including training, curriculum development, policy implementation and community development. It has proved impossible to devise a single, simple set of PIs to reflect the scope of these activities. It has been suggested [60] that useful PIs for health education are more likely to be developed at the local than the national level and that they will be linked to specific programmes or sets of objectives. This will help to clarify which objectives can be monitored by PIs and which, like 'fuzzies', are best assessed in some other way.

INDICATORS: A REVIEW

Throughout this chapter we have explored in some detail the range and variety of indicators of successful health promotion and education programmes. An attempt was made to demonstrate the theoretical elements contributing to various outcomes via individual decision-making and showing how these might be assessed by means of a 'chain' of indicators ranging from indirect through intermediate to outcome. It was also, hopefully, apparent that intermediate indicators might be considered outcome indicators of success for certain models of health education. For instance, in Figure 3.5, a measure of self-esteem might be an intermediate indicator for a preventively oriented cancer education programme but an outcome indicator for a personal/social education programme having as its goal self-empowerment. These points

Table 3.2 Taxonomy of indicators which may be used in evaluating health promotion/
health education programmes

Types of measure	Examples
Clinical/epidemiological measure	Measures of mortality and morbidity (incidence and prevalence rates); sickness absence rates; bed occupancy, etc.; disability indices; plaque index; serum cholesterol level; control of diabetes; blood pressure.
Subjective indicators/ measures of 'quality of life'/wellbeing	Level of reported satisfaction; Nottingham Health Profile; Bradburn Affect Balance Scale; Personal Competence Scale; Level of assertiveness; level of self-esteem.
Behavioural indicators	
Routines	Dietary behaviours; exercise; routine use of stress management skills.
Single time choices	Visit to doctor for cyto test; writing letter to MP about sports sponsorship by tobacco industry.
Skills (psychomotor)	Breast self-examination; cardio-pulmonary resuscitation
Skills (social interaction)	Assertiveness; resisting social pressure to smoke.
Intermediate indicators	
Awareness/attention	Paying attention to poster; awareness of TV public service advertisement about coronary heart disease.
Perception/interpretation	Correct interpretation of doctor's advice.
Recall of information	Remembering that saturated fats are unhealthy (but not necessarily understanding why).
Understanding	Understanding that cancer is not a single undifferentiated disease.
Decision-making skill	Making appropriate choice of heart healthy food in a supermarket.
Values	Valuing deferred gratification when superior pay-off to immediate gratification.
Beliefs	Belief in susceptibility to accident; belief that life after retirement may be productive and enjoyable.
Attitudes	Positive attitude to breastfeeding baby; feeling it is important to lose weight; satisfaction with doctor's communication.
Drives	'Addiction' to alcohol; dependence on tobacco.
Personality measures	Self-esteem; health locus of control; ego strength.
Indirect indicators	Number of leaflets distributed; teacher's attendance at course on new approaches to drug education; schools buy new health education teaching package; schools use teaching package correctly.

should be born in mind when considering Table 3.2 which lists and exemplifies various indicators in roughly ascending order of their approximation to 'distal' outcome indicators. It will be noted that the term 'personality measure' has been used as one variety of intermediate indicator – and this, perhaps, requires some explanation. It is clearly inappropriate here to venture into the field of personality theory – not is it particularly profitable since classic measures of personality type have little relevance to the evaluation of health promotion programmes.

It is difficult to draw a fine line between measures of personality and measures of other individual characteristics such as knowledge and beliefs. For the purpose of the present discussion, only those variables which define a relatively enduring personal attribute will be described as measures of personality (or which describe a cluster of characteristics more or less peculiar to the individual). Both self esteem and perceived locus of control could be viewed as personality measures or as an example of a value and a belief respectively. Similarly the notion of Ego Strength would legitimately be seen as a personality trait which would be part of mainstream personality theory (see Cattell's 16 PF Test, [61]) and also have relevance for health-related behaviour. For instance an increase in both self-esteem and ego strength would be expected to help individuals resist social pressure to engage in unhealthy behaviours.

Again, while not a recognized and standardized test of personality, profiles of smoking type would also qualify (although this might be a useful indicator for research in health education it would have no value as indicator of evaluation since it is presumably not desirable to change type of smoker – even if it were possible – but rather to achieve smoking cessation).

The various personality measures discussed above serve to illustrate nicely the point made earlier – that an indicator might be either intermediate or outcome depending on the health education model adopted. For instance, enhanced self-esteem and increased internality might be an entirely self-sufficient goal for a mental health programme or alternatively it could be only an intermediate point in a programme which considers these attributes as necessary precursors to a more distal goal of resisting social pressure to smoke or drink immoderately.

The present chapter has examined indicators of success and the theoretical framework which should help evaluators make appropriate choices. The remaining chapters will consider evaluative aspects of major strategies for delivering health education – in schools, health care contexts, via mass media, in the workplace and by means of various community interventions, including community development.

REFERENCES

1. Rosenman, R. H. (1977) History and definition of the type A coronary-prone behavior pattern, in: *Proceedings of the Forum on Coronary-Prone Behavior*, (ed. T. Dembroski) Dept. of Health, Education and Welfare, Pub. No. (NIH) 78-1451, Washington DC, pp. 13–18.
2. Warner, K. E. (1981) Cigarette smoking in the 1970s: the impact of the anti-smoking campaign on consumption, *Science*, 211, 729–31.
3. Tones, B. K. (1986) Preventing drug misuse: the case for breadth, balance and coherence, *Health Education Journal*, 45, 197–203.
4. Tones, B. K. (1987) Devising strategies for preventing drug misuse: the role of the health action model, *Health Education Research*, 2, 305–18.
5. Green, L. W. (1984) Health education models, in: *Behavioral Health: A Handbook of Health Enhancement and Disease Prevention* (eds J. D. Matarazzo *et al.*) John Wiley, New York.
6. McAlister, A. *et al.* (1982) Theory and action for health promotion: illustrations from the North Karelia Project, *American Journal of Public Health*, 72, 43–53.
7. Becker, M. H. (ed) (1984) *The Health Belief Model and Personal Health Behavior*, Charles B. Slack, Thorofare, New Jersey.
8. Janz, N. K. and Becker, M. H. (1984) The Health Belief Model: a decade later, *Health Education Quarterly*, 11, 1–47.
9. Fishbein, M. and Ajzen, I. (1985) *Belief Attitude, Intention and Behavior: an Introduction to Theory and Research*, Addison-Wesley, Reading, Mass.
10. Ajzen, I. and Fishbein, M. (1980) *Understanding Attitudes and Predicting Social Behavior*, Prentice Hall, New Jersey.
11. Baric, L., MacArthur, J. and Sherwood, M. (1976) A study of health educational aspects of smoking in pregnancy, *International Journal of Health Education*, Supplement to Vol. XIX.
12. Freidson, E. (1961) *Patients' Views of Medical Practice*, Russell Sage, New York, pp. 146–7.
13. Rotter, J. B. (1966) Generalized expectancies for internal versus external control of reinforcement, *Psychological Monographs*, 80.
14. Tones, B. K. (1987) Health Promotion, 'Affective Education and the Personal-Social Development of Young People', in: *Health Education in Schools* (2nd edn) (ed. K. David and T. Williams) Harper and Row, London.
15. Tones, B. K. (1987) Op. cit. [4].
16. Janis, I. L. and Mann, L. (1977) *Decision Making*, Free Press, New York.
17. Fishbein, M. (1976) Persuasive communication, in: *Communication Between Doctors and Patients*, (ed. A. E. Bennet) University Press, Oxford.
18. British Broadcasting Corporation (1983) *Understanding Cancer*, BBC Broadcasting Research Special Report, BBC Research Information Desk, London.
19. Rokeach, M. (1973) *The Nature of Human Values*, Free Press, New York.
20. Fishbein, M. and Ajzen, I. (1985) Op. cit. [9].
21. Baric, L. (1978) Health Education and the smoking habit, *Health Education Journal*, 37, 132–7.
22. Russel, M. A. H. *et al.* (1979) Effect of General Practitioners' advice against smoking, *British Medical Journal*, 2, 231–5.

23. McGuire, W. J. (1981) Theoretical foundations of campaigns, in: *Public Communication Campaigns*, (eds R. E. Rice and W. J. Paisley), Sage, Beverly Hills.
24. Rogers, E. M. and Shoemaker, F. F. (1971) *Communication of Innovations*, Free Press, New York.
25. Green, L. (1986) Health education strategies and approaches to evaluation in community and mass media, in: *Smoking Control: Strategies and Evaluation in Community and Mass Media Programmes*, (eds J. Crofton and M. Wood), Report of a Workshop, Health Education Council, London.
26. Hovland, C., Lumsdaine, A. and Sheffield, F. (1949) *Experiments on Mass Communication*, University Press, Princeton.
27. NACNE Report (1983) *A Discussion Paper on Proposals for Nutritional Guidelines for Health Education in Britain*, Health Education Council, London.
28. Popham, W. J. (1978) Must all objectives be behavioral? in: *Beyond the Numbers Game*, (eds D. Hamilton *et al.*) Macmillan, London.
29. Parlett, M. and Hamilton, D. (1978) Evaluation as illumination: a new approach to the study of innovatory programmes, in: *Beyond the Numbers Game*, (eds D. Hamilton *et al.*) Macmillan, London.
30. Mager, R. F. (1962) *Preparing Instructional Objectives*, Fearon Publishers, Belmont, Cal.
31. Bond, B. W. (1958) A study in health education methods. *International Journal of Health Education*, 1, 41–6.
32. Green, L. W. and Lewis, F. M. (1986) *Measurement and Evaluation in Health Education and Health Promotion*, Mayfield Publishing Co., Palo Alto, Ca, pp. 174–6.
33. Davies, I. K. (1981) *Instructional Technique*, McGraw Hill, New York, p. 22.
34. Mooney, G. H. (1977) *The Valuation of Human Life*, (Appendix C) Macmillan, London.
35. Cochrane, A. C. L. (1972) *Effectiveness and Efficiency: Random Reflections on the Health Service*, T. Rock Carling Lecture 1971, Nuffield Provincial Hospitals Trust, London.
36. Townsend, J. (1986) Cost Effectiveness, in: *Smoking Control: Strategies and Evaluation in Community and Mass Media Programmes*, (eds J. Crofton and M. Wood) Report of a Workshop, Health Education Council, London.
37. Bodmer, W. F. (1985) Understanding statistics, *Journal of Royal Statistical Society*, 148, 69–81.
38. Mather, H. F. *et al.* (1971) Acute myocardial infarction: home and hospital treatment, *British Medical Journal*, (7th August), pp. 334–8.
39. Colling, A. *et al.* (1976) Teesside coronary survey: an epidemiological study of acute attacks of myocardial infarction, *British Medical Journal*, 2, 1169.
40. Green, L. W. and Lewis, F. M. (1986), op. cit. [31].
41. Windsor, R. A. *et al.* (1984) *Evaluation of Health Promotion and Education Programs*, (Appendix C) Mayfield Publishing Co., Palo Alto, Ca.
42. Terris, M. (1981) The primacy of prevention, *Preventive Medicine*, 10, 689–99.
43. Green, L. W. (1974) Toward cost-benefit evaluations of health education: some concepts, methods, and examples, *Health Education Monographs*, 2, 34–64.
44. Laing, W. A. (1982) *Family Planning: the Benefits and Costs*, No. 607, Policy Studies Institute, London.

45. Smith, A. (1977) The unfaced facts, *New Universities Quarterly*, Spring 1977, 133–45.
46. Cohen, D. (1981) *Prevention as an Economic Good*, Health Economics Research Unit, University of Aberdeen.
47. Draper, P., Bert, G. and Dennis, J. (1977) Health and wealth, *Royal Society of Health Journal*, **97**, 121–7.
48. Hunt, S. M. and McEwen, J. (1980) The development of a subjective health indicator, *Sociology of Health and Illness*, **2**, 231–46.
49. Hunt, S. M., McEwen, J. and McKenna, S. P. (1985) Measuring health status: a new tool for clinicians and epidemiologists, *Journal of the Royal College of General Practitioners*, **35**, 185–8.
50. Briscoe, M. E. (1982) Subjective measures of well-being: differences in the perception of health and social problems, *British Journal of Social Work*, **12**, 137–47.
51. Hall, J. (1976) Subjective measures of quality of life in Britain: 1971 to 1975: some developments and trends, *Social Trends*, **7**, 47–60.
52. Bradburn, N. (1969) *The Structure of Psychological Well-Being*, Aldine, New York.
53. DHSS (1983) *First National Package of Performance Indicators for the NHS*, Press Release, London.
54. Birch, S. and Maynard, A. (1986) *Performance Indicators and Performance Assessment in the NHS: Implications for Efficiency and Proposals for Improvement.* Centre for Health Economics, University of York.
55. Klein, R. (1981) The strategy behind the Jenkin non-strategy, *British Medical Journal*, **282**, 1089–91.
56. Kushlik, A. (1975) Some ways of setting, monitoring and attaining objectives for services for disabled people. *British Journal of Mental Subnormality*, **21**, 85.
57. Patton, M. Q. (1982) *Practical Evaluation*, Sage, Beverly Hills.
58. James, M. (1987) Performance indicators for the National Health Service. *Health Trends*, **19**, 12–13.
59. DHSS (1983) *NHS Management Inquiry* (leader Sir Roy Griffiths), London.
60. Korner, E. (1984) *Steering Group on Health Services Information, Fifth Report to the Secretary of State*, HMSO, London.
61. Cattell, R. B. (1965) *The Scientific Analysis of Personality*, Penguin, Harmondsworth.

4

SCHOOL HEALTH EDUCATION

INTRODUCTION

Schools have been widely promoted as a major context for the delivery of health education. This is an acknowledgement of the importance of health as integral to the complete development of the individual; of the right to health knowledge for its own sake; and the perceived significance of the early learning of health-related knowledge, attitudes and behaviours for the present and future health of individuals and their families and communities. Schools, moreover, in many countries can reach a large proportion of the population over an extended period of time. The American Public Health Association [1] has recognized this:

> The school, as a social structure, provides an educational setting in which the total health of the child during the impressionable years is a priority concern. No other community setting even approximates the magnitude of the school education enterprise ... thus it seems that the school should be regarded as a social unit providing a focal point to which health planning for all other community settings should relate.

Given this importance of childhood and youth in the individual 'health career', ways also need to be found of reaching those children not able to attend school, a fact recognized in a recent policy statement from the International Union of Health Education [2]. Major documents, such as that of Alma Ata on Primary Health Care [3] and the American 'Healthy People' [4] have also focused on the importance of the school in the promotion of community health. Alma Ata [3] gave the education sector a major role in primary health care:

> Schools could provide the efficient means to attain all of the eight components of primary health care and could ensure that young people can be educated to have a good understanding of what health means, how to achieve it, and how it contributes to social and economic development.

In 1980 the USA developed a list of 227 objectives directed towards achieving Health for the Nation by 1990 [5]. This list was analysed by Kolbe and Iverson [6] who believed that approximately one third could be attained directly or indirectly through school activities.

While it is the concern of this chapter to address specific health education activity in schools, the contribution to health of education in general should not be overlooked. This contribution is recognized, for example, in one of the global indicators for Health For All by the Year 2000: the number of countries in which the literacy rate of both men and women exceeds 70% [7]. It has been shown, for example, that a child born to a mother with no education is twice as likely to die in infancy as a child born to a mother with only four years' schooling. The role of schools in achieving both education and health has been described [7] by Kolbe:

> Health and education are interdependent goals and schools provide one of the most universal and efficient means of achieving them both; in virtually every nation schools comprise existing systems, facilities and trained personnel to protect and improve the health of communities.

While the outcomes desired from school health education are a matter for debate, the goals proposed by Kolbe [8] are a good general reflection of expectations:

> First, we can expect school health education to increase understandings about the philosophy and science of individual and societal health;
> Second, we can expect school health education to increase the competencies of individuals to make decisions about personal behaviours that will influence their health;
> Third, we can expect school health education to increase skills and inclinations to engage in behaviours that are conducive to health;
> Fourth, school health education programs, strategically with other school and community health promotion efforts, can be expected to elicit behaviours that are conducive to health; and
> Fifth, we can expect school health education to increase the skills of individuals to maintain and improve the health of their families, and the health of the communities in which they reside.

This chapter continues by briefly outlining the development of health education in schools in the UK and the philosophical approaches which characterize it, prior to posing some general questions on its evaluation.

HISTORICAL BACKGROUND AND APPROACHES TO SCHOOL HEALTH EDUCATION

Chapter One discussed alternative philosophical approaches to health education and the outcomes associated with each. Having an educational brief, schools might be expected to adhere solely to educational and self-empowerment models. While there is undoubtedly considerable commitment to such models, much that takes place in schools also reflects preventive approaches to health education and a great deal of evaluative activity has focused on outcomes associated with the latter approach. Some brief comments on the development of school health education in the UK may serve as a useful background to understanding the mix of philosophical approaches in school health education.

From the mid 1960s particular energy has been devoted to the development of school health education but a slow development had been taking place since at least the beginning of the century. A difficulty in tracing this development arises in part from the general transition from definitions of health which narrowly emphasized physical health to multidimensional concepts. Earlier in the century, therefore, discussion of health education reflects the narrower concepts of health although at the same time educational literature in general often incorporated ideas which later came to be closely associated with broader concepts of health education. For example, the child-centred progressive philosophy of education had its roots in the 18th and 19th centuries in the writings of Rousseau, Froebel, Pestalozzi and others. It gradually made an impact on education in this century, particularly in the primary sector and the 1960s have been described as a highpoint of progressivism in British schools. The concepts of progressivism – child-centredness, autonomy and developmental approach to learning contributed to the climate in schools in which health education slowly developed. It was, however, the first of the general health education projects produced in the 'renaissance' [9] period of health education in the 1970s which fully incorporated these ideas.

Looking at the development of health education in England and Wales the first requirement for its inclusion (using the term hygiene rather than health education) came in 1904. According to Sutherland [10], the first actual mention of health education seemed to come with the setting up of the Central Council for Health Education in 1927 and he suggests that the term 'education' could have been used for the purpose of making health propagandism acceptable in schools. In the previous year the Hadow Report [11] provided only passing mention of hygiene but with its developmental perspective it contributed to, and reflected, the growth of a child-centred climate in education. This influence can be identified in the 1928 Board of Education *Handbook of Suggestions for Health Education* [12]. Revised in 1933 and 1939, it was a standard document on school health education. Although this document had a particular emphasis on hygiene and the promoting of healthy habits and many of the activities suggested were allied to a preventive model of health education there was also commitment to the development of health knowledge for its own sake around pupils' own interests. The document emphasized the need to regard health as more than a mere subject on the curriculum and also as more than the promotion of the routine practice of healthy habits. Health was an ideal, the inculcation of which was no less important than those of truth, goodness and beauty. A further handbook in 1957 [13] emphasized more broadly the importance of environmental improvements in securing health, health as a balance between humans and their environment, and the pursuit of positive health. The year 1964 has been noted as a particularly significant point in the general development of health education. The Cohen Report [14] of that year was concerned with health education in the National Health Service and also made some recommendations on health education in the formative years. This report preceded the foundation of the Health Education Council (HEC) and the growth of health education units within health authorities which together played a most important role in the subsequent developments of school health education. The period since 1964 has been one in which there has been considerable debate on the curriculum as a whole (as well as consideration of specific subjects, including health education, within the curriculum) [15, 16, 17, 18]. There has also been a parallel debate on prevention and health and publications from the Department of Health and Social Security (DHSS) [19, 20, 21, 22]. The debates in education emerged for a complex of reasons which can be identified but not analysed here. They included: the gradual erosion of the political consensus on education which had characterized the period since 1945; a questioning of the relevance of the curriculum in a period of rapid technological change; acknowledgement that the slow transition to comprehensive education in the secondary sector had been preceded by insufficient discussion of the curriculum as a whole; consideration of the needs of the less academic pupil in the Newsom Report [23] and the raising of the school leaving age (ROSLA). During the 1960s and the early 1970s a large number of curriculum projects were developed, mainly with the support of the Schools Council and the Nuffield Foundation. These were directed towards most subjects in the curriculum but with early attention to the sciences and modern languages. Some of these projects such as Lifeline (for moral education) [24] and the Humanities Curriculum Projects [25] addressed content and methodological areas common to the subsequent specific health education projects. The first of many specific health education projects was commissioned in 1973. Coming relatively late in the surge of curriculum development activity it was able to draw on lessons learned on development and dissemination.

Teasing out the commitment to differing philosophical approaches to health education in the period is not easy. Drawing on a variety of secondary sources such as educational documents, the *Health Education Journal* and accounts of school work, some tentative observations can be made. Preventive and educational approaches seem to have coexisted throughout the period. In the earlier part of the century statements such as 'learning healthy ways of living must precede learning about health' offer evidence of the existence of the preventive approach. At the same time discussion of the development of health knowledge around pupil interests using project and other activity-based methods [26], and the emphasis on health, not just as an end in itself but as a means to living life more abundantly, illustrate features of the educational approach. Health education, unlike other subjects in the curriculum, is one with a history of involvement by outsiders, frequently health professionals. The School Health Service is also part of the parallel curriculum. The commitment of health workers to the medical model would ensure a continuing influence on the use of preventive approaches in school health education. Teachers are also likely to adopt preventive approaches in accordance with personal preference, the age of children, the aspects of health in question and in response to particular school and community pressures. Evidence of the support of aims associated with both approaches can be seen in a fairly recent study by Charlton [27]. She reported on the aims of health education as seen by students and tutors in initial teacher training. Asked to rate each of a list of aims, the provision of information was consistently rated first, followed closely by influencing pupils' attitudes and influencing pupils' behaviours. Increasing decision-making skills was rated first by only a very small percentage of students but by a higher percentage of tutors.

The last 15 years have seen a growing sophistication of the educational model in health education and a broadening to become what this text has described as a self-empowerment approach. Ideas associated with child-centred education – self-esteem, developmental organization of health education and the enhancement of decision-making skills – feature strongly in projects such as My Body and the Schools Council Health Education Project (SCHEP 5–13) [28]. These ideas were reinforced by influences from the personal growth movement, and augmented by those of Freire and the writings of the post-industrial theorists [29, 30]. The fullest incorporation of a self-empowerment model can be seen in the new Healthskills Project [31] for teachers and pupils.

It is the radical–political model of health education which, arguably, has had the lowest profile in school health education to date. While the raising of awareness about social and environmental causes of ill health has not been ignored, it does not seem to rank highly in importance as an aim with teachers. In a recent survey in Welsh secondary schools [32], teachers rated topics in order of perceived importance. The environment and health were rated as very important by only 28% of respondents. Although the recent projects have given wider coverage to broader social and environmental issues there is only one, Health Careers [33], which addresses these centrally. This project, on available evidence [34] is little used in schools. Health Careers, while incorporating consciousness raising and consideration of health promoting strategies, does not go beyond the concepts of the educational approach to espouse all aspects of the radical–political model:

> The aim of the course is that young people develop a conception of health relating to the broader social and economic conditions that together with their responses to these conditions affect their health and that they actively explore some of the practical possibilities for changing these circumstances and their responses, with the object of enhancing health.

Health education in British schools appears to be informed therefore by a mix of the philosophical approaches identified in Chapter One. The categorization of approaches adopted here may not be articulated by practitioners themselves and it may not be usual for teachers to identify solely with any particular approach. In a small scale study Anderson [35] found only two teachers clearly identifying with a specific approach. Over-adherence to any one approach can have negative aspects. For example, the perfectly laudable observations on the victim blaming effects of much individualistic health education has led, in some instances, to disapproval of any individually focused work, whether conforming to preventive or educational approaches. Dorn [33] identified what he described as a false dichotomy between voluntaristic and deterministic approaches which was deeply entrenched in the mainstream of health education and impeded its development. He recognized the importance of both. Most of the major statements of aims for health education incorporate outcomes which derive from more than one philosophical approach. In evaluating practice it is necessary to assess the importance attached to particular aims as well as the success in achieving stated outcomes.

EVALUATING SCHOOL HEALTH EDUCATION – GENERAL DISCUSSION

While it is commonplace to note the paucity of evaluation in health education it can be suggested that schools in most countries have been particularly slow to fully evaluate all aspects of their work. Williams [9] commented on this shortcoming:

> Evaluation and assessment are words we need to hear more of. We must help teachers to evaluate and assess the gains they make with their pupils in terms of knowledge, attitudes and of course the influences on their decision-making skills and health behaviour. We also need more longitudinal and short-term studies of the effects of health education on schools, individual pupils and teachers.

A whole variety of reasons could have contributed to the shortcomings:

1. The general climate of evaluation in education as a whole. While formal assessment of pupil attainment, particularly in the cognitive domain, and informal appraisal of all features of the curriculum have always been school activities, more comprehensive formal evaluation of a range of outcomes has been slower to emerge.
2. Failure to recognize the importance of evaluating a subject which has generally held a low status within the curriculum.
3. A lack of skills to evaluate the range of objectives addressed by health education. Teachers are skilled in the assessment of cognitive areas but may be less so in assessing both attitudes and competencies such as decision-making skills and assertiveness.
4. A general shortage of time and other resources to support evaluation.
5. In the absence of an agreed set of aims for school health education, specifying outcomes to be addressed in evaluation can be difficult.

There are various changes in education which should contribute to a lessening of some of the barriers to evaluation. There is a growing pressure towards accountability. Although many reservations exist about innovations such as the regular testing of children in basic subjects, a general climate of accountability is likely to lead to an increase in some evaluation skills. Both the development of GCSE with its assessment of a wider spectrum of competencies [36] and the production of pupil records of achievement should also increase teacher expertise. Courses disseminating school health education projects emphasize evaluation and develop skills in it and many project materials include pupil evaluation sheets which act as a reminder to teachers. A full development of 'the teacher as researcher' [37] would, arguably, make the greatest contribution to an increase in evaluation.

There are probably no aspects of evaluation which are unique to schools but there are features which may be more of an issue in this context than others:

1. Delineating what is to be evaluated as health education. The broader the definition of health education the more difficult it becomes to differentiate it from education in general.
2. Health education can be organized in a number of ways in schools. In the secondary sector, for example, it may be provided through coordinated inputs from across a number of curriculum subjects such as biology, home economics and physical education; as a constituent strand of a personal and social education course; in the context of tutorial time; as a timetabled subject in its own right or various combinations of these and other arrangements (Figure 4.1). If attempting, for example, to evaluate sex education in the curriculum, identifying all the contributory elements from the formal curriculum can be difficult. If the additional elements of the curriculum are also considered evaluation becomes even more complex.

3. Where health behaviours are a focus for evaluation there are two particular issues. First, behaviours such as alcohol use, drug use and smoking which are perceived as very important by teachers typically occur outside the school environment and evaluators must rely on reported measures. Second, cause for concern may be the long-term adoption of behaviours or behaviours that do not occur for the first time until some time after leaving school; as indicated in Chapter Two, long-term evaluations are more difficult to carry out than short-term ones.

4. Decisions about who should plan and carry out evaluations. Where there is commitment to empowerment approaches pupils could participate in, rather than merely cooperate with, the evaluation process.

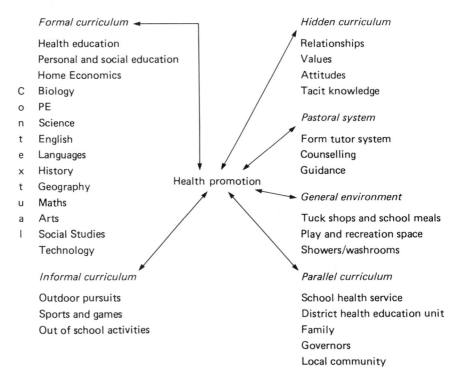

Figure 4.1 Health promotion in the school.

In evaluating school health education we can focus on any, or all, of five distinct, although overlapping and interacting levels.

1. Individual pupil: evaluation addresses learning outcomes of pupils achieved as the result of formal and informal health education activities within the total school curriculum (Fig. 4.1).

2. Individual school: health education of pupils occurs within the context of the total school environment. A second level of evaluation appraises the individual school as a health promoting environment.
3. Community: schools exist within communities. The immediate and longer-term effects of school health education on these communities can be assessed.
4. The school system: while effective health education may be demonstrated in small-scale studies with groups of pupils, or in individual schools as a whole, it is important to enquire about the extent to which the schools system as a whole in any country provides a satisfactory health education for all pupils.
5. National and local policy: a variety of policies related to education and to health can have a bearing on the development of appropriate, and successful, health education in schools.

Space precludes a systematic and comprehensive review of appropriate evaluations. The following discussion will address these five levels in order to offer general observations and highlight issues of particular interest.

EVALUATING SCHOOL HEALTH EDUCATION – SPECIFIC CATEGORIES

Individual Pupil

Much of the evaluation of health education in terms of pupil gains has focused on classroom activities offered within the formal curriculum. Studies have addressed any one, or combination of the indicators – whether outcomes, intermediate or indirect, discussed in Chapter Three. A substantial proportion of studies to date have focused on the intermediate indicators of knowledge, beliefs and attitudes and the outcomes of health and health behaviour. There appears to be a growing optimism that health education can be effective in addressing these particular variables. For instance, writing in 1981, Bartlett [38] concluded that the best developed school health education programmes were successful in increasing knowledge, somewhat successful in improving attitudes and infrequently successful in facilitating lifestyle changes. Only four years later, however, Mason and McGinnis [39], reporting on the School Health Evaluation Study, said:

> ... the study unequivocally demonstrates that school health education is an effective means of helping children to improve their health knowledge and develop healthy attitudes. It also shows that school health education can decrease the likelihood that children will adopt behaviours that are hazardous to health, such as cigarette smoking.

Others [40, 41] have concurred with this view although Reid and Massey saw progress as somewhat uneven and thought it desirable to consider results for different health topics individually. Attention has been directed to a fairly large number of health topics depending on what are seen as problems in any particular place or any specific time. Reid and Massey concluded from their review:

> ... given suitable methods used in appropriate contexts, schools can favourably affect teenage health-related behaviour in relation to smoking, oral hygiene, rubella immunization, and teenage fertility. There is also some evidence for potential success in the field of diet and exercise.

Two of these health topics, dental health and smoking, will be discussed in order to illustrate the kinds of successes which have been achieved. Rubinson has provided [42] a general discussion of the evaluation of school dental health education programmes in which she identified a shift of focus to a more careful examination and questioning of the behaviour portion of the knowledge – attitudes – behaviours triad. Natural Nashers [43] a health education programme for the early secondary school years has been subjected to thorough evaluation [44]. It is designed to be offered largely in the context of the biology curriculum in three approximately one-and-a-half hour sessions. There are also project suggestions and a home experiments diary. It is designed to develop a number of concepts and beliefs and the skills of disclosing and toothbrushing. The evaluation included both formative and summative elements and investigated changes in pupil knowledge and beliefs, changes in pupil oral hygiene, teacher opinions, pupils' reported behaviours and beliefs and parental responses. A sample of 2871 was used from schools randomly assigned to study and control categories. Using a pre-test/post-test questionnaire, significant differences in knowledge were obtained between study and control groups after teaching the programme. For questions checking knowledge on the age of eruption of permanent teeth, frequency of sugar intake and reasons for teeth, the results shown in Table 4.1 were obtained. For all three items the differences were significant at the 5% level.

The evaluation analysed results by class, gender and a number of other background factors: visiting the community dentist, attendance for regular checkups, and whether pupils had received a demonstration of toothbrushing and received dietary advice. On the three knowledge measures correct responses were more likely from girls, pupils from non-manual backgrounds and regular attenders. The results for beliefs were rather more mixed. While the project was successful in developing a new belief in the study group in the role of sugar in dental caries it was not so successful in changing the already held beliefs about the preventive action of toothbrushing on dental caries. A gingival index measure was used as an indicator of oral hygiene. No significant

Table 4.1 Changes in knowledge

	Eruption, first permanent		Frequency of sugar intake		Reasons for teeth	
	Study	*Control*	*Study*	*Control*	*Study*	*Control*
Pre (%)	13	13	18	19	53	51
Base	1399	1453	1401	1419	1613	1636
Post (%)	29	17	46	25	82	57
Base	1373	1319	1364	1275	1460	1435
	$z = 4, p < 0.05$		$z = 6.33, p < 0.05$		$z = 8.33, p < 0.05$	

differences were found between study and control groups. In discussing the results from the evaluation the reliance on criteria of immediate behaviour change as a measure of the effectiveness of a programme was questioned. The interests of the sponsors of the study were seen as lying in evidence of success in achieving clinical outcomes. It was felt however that the children had other needs such as lack of dental knowledge which were being met through involvement with Natural Nashers. This was quite probably the case but it is perhaps appropriate to question the financial costs of this project associated with achieving such knowledge gains.

In a questionnaire survey of 106 teachers involved in teaching the project 93% felt that Natural Nashers was an effective way of bringing health education into the curriculum, 71% that it was effective in teaching aspects of biology, and 83% thought it motivated adolescents to look after their teeth. Most felt that Natural Nashers aided their teaching (98%), did not erode their freedom in the classroom (78%) and did not make their teaching too mechanical (83%).

This programme was particularly interesting for the very thorough and reflective consideration to which it was subjected at all stages of its development, dissemination and evaluation. Discussing the project, Craft [46] said:

> ... an appropriate programme will contain accurate messages, include activity but avoid victim blaming: an acceptable programme will take user values into account and recognize the background of teachers. An appropriate evaluation will be matched to the nature of the programme and information needed whilst to be acceptable it must take into account the needs of sponsors, developers and mediators. In the area of dissemination, to be appropriate implies recognizing local area needs and the desirability of developing a support structure.

Acceptability in turn may rest upon involving all significant interest groups and encouraging both local interest and growth.

While the gains reported in the above study were relatively modest there is a general view that some very real success can be claimed for smoking education in schools. In a recent review Reid and Massey [40] concluded that, although occasional negative findings occurred, the overwhelming majority of reports from North America, Europe and Australia indicated that schools had a potentially major role to play in preventing smoking. It is acknowledged that although the bulk of success has been with 11–13 year olds, long-term effectiveness is not so clear, neither is the effect on recruitment in later teenage years, on girls compared with boys and on different class groups. The successes can be illustrated by referring to the School Health Curriculum Project (SHCP) in the USA and the My Body project developed from it in the UK [46, 47, 48]. The SHCP was one of four projects assessed in the School Health Evaluation study which involved 30 000 children in the USA in grades four to seven (9–13 years). In the SHCP study, using a post-test questionnaire significant differences between study and control groups were found for knowledge items and smoking-related attitudes. On a self-reported measure of smoking used with 7th grade pupils, 12.7% of control students reported smoking against 7.7% who had received SHCP [49]. It was estimated that if these results were extrapolated nationwide 146 000 7th graders would delay the onset of smoking. Evaluation of the My Body project reported gains in knowledge, changes in attitude and a probable halving of the rate of experimental smoking [50]. A longer term follow up of this project offered evidence on an aspect of smoking of current concern – the smoking of girls and women. Four hundred children in seven junior schools were taught the programme in the winters of 1977/8 and 1978/9. In the springs of 1980 and 1982 they, together with age-matched controls, completed a questionnaire on knowledge, attitudes and reported behaviours. A weakness of this study, recognized by the researchers, was the failure to incorporate controls from the start. The programme appeared to have a differential impact on boys and girls. Boys who were taught the programme were less likely than boys in the control groups to smoke subsequently while girls taught the programme were more likely than controls to adopt smoking. When allowance was made for the effect of parental and sibling smoking the differential effect persisted [51]. The purpose of the My Body project is to provide children with a thorough understanding of personal health and to 'inoculate' them against pressures to smoke after entering secondary school. This appeared to have been successful with the boys. With the boys the intention to start smoking at 11–12 years of age was a good predictor of behaviour two years later. It was concluded that the My Body project had been taught at an age which would have maximum impact on smoking incidence among boys. In the case of the girls, whose smoking careers lagged behind those of the boys, the intervention had come too early. Charlton [52] also reported differential effects on the two sexes using a two lesson smoking topic directed at children and their parents. Significant impact on boys and their fathers occurred but there were less positive results among girls and their mothers. The two most effective factors about these teaching materials were that they appeared to delay the recruitment of boys to smoking and to influence fathers to stop. It can be suggested that, to date, the psycho–social factors influencing the smoking of girls and women have been less well recognized than those influencing boys and men. Smoking education evaluations depend on reported measures with the known tendency of respondents to under report. More objective measures have been developed. The measure of thiocyanate ions in saliva is an example and the use of the test is said to corroborate self-reporting [53]. Prior knowledge of the possibility of an objective test increases levels of reported smoking. Gillies [54] has argued that thiocyanate estimation appears to have limited value at low smoking levels. She also raises the ethical issues connected with the use of the test or suggested use of it:

> It is arguable whether or not it should be acceptable for researchers in schools to use methods which assume that children will lie about something if asked. Such an assumption about lack of truthfulness could undermine the trust built up between teachers and their pupils.

Smoking behaviours and the influences on them in young people have been subject to considerable scrutiny and a variety of methodological approaches have been adopted in smoking education. Of particular interest in the last 10 years has been the use of methods which address the social influences on smoking. Evans [55] identified peers, parents and the media as major sources of pressure and in response attempted to familiarize children with these pressures and with ways of dealing with them. McAlister and others [56, 57] developed the ideas further and added the use of peer leaders as educators, activities to increase social commitment not to smoke, and the role-playing of situations that needed resistance to social pressure. A number of studies have reported significant results using these approaches [58, 59] but comparisons between them are not easy because the precise elements and their organization vary. It is also difficult to deduce which elements are of particular significance as noted by Flay [60] in a review of this literature. Smoking education was discussed comprehensively by Reid [61] who observed:

> There has been such a remarkable reversal since Thompson concluded in an earlier review of smoking that most methods had shown little success. One can almost claim that most methods have been highly successful in the short term.

Even approaches based largely on giving information have been successful. Some of the reasons suggested to account for these successes are: the fall in prevalence of smoking in the adult population and the consequent changes in the social environment in which smoking choices are made; the use of non-didactic approaches with an emphasis on discussion and active finding out from films and books; and an emphasis on immediate effects of cigarette smoke as opposed to the long-term hazards.

While the gains in dental health and smoking education and for other health topics not discussed here have been welcomed three questions can be asked:

1. Should school health education be pursuing health behaviour change? While philosophical positions will affect the answer to this question there appears to be some broad general support among teachers, as noted earlier, for preventive approaches [27]. It is the balance between approaches which has to be given particular attention.

2. Accepting some level of commitment to behaviour change, are the successes to date good enough? The assumptions of the criticized knowledge – attitudes – practice (KAP) model continue to inform much work: given the development of an appropriate body of knowledge, favourable attitudes and subsequently desired behaviours are expected to follow. As Parcel [62] has said, this can be a backwards approach; if behavioural outcomes are the desired ones, he notes: 'It may be more effective to start by thoroughly identifying the behaviours and then work backwards, identifying the knowledge and skills needed to develop the behavioural capability for practising those behaviours'.

   He stresses that more emphasis and importance needs to be given to utilizing sophisticated conceptualizations and theoretical models in the design of school health education interventions if greater successes are to be achieved.

3. Do health topic focused projects have general as well as specific benefits? The adoption and implementation costs of some health topic focused projects can be considerable and adequate resources may not be available to support education related to all health topics of concern. Projects could be assessed by broader educational criteria as well as the specific health behavioural ones. Parcel [62] says that focused programmes such as the 3 R's High Blood Pressure Project (evaluated in the School Health Education Evaluation (SHEE)) are likely to effect targeted outcome in their specific area, but they are unlikely to be generalizable to broader outcomes for school health education. The My Body project on the other hand, which as noted earlier incorporates active learning methods, is likely to have broader outcomes.

The development of knowledge is common to all approaches to health education. Further to the third question above some comments can be made on the knowledge component of health education. For maximal impact on specific health behaviours knowledge may need to be very specifically focused – for example, the knowledge of frequency of sugar intake as a preventive measure in dental caries. We need to ask, however, if pupils develop that knowledge in ways which leave them open to reassessing it in the light of later developments. Health education can offer many examples of adherence to educational messages of the past, now superseded. If this is to be prevented, school health education would be better developing the general skills of acquiring and appraising knowledge rather than delivering current wisdom even if this is at the expense of short-term behavioural change. This point was recognized in the document *Health Education from 5 to 16* [63] which emphasized as one of the objectives of health education that pupils should know how to distinguish between fact, promotion and polemic, and how to weigh and interpret information about health from a variety of sources. Brierley [64] had earlier observed that the experience of weighing evidence on diet, smoking, immunization, fluoridation and other health issues was rather thin in health education.

Up to this point the discussion has been dominated by evaluations addressed to health behaviours and related factors. To examine these prior to the goals of the self-empowerment model may appear to underrate the latter. This was not the intention and the writer shares the view [40] that

> ... the need for personal growth and skill enhancement leading to the development of responsible, autonomous and assertive young people, capable of making rational and well informed decisions about their health is the foundation of successful health education.

The order of discussion was chosen to reflect the balance of literature evaluating school health education and also to examine initially those goals which could be seen as more clearly specific to health education alone rather than generally shared with personal and social education or education in general. Bartlett [38] in his 1981 assessment of school health education said that its effects on such pupil outcomes as decision-making and social interaction abilities have seldom, if ever, been measured. As with the other goals already discussed there has been progress since this was written but it remains the case that goals associated with the empowerment model have received less detailed attention. Evaluation may focus on a variety of personality variables such as self-esteem or locus of control or on skills such as decision-making, assertiveness and resisting social pressures. A number of studies have addressed the personality variables, either singly or in the context of a battery of measures. Using an experimental design (with informed consent) with a small group of 5th grade children Blazek and McLellan [65] reported a significant increase in locus of control measures after participation in self-care instruction rather than a general health discussion. The measures were taken immediately at the end of the study and the need for longer term follow-up was recognized. In a longer term evaluation of the School Health Curriculum Project (SHCP) using a post-test only experimental design, Hillman *et al.* [66] concluded that taking part in the project had a positive effect on locus of control. Both these studies used the Children's Health Locus of Control Scale. Botvin's evaluation of a lifeskills approach to smoking education [67] included a number of personality variables (locus of control, anxiety, self-image, susceptibility to social influence, need for acceptance and peer identification). Using an experimental design with children in grades 8–10 (14–16 years) and a pre-test post-test questionnaire Botvin found significant differences in several of the variables although those affected differed between grades. Botvin suggested that different aspects of his programme could have been salient for children of varying ages. He also raised the point [67] about the wider benefits of his programme:

> The emphasis on self-empowerment and acquisition of basic coping skills not only makes the programme intrinsically interesting to students but indirectly addresses other important areas of health. Such a programme may serve as a core around which an entire health education curriculum might be developed.

Decision-making is a skill which has been rated highly in statements of aims of health education and it has been addressed in one way or another in the majority of curriculum projects. How successfully decision-making skills have been developed is difficult to judge as there are few studies to draw upon. Developing measures for assessing these skills is more difficult than for knowledge or attitudes. It is necessary in the first place to define an act of decision-making. People do not make decisions in the same way on all occasions – strategies vary according to the choice in question, situational factors and characteristics and competencies of the actual decision-maker(s). Much decision-making education is directed towards the development of a rational, or what Janis and Mann describe as a 'vigilant' decision-making strategy [68]. Briefly, this requires the decision-maker to be able to recognize a choice situation, generate the alternatives available, collect and appraise information on each alternative, clarify values related to each alternative, order alternatives and make the choice. A number of personal and social skills are often needed to implement a decision. Teaching activities may either address individual elements of the whole skill or coherent decision-making acts. Skills may be taught in a general sense or be related to a whole variety of health decision-making situations, and there may be varying emphases on the cognitive act of decision-making and the personal competencies to use skills when required. Evaluation may include objective and subjective measures of elements, or the whole of, decision-making acts. The degree of importance attached to objective measures as opposed to subjective ones will depend, yet again, on the philosophical approach of the evaluator. Feelings of self-empowerment may result from active involvement in decision-making. This development may be held to be more important than objective measures of skill. In many cases, of course, there is likely to be a correlation between objective and subjective assessments. The literature includes more evaluations of elements of decision-making than of coherent acts.

Lammers *et al.* [69] assessed the effects of the School Health Curriculum Project (SHCP) on health knowledge and selected cognitive dimensions of decision-making skills with reference to smoking. Using the Health Decision-Making Index, the focus was on the generation of reasons for and against smoking, identifying the three most important, and developing a behavioural intention. At the post-test there was a significant difference between experimental and control pupils. The former produced a higher total number of reasons. This study replicated the findings of an earlier study by Duryea [70] and concluded that the SHCP has the potential to affect the cognitive dimension of the decision-making process. Duryea considered that the greater the number of alternatives considered for a given decision the greater the possibility the decision would be a rational one. Botvin's lifeskills training approach discussed earlier [67] included two sessions related to the decision-making process. In the first, students discuss how they make important decisions and a strategy for making decisions is suggested. There is a focus on the tactics others may use to influence decisions and how persuasive influences may be resisted. The second session deals with techniques used by advertisers to influence consumer decisions. Evaluation of the approach as a whole in a number of studies indicated that new cigarette smoking among junior high school students was reduced by at least 50% after training. Although as we noted earlier significant gains on a number of other variables have occurred there appear to be no specific reports on decision-making competence. The large-scale School Health Evaluation Study included three practice elements in its evaluation questionnaire: social adaptability, personal health practices and decision-making skills. In considering decision-making it focused attention on information gathering and techniques of logical decision strategies. Using self-reporting scores on all three, health skills were significantly greater in the experimental group than the control with the biggest differences being recorded for decision-making skills. An early evaluation of decision-making skills as a whole took place in 1975–6 in 20 English and 10 Danish schools [71]. Following a 5–10 hour course on drug choices pupils completed a questionnaire on knowledge and decision-making skills in relation to legal and illegal drugs. In addition teachers were interviewed before and immediately after the teaching and again three months later and they also kept a diary of the lessons. Both knowledge and decision-making scores were higher in the experimental groups than the matched control groups in the post-test administered three months after the teaching. The differences on the decision-making measure were, however, very small and were related to the goals of the teachers. When the teacher endorsed the decision-making goal the pupils learned more. The teachers all used the prepared manual for the course but had no further special training. In the field of drugs education there is a general concern that teaching should not lead to an increase in experimentation. This particular evaluation reported that there was no evidence of an increase in experimentation with legal or illegal drugs associated with the teaching of the course: changes in experimentation were the same in experimental and control groups. The researchers commented that it was not surprising that the decision-making goal, a less familiar and more difficult one than that of increasing knowledge, was attained only to a moderate extent. They hoped that in the future teachers' greater familiarity with the decision-making goal and enhanced confidence in teaching the skills combined with improved teaching strategies would lead to more substantial gains in pupil performance. In the intervening period there has been an increase in familiarity with the decision-making goal and greater availability of teaching materials incorporating decision-making activities. There are, however, still too few studies evaluating the success of health education in achieving this central goal.

Earlier in this section comment was made on the current comparison of knowledge-based and psycho–social approaches to smoking education. Another area in which there has been ongoing interest in the effects of alternative teaching methods has been that of drugs education. In a recent review [72] Dorn has stated:

> One of the key questions about drug education, and about broader approaches to health and social education, is whether or not any approaches are known to reduce the chances of children beginning to experiment with drugs.

A very particular interest has been in the use of scare tactics and the reviewer concluded:

> On the basis of knowledge of the drug education literature of 300 articles and in the light of the most scientifically sound parts of that literature, we conclude that scare or horror warning approaches to drug education do not reduce, or even restrain, drug use.

This conclusion was in line with recommendations of the Advisory Council on Misuse of Drugs [73] that:

> Drug education should not focus solely on factual information about drug misuse, even less present such information in a way that is intended to shock or scare ... a balanced approach is needed which focuses more on social and cultural factors.

This conclusion is pertinent to the current concern with AIDS education – a topic also open to the use of scare tactics.

Finally a comment on an indicator which does not emerge as strongly from evaluative studies as perhaps it might – the satisfaction of young people with the content and delivery of health education. Undoubtedly much informal evaluation takes place and many of the health education projects contain good suggestions for monitoring pupil views. More results might be formally reported. In a recent evaluation of the personal and social development curriculum (including health education) in a comprehensive school, Hucker [73a] interviewed twenty pupils from each of the three years involved in the programme. The researcher commented on the responses and thoughtful answers of those who had completed all three years. Their observations will be drawn on in restructuring the course. It is not easy to find evidence of the degree to which young people are involved in deciding on the content and organization of health education curricula. Where this is practised teachers (personal communication) have reported that the areas selected by pupils are usually much the same as they might have selected themselves but pupils were much more committed to a curriculum which belonged to them and was seen to meet their needs.

The School as a Health-promoting Environment

The school supports the health education of its pupils in two main ways: by offering appropriate programmes of teaching within the formal curriculum and by ensuring that the school environment as a whole supports the classroom work. While there has always been some recognition of the fact that features of the school environment can be antagonistic to health education in the curriculum, the 1980s have seen a more concerted focus on the school as a health promoting environment. There is also a growing recognition that the health promoting school is concerned to promote the health of all its members – students, teachers and support staff. For example, in the American state of Oregon school personnel [74] have been asked to adopt a different philosophy of health education and to promote their own health before trying to promote the health of their students, and school administrators have been charged with making schools healthier places in which to live and work. Stevens and Davis [74] have looked at the characteristics of schools in Oregon and the activities in them which differentiated those with exemplary health promotion climates. They defined two types of school district: 'hot' ones with strong health promotion attributes and 'cold' ones lacking the attributes. Hot districts had modified some of the traditional norms of school health education and were addressing social and organizational factors, staff development was a primary target, consideration was given to food in schools and health education services were extended beyond the classroom. On the other hand, both hot and cold districts had similar educational programmes for students and only one hot district had a comprehensive health education programme. Administrators in hot districts when questioned on the lack of comprehensive programmes said that they thought it was more important to use their efforts and resources to demonstrate a commitment to healthy concepts before investing in a revision of the curriculum. Overall the greatest difference between hot and cold districts existed in the number of health-related staff services and the smallest differences were in the use of buildings, student educational programmes and student services. The researchers concluded that hot districts have changed not only the context of their schools, but also their ability to directly influence a greater number of Health Objectives for the Nation [5].

It has not been usual to include schools in workplace education. The Carolina Healthstyle Program, however, which was established [75] in 1982 for 20 000 state employees was broadened to include all school district employees in 1985. In this initiative the school setting was seen as offering an ideal opportunity to endow students with health promotion knowledge and skills. Three components: school health services; a healthy school environment; and health education should, it said, 'each be included in a comprehensive school health promotion program to maximize the potential for making the school an agent for community health behaviour change'. A pilot worksite wellness programme was implemented in one school district in 1985 and followed up with programmes in four more districts in 1987. The programme has a formal structure with a programme coordinator at district level, a steering committee at school district level and a smaller Healthstyle committee in each school building. This last committee plans and implements a wellness or health promotion programme for its school building which:

1. Determines employees' needs and interests in health promotion programmes;
2. Determines what facilities, health services and other resources are available within the worksite;
3. Develops plans or commitments to conduct certain activities over the year;
4. Implements plans, evaluates and modifies for the next year.

In the pilot district employees paid $5.00 to join the programme and 75% participation occurred. There are no reported results to date from this pilot district. It is envisaged that teachers and staff involved in the programme will influence students in the classroom by role modelling good health behaviours, raising awareness of health issues and supporting comprehensive health education in the school curriculum. In the UK training workshops for coordinators of school health education carried out as part of the dissemination of the Schools Health Education Project (SHEP 13–18) [76] included an activity designed to enable school staff to think about the health promoting features of their schools. The new Healthskills Project [31] which provides for staff development prior to classroom work also strongly emphasizes the importance of the school context:

> To have an effect it is essential that self-empowerment is part of an approach and philosophy applied through the whole school – not just something that happens on Friday afternoons in personal, social and health education lessons.

We might expect to record the development of whole school general health promotion policies. In actual fact the trend to date seems to have been more towards the development of specific policies for areas such as smoking and nutrition. In the case of nutrition this can be seen as a response within schools to the long-standing recognition that school meals and tuckshops can counteract classroom education and in the case of smoking to a recognition of the influence of teachers as role models in the smoking career. The focus on both of these topics may also have been influenced from outside schools by the existence of district smoking and nutrition policies. In a recent survey of one third (n = 74) of Welsh secondary schools 71 (83%) had a policy on smoking directed towards pupils but only 25 had a policy regarding smoking by staff in school. However, 55 did have a restriction on smoking outside the staffroom with 43 specifying that no teacher should smoke in the presence of children. The basis for the smoking policies generally seemed to be narrower than would be expected of a fully-fledged health promotion policy; as Nutbeam *et al.* [32] commented:

> Although most schools reported having policies which addressed pupil smoking many regarded smoking as mainly a disciplinary issue. Very few schools had explicit policies which addressed smoking by teachers – an issue which needs to be more formally approached in Welsh schools.

A long term follow-up of smoking in Derbyshire schools by Murray, Kiryluk and Swan offers some evidence of the impact of teacher smoking. They found that more boys smoked in schools where the headteacher smoked and more girls in schools where female assistant teachers smoked. The effects appeared to persist after pupils had left school although the writers urged caution in inferring causal relationships [78]. Bewley [79] had earlier shown the impact of male teachers' smoking on male pupils. Teachers' attitudes and behaviours are both important in ensuring that smoking education in the classroom is supported by the environment as a whole. A study by Nutbeam [80] in 29 primary and secondary schools in the south of England addressed teacher attitudes and behaviours. Twenty-two per cent (n = 192) of the men and 15% (n = 196) of the women were smokers which compared favourably with the norm for smoking in the socio-economic group to which teachers belonged (29% in 1984). It was found that 70% of teachers in the sample accepted their exemplary role in relation to smoking and over 80% agreed that they had an active role in influencing children's health behaviour as it related to smoking. There was a general consensus on the need to provide a smoke-free environment for non-smokers but less agreement on efforts to restrict smoking by teachers. Nutrition policies in schools are also on the increase although in the Welsh study only a minority of schools had a formal nutrition policy. More than a half of the respondents reported the existence of nutrition policies in their local education authorities although at the time of the survey none actually existed. Six of the 46 schools with tuckshops had policies on these. Discussions of schools as health promoting institutions frequently emphasize those factors, such as smoking by teachers, which have an influence on health topic work in the classroom. If the emphasis is on a self-empowerment approach to health education there is little in the school environment which does not have some bearing on its health promotion standing. Brief comments can be made on two aspects of the school environment: the support of the school for decision-making, and the promotion of equality. Anderson [77] in a discussion of the Healthskills project comments on the first of these:

> An important component of staff development workshops is to provide an opportunity to discuss and examine the ways in which the school presently empowers or depowers its students and staff, and to look at how it might change. Without this step, the notion of informed decision-making, so important to health education, but requiring a degree of personal autonomy and self belief, is likely to remain nothing but a notion.

Schools have a commitment to equal opportunities but can fall far short of fulfilling this aim in practice. Very many factors can be considered in evaluating a school's success in this respect: the appropriateness of the curriculum as a whole and of health education in particular to a multiracial society; respect for cultural diversity; proper integration of young people with special needs; avoidance of racism and sexism; and appropriateness of teaching methods and resources. The Schools' Council has produced a number of documents to assist schools in carrying out appraisal of the curriculum in a multiracial society and of sex stereotyping in teaching materials. Some schools have developed 'user friendly' statements of the schools' policy on equalities which are given to all newcomers.

Although there is greater awareness of the importance of the school environment as a background to classroom health education the comment by Stevens and Davis [74] remains pertinent:

> As educators, it is time we gave serious consideration to efforts that affect not only behaviour, but the political, social and organizational factors that are often antagonistic and inconsistent with instructional and behavioural interventions.

School Health Education and the Health of Families and Communities

The California Worksite Program [75], discussed in the previous section, concluded by saying:

> Schools are also potential community wellness centres that reach the whole community through involvement of parents in school activities and community involvement through adult continuing education. Through the network of persons connected to the schools setting a health program is able to influence a large proportion of people.

In the long term it is hoped that children who have received a comprehensive health education course in schools will have a positive influence on their own families and communities. Increasingly, however, the immediate impact that school health education can have on children's families and communities is being considered. Schools are also looking at ways the community can contribute to health education in school. When he reviewed the development of school health education in 1986 Williams [9] said that remarkably little attention had been paid to the effects of school health education on families. A number of studies have begun to look at these effects, often as a component of more comprehensive evaluations. Wilcox *et al.* [81] on evaluating the My Body project reported considerable discussion between parents and children following lessons in primary schools. Murray, Swan and Clarke [51] in the long-term evaluation of the same project examined the smoking practices of children's parents as reported by the children. They found that the overall prevalence of parents' smoking was slightly lower in the intervention group and the general decline between 1980 and 1982 was slightly more apparent in that group. A higher proportion of the parents of the girls than of the boys stopped smoking between 1980 and 1982. Of those parents changing their smoking behaviour the proportion giving up was consistently greater in the parents of those in the intervention group. Again on the subject of smoking, Charlton's study [52], discussed earlier, was designed to influence parental smoking. The Natural Nashers project also included a small evaluation of its impact on families. It studied 35 families whose children had received the programme and 35 which had not. Twelve of the study families reported changes in behaviour compared with seven of the controls. Twenty-two of the study families reported having received new information and in 18 of these the source was the young person who had been taught the programme. Finally, the 3R's High Blood Pressure Program was developed in Georgia as a response to high blood pressure as a major health problem in that state. The project was based on the proposition that 6th grade students could be taught practical information about high blood pressure. They could then facilitate the health education of families and peers and help effect blood pressure control within the community [82]. The Child to Child project [83] was developed to operate in a similar way. It is an international programme designed to teach and encourage school age children to concern themselves with the health of their younger brothers and sisters. Adopted particularly in developing countries the programme teaches children simple prevention and curative activities which they pass on to other children and their families. An example of the use of this approach was in the context of an oral health programme in Thailand. Teachers of the youngest children were keen to organize toothbrushing exercises but the interest declined among teachers of the older children. This was seen as an occasion to promote child to child activities and train the higher grade students (10–11 years old) to become 'oral health leaders' and supervise the younger grade students. Although the programme was well received no objective data are provided in the report [84].

Rather than children taking their knowledge to the community the reverse can happen. There is a long history of bringing members of the community to contribute in various ways to health education in the classroom. In the Welsh survey [32] already cited, schools were asked about the involvement of parents and outside agencies in the planning and teaching of health education. A wide variety of people and agencies were listed – headed by the health education service and other community health services. Fifty-seven schools (78%) reported involving parents and half of the schools consulted parents in the development of health education programmes – although in relatively passive ways. One quarter of the schools teaching health education neither consulted or informed parents. Finally, schools can develop links with community health initiatives and those designated as community schools may have a variety of activities which contribute to community health.

The Education System as a whole and its contribution to Health Education

The various evaluative studies, some small-scale, and some large-scale, have provided evidence of effective ways of achieving the outcomes and intermediate and indirect indicators associated with the different approaches to school health education. If we are concerned with the population as a whole we want to know how far the outcomes we value can, and have been achieved with this larger group. Irrespective of what it is hoped that school health education will accomplish, if success is to be possible appropriate programmes of education have to be provided. In England and Wales a survey in 1981–82 offered evidence of the extent of provision [85]. Eighty-five per cent of secondary schools and 87% of primary schools provided some formal health education. The amount of this provision was variable, with less than one third of the primary and less than two thirds of the secondary schools offering a planned programme. Forty-eight per cent of the secondary schools had someone responsible for health education [78]. In the Welsh survey [32] carried out more recently 72 of the 76 schools who responded reported that health education was taught and 59 (78%) had a planned programme. Fifty-nine schools also reported having a person designated as responsible for coordinating health education and in 43 schools this person had undergone specific in-service training. A survey of this kind only provides fairly simple descriptive information but the researchers pointed out that it did indicate that in schools where planned programmes existed coverage fell short of the ideal. Relatively few schools offered health education to all pupils in all years and a higher proportion timed inputs for the later years rather than the arguably more important earlier years. Countries with a prescribed national curriculum are able to require that all children follow a comprehensive health education curriculum. The timing, organization and support of such a programme in order for it to be maximally effective has then to be decided.

The difficulties of providing evidence of the overall success of health education are recognized. As Newman [86] has pointed out, schools are organized to facilitate learning not to conduct evaluative research. The major study, referred to above, [87] has been widely acknowledged as especially important because it has addressed the effectiveness of school health education in general. This study, the School Health Education Evaluation (SHEE), has been used in the USA to argue for health education in the face of the 'back to basics' movement. To recap, this was a study of four different health education programmes in 20 states in the USA involving 30 000 children. It had as its primary purpose the breaking of what has been described as a 'poverty cycle' in evaluation [87]:

> Even if resources for appropriate evaluation are available results could be disappointing because the programme being evaluated did not have adequate resources to be implemented correctly.

As an evaluation it addressed the issue of the need for experimental studies of teaching carried out in exemplary fashion and also the need for representative studies of the curriculum in natural surroundings. It therefore incorporated a representative study of the four curricula in normal classroom situations and an experimental study of the School Health Curriculum Project (SHCP). Reviewing the SHEE study Cooke and Walberg [88] described it as of the highest quality with respect to inferences about causal connections and the generalizations that it promotes. Health educators now had, they said, a large scale credible study to use of support their advocacy. The evaluation was made using a pre-test/post-test questionnaire. This test instrument was not tied to the aims of any one of the four health education projects being assessed but addressed those learning objectives that experts and parents stated to be the most important in grades 4–7. These objectives included 10 knowledge areas, four attitude areas and three practice areas.

The evaluation reported significant increases in knowledge for study classrooms when compared with controls. Smaller but still significant increases were also found for attitudes and self-reported practices. The effectiveness of programmes was linked to the extent to which the projects in question were fully implemented. When results obtained with full implementation were compared with the results for the programme sample as a whole, higher scores were obtained in all three domains in the study group. The impact of full implementation was, however, considerably less on knowledge items than on attitude and practice ones. In other words, teachers appeared to be quite effective at meeting the specific knowledge-related objectives while only partly implementing programmes. The objectives involving attitudes and practices were not as clearly realized with partial implementation.

The amount of in-service training received by teachers was also related to programme implementation measures: the fully trained completed a greater percentage of the programmes with greater fidelity than the partly trained who were, in turn, better than the untrained. Interesting evidence on the cumulative impact of repeated instruction was offered for one of the projects (SHCP). Student performance was tracked through two consecutive years to provide an estimate of the benefits of cumulative exposure. For all three classes of variables, groups with two units of exposure performed better than those with one, regardless of grade levels.

Finally, some consideration of the costs of adoption and implementation were provided. Of the four projects it was only the SHCP where adoption costs were a significant proportion of total costs. The average costs associated with each project were also highest for the SHCP. While adoption costs are a small percentage of total costs they are the most visible percentage. A commitment to teacher training and support materials may be crucial in fostering teacher acceptance and ensuring that administrative commitment is carried in to the classroom. The results of the study [89] have been summarized:

> The study shows, in general, that health education does make a difference, that it works better when there is more of it, and that it works best when it is implemented with broad scale administrative support for teacher training, integrated material and continuity across school years. It works best where there is attention to the building of a foundation of basic health knowledge, rather than starting with categorical health problems later in the academic course of pupils [89].

Although received with some enthusiasm the School Health Evaluation Study does have its limitations. On its own admission the study sample was mainly white and middle class although it is not made clear why this was the case in such a large-scale study. The follow-up period was not as long as would have been liked and the study was addressed only to younger children. Although it did focus on some of the outcomes associated with the empowerment approach it offered no comprehensive assessment of these outcomes. Many are associated with the success of education as a whole and should, in part, be assessed in this wider context. The development of GCSE in the UK with its greater attention to problem solving and decision-making offers an opportunity for some national assessment of these skills. Outcomes associated with the empowerment approach can also be incorporated in profiling and records of achievement. The specific contribution of health education to empowerment goals needs further and sustained evaluation.

Policy and other influences on School Health Education

The final, and somewhat distinct element that can be addressed in a complete evaluation of school health education is the combination of policies and other activities which in varied ways serve to influence its development and maintenance within the curriculum. These can include: policies and general debates on the curriculum as a whole or on health education and personal and social education in particular; various aspects of initial and continuing education for teachers; and the influence of the NHS and the health education service in the community. Where curriculum policy is concerned, evaluators can consider both the nature of policy and its implementations. Many countries have a nationally prescribed curriculum and where this is the case it is possible for health education to be a required element within it. In the UK in the period since 1945 schools have only been required by law to provide religious instruction and Lawton has commented [90] that from 1945 until 1970 there also seemed to be no central policy on the curriculum. As noted earlier since the 1970s there has been considerable debate on the curriculum and this has culminated in the 1988 Education Reform Act which specifies a national curriculum. Up to this point, therefore, UK schools have been in a position to structure their own curricula within a network of constraints: examination boards, school governors, parents, local education authorities, universities, etc. Schools have been exhorted to develop the curriculum by competing interests, amongst which has been the lobby for health education. Most of the educational reports from the 1970s onwards have encouraged the development of health education and in this time the Department of Education and Science has produced two discussion documents [16, 63]. Despite this support neither health education nor personal and social education have been listed as core or foundation subjects within the new national curriculum although health education has not gone unmentioned. The Consultative Document [91] said:

> In addition, there are a number of subjects or themes such as health education which can be taught through other subjects. For example, biology can contribute to learning about health education, and the health theme will give an added dimension to teaching about biology.

Although the organization of health education through other curriculum subjects is in line with a widely recommended way of providing for it, criticism has been expressed of the narrow view of the subject which comes from the document. To ally health education so clearly with biology seems to present a somewhat limited conception and to overlook the growing tendency, particularly in secondary schools, to offer health education as part of a broad strand of personal and social education. From later comment by the Secretary of State for Education it does appear that health education is expected to continue much as at present. It is too early to say if the pressures of providing the required elements of the formal curriculum and meeting the new demands for regular assessment will have a detrimental impact on health education. In addition to the national documents on the curriculum local education authorities may also produce guidelines on health education. The impact they have on schools varies considerably but they can be of particular use for triggering a discussion with schools on their health education.

The School Health Evaluation Study [87] pointed out the importance of in-service teacher training in securing the full implementation of curriculum projects. Evaluation of teacher training could examine the extent and nature of the provision of health education within initial and continuing education of teachers. A survey of schools and teacher training institutions in England and Wales reported that 98% of teachers felt that teacher training should incorporate a core course of health education and 75% of student teachers wanted to teach health education. At the time only 25% of institutions offering B.Ed. courses and 10% of those with postgraduate certificate in education (PGCE) courses offered students a core course in health education. While the survey offered only a general overview it can be said that it represented a high level of perceived responsibility for health education on the part of teachers and students and insufficient response by the institutions. A major contribution to in-service education for teachers has come from the dissemination activities associated with all the main health education curriculum projects. For example the SHEP 13–18 Project ran six-day workshops for coordinators of health education in 52 education/health authorities. A follow-up survey reported that the dissemination programme had been well received and some 10 authorities had gone on to run further programmes on the same lines. In this survey it emerged that most authorities had run three or more health-related in-service courses – most commonly on SHEP 13–18, Teacher's Advisory Council on Alcohol and Drug Education (TACADE) materials and the Active Tutorial Work project [92]. Finally, preliminary observations indicate that many schools are using some of the newly required in-service training days to review personal, social and health education.

As previously mentioned both the Health Education Council (now replaced by the Health Education Authority) and health education units have initiated and supported curriculum development of health education. In addition Reid and Massey [40] have pointed out that up to nine out of ten local education authority in-service courses receive substantial NHS financial support. The other major contributor to the curriculum development of health education has been TACADE, both in the area of in-service teacher education and in the production of teaching materials. Finally, health education units based in district health authorities have provided, in a variety of ways, sustained support for the health education in their local schools.

CONCLUSIONS

Schools are widely seen as having a key role in health education whether the desired outcomes of such activities are changing behaviours or the personal and social skills associated with self-empowerment. In the UK there has been a gradual development of health education in the curriculum with a recent trend towards viewing it, and providing for it, as part of a broader programme of personal and social development. As in other contexts where health education takes place, debates over its aims have occurred and influenced the type and extent of evaluation. There is now a considerable body of literature which has evaluated outcomes of health education: individual knowledge, attitudes and health-related behaviours. There is rather less relating to the goals concerned with the self-empowerment approach. A newly published study of personal and social education carried out by Her Majesty's Inspectors has said that this area suffered from minimal evaluation [93]. It is difficult to decide on the limits of what is to be evaluated as health education – the broader the aims of health education become, the more evaluation could be addressing the educational process as a whole. Green [41] has cautioned against attempting too much in health education, and also too little:

> Grandiose expectations of some advocates and practitioners will slate health education unnecessarily for failure. The limited expectations of others will relegate it to activities which are trivial at best, wasteful at worst.

Reviewers have all noted successes in achieving certain outcomes. Kolbe [41] reviewed 15 meta-evaluations published between 1980 and 1985 which together synthesized the findings of several hundred studies conducted to determine the effectiveness of school-based interventions related to nine specific areas. The most important generalization from these was that school-based health education programmes consistently improve targeted health knowledge, attitudes and skills and inconsistently improve targeted health behaviours. Reid and Massey's review which reported successes also noted areas such as alcohol and drug abuse where effects of health education were uncertain and some cases (e.g. solvent abuse) where specific school health education may actually be counterproductive. The successes which Kolbe and the reviewers of the School Health Evaluation Study have also noted have been welcomed, both as achievements in their own right, and as potentially useful when seeking resources for health education. Newman [86] has stressed that:

> At a time when the efficacy and efficiency of all education is under scrutiny and the public is encouraging schools to 'return to basics', supporters of subjects like health education, thought by some not to be basic, need to show the effectiveness of health instruction.

While the value of demonstrating such successes should be recognized it is also important that they are not used to channel health education in one specific direction. The outcomes associated with the empowerment approach are more difficult to evaluate and successes not so easy to 'chalk up' but their importance is greater if we believe in working to promote positive health for all.

In this chapter discussion has focused on five levels at which school health education can be evaluated. Such a division can be at the expense of emphasizing the interaction between levels in practice and the need to focus on such integration as part of evaluation. What is increasingly recognized and emphasized is the importance of viewing classroom activities against the background of the school as a health promoting environment which, in turn, is part of a local community. School health education can influence, and be influenced by, its local community. A weakness of school health education has been its relative slowness to consider the social and environmental causes of ill health and to debate collective as opposed to individually focused solutions to problems of ill health. In discussing the five expectancies of health education (listed in the introduction) Kolbe [8] has said:

> ... we can expect health education delivered in the school to increase the abilities of individuals to analyse the forces of government, economics and social organisations that can influence health. In participatory democracy it is vital for people to understand the complex issues that surround existing or proposed social actions to protect and improve the health of populations. We can expect schools, perhaps better than any other delivery setting, to increase the desires and abilities of individuals to participate effectively in such civic decisions and civic activities that ultimately influence their personal health, the health of their families, and the health of the communities in which they reside.

Finally, if the range of expectations of health education outlined in the introduction is to be achieved schools need to offer comprehensive, coordinated programmes, backed up by adequate resources, teacher training, and continuity throughout the school years. Last, but perhaps most important of all, health education should be responsive to young people's expressed needs and they should also be able to play participatory roles in the evaluations which take place.

REFERENCES

1. Allensworth, D. D. and Wolford, C. A., (1988) Schools as agents for achieving the 1990 health objectives for the nation, *Health Education Quarterly*, **15**, pp. 3–15.
2. International Union for Health Education (1987) Policy statement on health education for the school aged child, *HYGIE*, **VI**, 5–6.
3. World Health Organization (1978) *Primary Health Care: Report of the Conference on Primary Health Care*, WHO, Geneva.
4. US Department of Health, Education and Welfare (1979) *Healthy People: The Surgeon General's Report on Health Promotion and Disease Prevention*, US Government Printing Office, Washington, DC.
5. US Department of Health and Human Services (1980) *Promoting Health/Preventing Disease*, US Government Printing Office, Washington, DC.
6. Iverson, D. C. and Kolbe, L. J. (1983) Evaluation of the national disease prevention and health promotion strategy: establishing a role for the schools. *Journal of School Health*, **53**, 294–302.
7. Kolbe, L. J. (1987) International policies for school health programmes. *HYGIE*, **VI**, 7–11.
8. Kolbe, L. J. (1982) What can we expect from school health education? *Journal of School Health*, **52**, 145–51.
9. Williams, T. (1986) School health education 15 years on. *Health Education Journal*, **45**, 3–7.
10. Sutherland, I. (1979) Health education, the school system and the young, in: *Health Education Perspectives and Choices*, (ed. I. Sutherland), George, Allen and Unwin, London.
11. Board of Education (1926) *Hadow Report: Report of the Consultative Committee on the Education of the Adolescent*, HMSO, London.
12. Board of Education (1928) *Handbook of Suggestions on Health Education*, HMSO, London.
13. Department of Education and Science (1957) *Health Education*, HMSO, London.
14. Ministry of Health/ Central Health Services Council/ Scottish Health Services Council (1964) *Health Education: Report of a Joint Committee of the Central and Scottish Health Service Councils*, HMSO, London.
15. Department of Education and Science (1977a) *Education in Schools: a Consultative Document*, HMSO, London.
16. Department of Education and Science (1977b) *Curriculum 11–16*, HMSO, London.
17. Department of Education and Science (1980) *A Framework for the School Curriculum*, HMSO, London.
18. Department of Education and Science (1981) *The School Curriculum*, HMSO, London.
19. Department of Health and Social Security (1976a) *Prevention and Health, Everybody's Business*, HMSO, London.

20. Department of Health and Social Security (1976b) *Priorities for Health and Personal Social Services in England*, HMSO, London.
21. Department of Health and Social Security (1977) *Prevention and Health*, HMSO, London.
22. Department of Health and Social Security (1981) *Care in Action: A Handbook of Policies and Priorities for the Health and Personal Social Services in England*, HMSO, London.
23. Central Advisory Council for Education (1963) *Half Our Future*, HMSO, London.
24. Schools Council (1972) *Lifeline, Moral Education Project 13–16*, Longman, London.
25. Schools Council (1970) *Humanities Project 14–16*, Heinemann, London.
26. Ellis, H. (1947) Organising a health week, *Health Education Journal*, 5, 129–33.
27. Charlton, A. (1980/1) An experimental methodology for HE in teacher training: a baseline survey with reference to cancer. *International Journal of Health Education*, Vol. XXIII, pp. 25–34.
28. Schools Council/HEC Project (1977) *Health Education 5–13*, T. Nelson and Sons, London.
29. Bell, D. (1973) *The Coming of Post-Industrial Society*, Heinemann Educational, London.
30. Touraine, A. (1971) *The Post-Industrial Society*, Random House, New York.
31. Anderson, J. (1988) *HEA Health Skills Project: Training Manual*, Counselling and Career Development Unit, University of Leeds, Leeds.
32. Nutbeam, D. *et al.* (1987) The health-promoting school: organisation and policy development in Welsh secondary schools. *Health Education Journal*, 46, 109–15.
33. Dorn, N. and Nortoft, B. (1982) *Health Careers*, Institute for the Study of Drug Dependence, London.
34. Jones, A. (1986) *SHEP 13–18: Some Years On*: A Report for the Health Education Council, University of Southampton.
35. Anderson, D. C. (1979) The classroom as a context for health education, in: *Health Education in Practice* (ed. D. Anderson), Croom Helm, London.
36. Department of Education and Science/Welsh Office (1985) *GCSE: The National Criteria: Home Economics*, HMSO, London.
37. Stenhouse, L. (1975) *An Introduction to Curriculum Research and Development*, Heinemann, London.
38. Bartlett, E. E. (1981) The contribution of school health education to community health promotion: what can we reasonably expect? *American Journal of Public Health*, 17, 1384–91.
39. Mason, J. O. and McGinnis, J. M. (1985) The role of school health, *Journal of School Health*, 55, 299.
40. Reid, D. and Massey, D. (1986) Can school health education be more effective? *Health Education Journal*, 45, 7–13.
41. Kolbe, L. (1985) Why school health education? An empirical point of view. *Health Education*, 16, 116–20.
42. Rubinson, L. (1982) Evaluating school dental health education programs, *The Journal of School Health*, 52, 26–8.
43. HEC/Dental Health Study (1984) *Natural Nashers*, HEC, London.
44. HEC Dental Health Study (1986) *Natural Nashers Dissemination 1984–6*, HEC, London.

45. Craft, M. (1984) Research in dental health education methods. *Journal of the Royal Society of Health*, **104**(1), 37–9.
46. Owen, S. L. *et al.* (1985) Selecting and recruiting health programs for the school health education evaluation. *Journal of School Health*, 55, 305–8.
47. Health Education Council (1983) *My Body*, Heinemann Education, London.
48. Noble, M. (1984) The 'My Body' Project: its development to date and plans for the future, in: *Health Education and Youth*, (ed. G. Campbell), Falmer Press, London.
49. Connell, D. B., Turner, R. R. and Mason, E. F. (1985) Summary of findings of the School Health Education Evaluation: health promotion effectiveness, implementation and costs. *Journal of School Health*, 55, 316–20.
50. Murray, M., Swan, A. V., Enock, C. *et al.* (1982) The effectiveness of the HEC's 'My Body' school health education project, *Health Education Journal*, **41**, 126–32.
51. Murray, M., Swan, A. N. and Clarke, G. (1984) Long term effects of a school based anti-smoking programme. *Journal of Epidemiology and Community Health*, **38**, 247–52.
52. Charlton, A. (1986) Evaluation of a family-linked smoking programme in primary schools, *Health Education Journal*, **45**, 140–4.
53. Evans, R. I., Hansen, W. B. and Mittlemark, M. B. (1977) Increasing the validity of self reports of smoking behaviour in children. *Journal of Applied Psychology*, **62**, 521–3.
54. Gillies, P. (1986) Accuracy in the measurement of the prevalence of smoking in young people. *Health Education Journal*, **44**, 36–8.
55. Evans, R. I. *et al.* (1978) Deterring the onset of smoking in children: knowledge of immediate physiological effects and coping with peer pressure, media pressure and parent modeling. *Journal of Applied Social Psychology*, **8**, 126–35.
56. McAlister, A., Perry, C. and Maccoby, N. (1979) Adolescent smoking: onset and prevention. *Paediatrics*, **63**, 650–8.
57. Botvin, G. J. and Eng, A. (1980) A comprehensive school based smoking prevention program. *Journal of School Health*, **50**, 209–13.
58. Luepker, R. V., Johnson, C. A., Murray, D. M. and Pechacek, T. F. (1983) Prevention of cigarette smoking: three years follow up of an education program for youth, *Journal of Behavioural Medicine*, **6**, 53–62.
59. Ledwith, F. and Oswin, L. (1985) The evaluation of a secondary school smoking education intervention. *Health Education Journal*, **44**, 131–8.
60. Flay, B. R. (1986) Psychosocial approaches to smoking prevention: a review of findings. *Health Psychology*, **4**, 449–88.
61. Reid, D. J. (1985) The prevention of smoking among schoolchildren: recommendations for policy development. *Health Education Journal*, **44**, 3–12.
62. Parcel, G. (1985) Comments from the field. *Journal of School Health*, 55, 345–7.
63. Department of Education and Science (1985) *Health Education From 5–16*, HMSO, London.
64. Brierley, J. (1983) Health education in secondary schools, *Health Education Journal*, **42**, 48–52.
65. Blazek, B. and McClelland, M. S. (1983) The effects of self care instruction on locus of control in children. *Journal of School Health*, **53**, 554–6.
66. Hillman, K. S. *et al.* (1985) A retrospective assessment of the long range effects of the fifth and sixth grade units of the School Health Education Project. *Health Education*, **16**, 21–7.

67. Botvin, G. J. Eng, A. and Williams, C. L. (1980) Preventing the onset of smoking through lifeskills training. *Preventive Medicine*, **9**, 135–43.

68. Janis, I. and Mann, L. (1977) *Decision Making*, Free Press, New York.

69. Lammers, J. W., Kreuter, M. W. and Smith, B. C. (1984) The effects of the SHCP on selected aspects of decision making among 5th graders, *Health Education*, **15**, 14–18.

70. Duryea, E. (1983) Decision Making and Health Education. *Journal of School Health*, **53**, 29–32.

71. Institute for the Study of Drug Dependence (1982) *Facts and Feelings About Drugs but Decisions About Situations*, ISDD, London.

72. Dorn, N. (1985) Can drug education reduce drug experimentation? *Health at School*, **1**, 66–8.

73. Advisory Council on Misuse of Drugs (1984). *Report on Prevention*, Home Office/ HMSO, London.

73a. Hucker, J. (1988) *An Evaluation of the Implementation and Development of a Personal and Social Development Course.* Unpublished dissertation, Leeds Polytechnic.

74. Stevens, N. H. and Davis, L. G. (1988) Exemplary school health education: a new charge from HOT districts. *Health Education Quarterly*, **15**, 63–70.

75. Maysey, D. L., Gimarc, J. D. and Kronenfeld, J. J. (1988) School worksite wellness programs: a strategy for achieving the 1990 goals for a healthier America. *Health Education Quarterly*, **15**, 53–62.

76. Schools Council/HEC Project (1982) *Health Education 13–18*, Forbes Publications, London.

77. Anderson, J. (1986), Health Skills: the Power to Choose, *Health Education Journal*, **45**, (1), 19–24.

78. Murray, M., Kiryluk, S. and Swan, A. V. (1981) School characteristics and adolescent smoking; results from the MRC Derbyshire Smoking Study 1974–8 and from a follow up in 1981. *Journal of Epidemiology and Community Health*, **38**, 167–72.

79. Bewley, B. R., Johnson, M. D. and Banks, M. H. (1979) Teacher's smoking. *Epidemiology and Community Health*, **33**, 219.

80. Nutbeam, D. (1987) Smoking among primary and secondary schoolteachers. *Health Education Journal*, **46**, 14–21.

81. Wilcox, B., Gillies, P., Wilcox, J. and Reid, D. J. (1981) Do children influence their parents' smoking? *Health Education Journal*, **40**, 5–10.

82. Davis, R. L. *et al.* (1985) Comprehensive school health education: a practical definition. *Journal of School Health*, **55**, 335–9.

83. Aarons, A. (ed) (1979) *Child to Child*, Macmillan, London.

84. Anumanrajadhon, T. and Infirri, S. (1986) Oral health: a quiet revolution. *Education For Health*, No. 1, pp. 25–36.

85. Williams, D. T. and Roberts, J. (1985) *TEP Survey Report: Health Education in Schools and Teacher Education Institutions.* Health Education Unit, Southampton.

86. Newman, I. (1985) Comments from the field. *Journal of School Health*, **55**, 343–5.

87. Gunn, W. J., Iverson, D. C. and Katz, M. (1985) Design of the school health evaluation. *Journal of School Health*, **55**, 301–04.

88. Cooke, T. D. and Walberg, H. J. (1985) Methodological and substantive significance. *Journal of School Health*, **55**, 340–2.

89. Greenberg, J. S. (1985) Comments from the field. *Journal of School Health*, **55**, 350–2.

90. Lawton, D. (1980) *The Politics of the School Curriculum*, Routledge and Kegan Paul, London.

91. Department of Education and Science (1987) *National Curriculum 5–16: Consultative Document*, HMSO, London.

92. Baldwin, J. and Wells, H. (1980) *Active Tutorial Work*, Basil Blackwell, London.

93. Department of Education and Science (1988) *A Survey of Personal and Social Education Courses in some Secondary Schools*, HMSO, London.

5

HEALTH CARE CONTEXTS

INTRODUCTION

In 1974 the President's Committee on Health Education in the USA described health education as an integral part of high quality health care [1]. Hospitals and other health care institutions were focal points of community health care, it said, and had obligations to promote, organize, implement and evaluate health education programmes. This chapter will examine health education in primary care and hospital care around themes already addressed in this book: the conceptions of health education held in these contexts, the debates on philosophical approaches, the organization and delivery of health education and the types of evaluation carried out. As in the previous chapter it is not intended to provide comprehensive reviews of evaluative studies, of which several already exist [2, 3, 4] but to highlight some of the issues which have arisen. While the immediate focus of concern is the health care service in the UK, much should be relevant to other countries. The chapter as a whole will draw quite heavily on literature from the USA since it was there that education in health care (especially in hospitals) developed more rapidly than in other countries.

TERMINOLOGY

Some initial comment is called for on terminology. The literature includes a variety of terms to cover educational activities in hospitals and primary care: health education, patient education, patient counselling, health promotion, patient teaching and more. There is some consistency in the use of terms but also confusion. Recently the journal *Patient Education and Counselling* carried out a Delphi exercise on terminology [5]. It adopted the twin terms of 'patient education' and 'patient counselling' to describe activities which it saw as involving an interactive process and which assisted patients to participate actively in their health care. **Patient education** was agreed to be 'a planned learning experience using a combination of methods such as teaching, counselling, and behaviour modification techniques which influence patient knowledge and health behaviour'. **Patient counselling**, in turn was an 'individualized process involving guidance and collaborative problem solving to help the patient to better manage the health problem'. The journal now assumes that authors will employ these definitions unless they state otherwise. In reporting this exercise the journal described differences of views in participants on such matters as behaviour change and 'planned experience' (if this implied the use of patient education protocols) and reported the wishes for more outcomes such as beliefs, attitudes and decision-making skills to be specified.

These definitions are broadly directed to only one part of what may be seen as health education activity in health care – work with patients or their families. This activity may be concentrated at the tertiary stage of prevention of the health condition which led to becoming a patient, together with variable emphasis on primary and secondary prevention of recurrence. In addition patients may also participate in general health education activities not immediately related to the current condition. Primary health care also offers education to those who are on practice lists and patients in one sense but who, at the time, have not initiated a consultation and accepted the 'patient role'. Much health visitor work can be seen as general health education with the well population and primary health care centres increasingly offer individual and group activities directed towards prevention or, more rarely, positive health. With the growing emphasis on health promotion as conceptualized in Chapter One, health care contexts may be offering activities directed towards the support of health promotion policy initiatives. One way of distinguishing the different educational activities is shown in Table 5.1. The distinction in the table are not consistently made in the literature and the activities associated with each of the terms may vary considerably. In general, there needs to be an awareness of changing terminology and a checking out of the practice associated with terms. As Wilson-Barnett has said recently [6] in exploring the relationship between patient teaching and patient counselling:

> Careless or confused use of terms such as information giving, teaching and counselling may lead to inadequate understanding and practice.

In this chapter the distinction between patient and health education in Table 5.1 will be broadly adopted except when referring to particular studies when the use of terms within them may be adopted for sake of convenience.

Table 5.1 Health promotion in health care

Patient education	General health education	Health promotion policy
Condition-specific education with patients. Frequently focused on tertiary levels of prevention but includes activities directed to primary and secondary prevention.	Aimed at primary prevention and promotion of positive health. For hospital patients and hospital workers. For patients in GP consultation in primary care. For all people on GP practice lists.	General or specific health promotion policies. Focused on health care institutions or local communities.

PATIENT EDUCATION

As in other contexts, a diversity of philosophical approaches to education exists in health care. A longstanding dominance by advocates of preventive approaches has been strongly challenged by those preferring educational ones. Fahrenport [7] has commented on the current scene:

> In sum the call for patient education or information comes from two different directions – a patient-centred one in which autonomy is the key word and a medico-centred one in which compliance still reigns.

These two calls for patient education have generated what can be seen as two literatures using different languages, different arguments for providing education, different criteria for assessing outcomes and so on. The language of the two approaches is illustrated in Table 5.2. Rather than present positions in

Table 5.2 Language and meaning associated with approaches to patient education

Medico-centred	*Patient-centred*
Compliance	Autonomy
Adherence	Patient participation
Planning for patients	Planning with patients
Behaviour change	Decision-making/empowerment
Passive patient	Active ('activated') patient
Dependence	Independence
Professionally determined needs	Patient defined needs
Patient	Client

such a polarized form it may be more helpful to see them as points on a continuum:

Medico-centred   Patient-centred

$\longleftarrow \qquad\qquad\qquad\qquad\qquad\qquad\qquad\qquad \longrightarrow$

Preventive   Simple educational Self-Empowerment
approach   approach   approach

In actual health care contexts individuals or specific occupational groups may either adhere fairly consistently to one approach or there may be variation according to client group, health condition, preferences expressed by patients, etc. These differences of approach can give rise to conflicts: between professional groups; within professional groups; between health professionals and patients and between patients themselves. The commitment of Dr Wendy Savage [8] to women's participation in childbirth decisions illustrated conflict between doctors, while Holohan [9] provides a nice example of lack of support by other patients for her attempt to assert her right to an active part in decision-making:

> The evening before my operation I was presented with a document which I had to sign authorizing the anaesthesia and also a mastectomy if biopsy proved unsatisfactory. I found this suggestion repugnant and a complete abrogation of my rights as an individual ... I felt that the decision to operate should be agreed on when I was conscious and in full possession of the facts ... It was then that I was aware of disapproval emanating from the other patients. I looked around the ward and everyone appeared silent with gaze averted. I was being isolated. Each of their movements was subtle but corrective. I was 'out of line' and they were willing my acceptance of the medical decision. In the face of this informal social control I signed the document.

There have been advocates of both preventive and educational approaches throughout the history of patient education. Early demands for patient education were a response to the acknowledged lack of compliance with medical regimens and the need for education to secure behavioural change in the prevention of major contemporary chronic diseases. The term 'compliance' fits in with the classic Parsonian model of the patient role – cooperating with the doctor, passive and dependent and an unequal partner in the relationship. With the recognition that in many chronic conditions the individual needed to be more fully involved in the working out of lifestyle changes and adherence to complex regimens, Szasz and Hollender suggested [10] that in addition to the guidance–cooperation model of the doctor–patient relationship a mutual participation model also existed. Although this may use patient-centred language (Table 5.2) its underlying implication is thay patients will comply with rational behaviour as defined by the professional. As will be discussed further, health services have been persuaded of the value of patient education because of its reported successes in improving compliance, increasing patient satisfaction and in various ways contributing to a reduction in costs. From the 1960s onwards a number of social movements developed which had general and specific influences on thinking about health care. These included the women's civil rights, consumer and self-care movements. More recently there has been the primary health care movement associated with Health For All by the Year 2000 (World Health Organization). Common to these influences are ideas of self-determination and active participation and these were expressed in health care in debates about such issues as informed consent and management of childbirth. Rights to information and to an active role in health decision-making were central concerns. The language of compliance was rejected and there was some preference for the use of the term 'client' rather than patient.

There can be no surprise at the prominence of preventive approaches to education in systems of health care committed to the medical model. It is interesting to question, however, the extent to which it is possible, or even desirable, to reject this model and wholeheartedly embrace educational and self-empowerment models. These questions have been discussed by Fahrenport [7] and Steele *et al.* [11]. After outlining the background to the active patient concept and reviewing research literature, Steele *et al.* made the following observations:

1. Patients in general want to be informed about their illnesses and the treatment options open to them;
2. Information that permits patients to anticipate and prepare for an experience can be a potent resource for coping with distress and the discomfort of illness and treatment;
3. Information interacts with patient preferences and personality traits in producing outcomes;
4. While there is evidence that some patients desire an active role in decision-making and many benefit from such a role, there is little evidence that this is sought by most patients in most situations;
5. Links between patient autonomy and clinical outcomes tend to be weak, ambiguous or mediated by unexamined variables;
6. Clinicians are often poor judges of patients' information needs and participation preferences.

They concluded that their observations did not lead to support for an across-the-board application of an 'activated' patient approach. They also called for more research based on standard definitions of the active patient concept and reliable measures of patient's participation preferences.

Fahrenport identifies a gap between theoretical views promoting emancipation and the self-empowerment of patients built around the philosophy of Paulo Freire, and the possibilities of achieving them in practice. She finds examples of humanistic patient centredness, more often in nurses than doctors, but this she sees as a long way from incorporating what Freire describes as dialogue. This would imply not simply two-way communication in which doctors took notice of patients and their needs but would require a conviction on the part of doctors that the patient's own knowledge was as relevant to the situation as medical knowledge. In actual practice, she contends, medical knowledge remains the norm in the hospital situation and is consolidated in two ways: through the assumption that it is medical knowledge that is to be disseminated to patients and through patients' own efforts to gain power in the situation by appropriating medical knowledge. In the process patients become 'lesser' doctors but the real doctors remain the guardians of the knowledge that is imparted in efforts to educate. Considerable practical barriers exist to establishing true dialogue: time and effort are needed in situations such as the hospital where people may not be present for more than a short time. Were success to occur it could not survive sanctions from medical practitioners towards truly autonomous patients. She concludes that patient education in hospitals is not the royal road to emancipation. Humanistic, patient-centred education is feasible and probably as far as we can go. Roter [12] in an examination of models for patient education offers a 2×2 model of decision-making in provider–client encounters which can be seen in Figure 5.1. She favours the Active Participation Model as one which gives better justice both to the realities of therapeutic encounters and also to ethical and philosophical concerns. This model assumes that the interaction should at minimum provide the client with a basis for effective participation in sound decision-making. She sees this as different from Szasz and Hollender's mutual participation ideas in being more consistent with a melding of patient and physician perspectives. She herself sees the Active Participation Model as consistent with Freire's thinking but her interpretation of his ideas is probably less purist than that of Fahrenport. Both Fahrenport and Roter offer similar recommendations for the practice of patient education.

To summarize, there has been debate between supporters of the different approaches to education in health care contexts with a growing importance attached to approaches advocating active patient participation. Often there

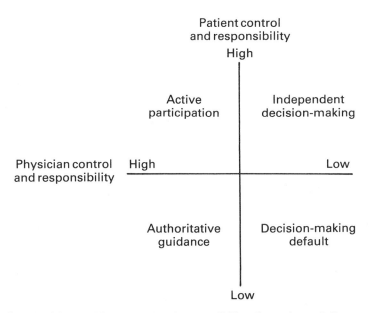

Figure 5.1 Decision-making control and responsibility dimensions of client–provider relations.

may be lip service paid to autonomy but little fundamental change from the objective of securing compliance. The degree to which full autonomy for patients is feasible has been questioned. There is a need for better models of the doctor–patient interaction. For instance, the model offered in the classic Parsonian analysis poses problems for understanding preventive activities – while the operationalization of concepts allied to self-empowerment models is seen to need more development. Finally, the growing health promotion movement is leading to changes in thinking about health care and towards a greater emphasis on positive health. This could lead, in hospitals and primary health care, to a change from a predominance of education related to specific conditions and general health education aimed at primary prevention towards a fuller commitment in theory and practice to education for positive health. While the debate about approaches can be pursued at a theoretical level, for those involved in day to day work in health care the lack of consensus leads to dilemmas which have to be resolved. For example:

1. Should education be in response to the needs expressed by the patient or should it be professionally determined?
2. Should a major aim be to achieve health-related behaviour change and associated health outcomes?
3. How far should education be directed towards achieving outcomes with demonstrable economic benefits?
4. In institutions where a number of professional groups contribute to education how can differences between them be resolved?
5. Is it acceptable to let patients make their own decisions if these turn out to be contrary to professionally recommended ones?
6. Can health services accept working to outcomes determined by patients?

EVALUATING PATIENT EDUCATION

Bartlett [13] in a recent editorial said that patient education can accomplish many things – improve patient satisfaction, improve appropriate utilization, control the malpractice threat and enhance the quality of care. For some it is primarily a means to increase patient adherence to regimens and management of conditions while for others it is a tool for enhancing patient participation in care and diminishing the power difference between patients and professionals. In reviewing evaluations it is necessary to ask if the diverse outcomes which professionals and patients have looked for have been achieved. A distinction between outcomes, intermediate and indirect indicators has been used in earlier chapters. This broad division will be adopted here although in the terms of one approach a measured variable may be an outcome while in another approach it can be an intermediate indicator. For example, within the preventive model, decision-making skills are intermediate to making responsible decisions associated with desired health outcomes but within the self-empowerment model the decision-making skills are the outcome itself. Similarly if an educational programme is responding to a patient's expressed wishes for information, patient satisfaction can be an outcome measure, but where patient satisfaction is believed to motivate desired behaviour change, satisfaction measures become an intermediate indicator. Table 5.3 gives examples of measures which can be adopted in evaluating education and counselling in health care contexts.

In the previous chapter a number of features of schools which had a bearing on evaluation were outlined. In the same way there are features of health care contexts which have a bearing on education and evaluation:

1. In contrast to schools (where the one professional group, teachers, are involved in the educational process) several professional groups have roles to play in both hospitals and primary health care;
2. The particular dominance of the medical profession in health care has

Table 5.3 Evaluating success

Outcomes	Intermediate indicators	Indirect indicators
Behaviours, e.g. adherence to medication, dietary change, smoking	Beliefs	Patient education libraries
Decision-making skills	Attitudes	Closed-circuit television provision
Active participation	Decision-making skills	Uptake of leaflets
Campaigning for services	Closed-circuit television use	Provision of leaflets
Development and implementation of health promotion policy	Self-esteem	Shared records
Cost-savings	Locus of control	Professional collaboration
Health: mortality, morbidity and subjective health measures	Knowledge	Health education in professional training
Medication use	Informed consent	Co-ordination
Personality measures: self-esteem, locus of control, autonomy	Behaviours	Education policy
Anxiety		Planned programmes of patient education
Patient satisfaction		Informed consent legislation
Professional satisfaction		Professional motivation
		Professional collaboration
		Co-ordination of patient education activities
		Sharing patient record

significance for an activity such as health education which depends on inter-professional collaboration for its full success;

3. The education of patients may increasingly be seen as an activity where nurses have the predominant role;
4. The barriers to acceptance and implementation of educational and self-empowerment models are greater than in schools;
5. In the current economic climate the pressures to demonstrate the effectiveness of education in cost-saving terms may be considerable;
6. In contrast to schools where education is a central activity it can be secondary to more immediate concerns in hospitals and primary care.

In considering the success of education in health care we can focus on outcomes for patients (as individuals or groups) or institutional factors which in various ways have a bearing on the former. What can be achieved in educational terms from health care is also influenced by policy developed outside any individual institution. Measures which can be applied at these three interacting levels are listed in Table 5.4.

As in the previous chapter it will not be possible to comment on all the outcomes and indicators listed. The intention is to focus on a number which reflect concerns of the main philosophical approaches and which highlight some issues in developing effective education in health care contexts. For this purpose three outcomes have been selected. The first, **compliance**, as previously noted, characterizes a medico-centred approach. While it is an outcome which may be unpalatable to some patient educators it has,

Table 5.4 Levels of activity

Individual	*Institution*	*Policy*
Compliance and adherence	Patient education	Health education in
Health measures	co-ordinators	initial training for all
Personality measures	Education as routine	health professionals
Satisfaction	part of consultation	Appointment of patient
Decision-making skills	in primary care	education co-ordinators
Active participation	Patient education in	In-service education
Compliance	care of hospital patients	Health promotion policy
Health-related behaviours	Provision of audio-visual	in NHS
	material, leaflets and	
	other resources	
	Health education for	
	at-risk groups in primary	
	care, etc.	
	Smoking policy	

nonetheless, been the subject of considerable research activity and in a time of focus on costs and benefits in health care is likely to remain of interest. The second outcome, **information exchange**, is integral to promoting compliance but is also central to achieving success in promoting the active participation of patients in health care. Finally there will be some consideration of studies which have focused on achieving **active participation** of patients. Small-scale intervention studies which demonstrate that outcomes, singly or in combination, can be achieved are of importance. If, however, patients as a whole are to benefit, knowledge of effective strategies needs to be widely accepted and applied. The final part of this chapter will look more generally at health education activities in primary care and hospital situations, noting some studies and discussing briefly some of the organizational and institutional factors which support effective patient education.

COMPLIANCE

It is a widely acknowledged fact that as many as 50% of patients fail to comply fully with their therapeutic regimens [14]. As Leventhal [15] recently noted, less attention has been paid to variability in non-compliance, this variability suggesting that non-compliance is a multifactorial problem influenced by characteristics of disease, treatment regimen and setting, together with stable and variable dispositions in participants. As observed earlier the awareness of non-compliance was one important trigger in the developments of educational inputs to health care. Haynes [16] suggests that activity in compliance research has been linked with new medical treatments. Particular 'pushes' have been associated with tuberculosis, the psychoses, rheumatic heart disease and, most recently, hypertension. Introducing [16] a review of compliance research, he believed that there had been no recent breakthroughs although much consolidation of earlier findings had occurred. The appearance of AIDS, it was believed, would act as a new stimulus to understanding compliance. Organizational and behavioural compliance interventions had certainly, he believed, increased the benefit of modern treatments. For example, hypertension studies of more than 10 years ago had shown less than one fifth of patients under good blood pressure control [17] whereas new studies showed up to 70% with good control [18].

Compliance literature has addressed health and behaviour outcomes and intermediate indicators as exemplified in Table 5.5. Various reviews of this literature have been offered: on compliance with prescribed medication [20], adherence to health behaviour change [19], theoretical approaches [15] and general reviews [21]. Criticism has been made of the weakness of theory associated with designing interventions and the understanding of non-compliance. Leventhal [15] has said that: '... theoretical analysis of the compliance problem is essential for forward movement'.

Table 5.5 Compliance with behavioural regimens. (After Cameron and Best [19])

Intervention	*Participation*	*Behaviour change*	*Risk reduction and health outcomes*
Information	Acceptance of intervention	Adherence to regimen: short term and long term	Change in markers, e.g. blood pressure, morbidity, mortality and quality of life measures
Counselling	Commitment to attempt change		
Instruction	Level of attendance Adherence to initiation procedures, e.g. monitoring		

A number of observations were made by Green [21] on a sample of evaluative studies of compliance. Most behavioural changes were, he said, measured by self-reporting with the attendant problems of memory and truth telling. Where intermediate measures were chosen other criticisms were levelled. Attitudes which were assessed were more often directed towards the intervention than to the behaviour which was the focus of the intervention. Underlying many of the studies was an implied causal pathway from education through to behaviour change.

Patient education -→ Patient satisfaction -→ Behaviour change

Many articles were criticized for failing to describe the educational and behavioural techniques employed. Green's main criticism appeared to be of the oversimplification of the analysis of behavioural tasks. Often, little attention was given to reviewing and differentiating the behavioural and non-behavioural determinants of a health problem or to giving priority to health behaviours on the basis of a critical assessment of their relative importance and changeability. A tendency to oversimplify the multiple influences of attitudes, beliefs, values, perceptions, social support, physical and financial barriers and the behaviour of health providers on patient's health behaviour also existed. These omissions and oversimplifications resulted in resources being concentrated equally on trivial and important behaviours, simple and complex behaviours and on rare and prevalent attitudes and beliefs. The result is an indiscriminate allocation of scarce educational resources resulting in a poor return in outcomes relative to apparent investment of effort. Epstein and Class [22] concluded that:

... the overwhelming majority of clinical compliance research is atheoretical, with the major goal being the technological solving of specific compliance problems. Few individual studies have had a psychological rationale for the development of their treatments.

Haynes *et al.* in their review of studies of compliance with medication published in the last 10 years [16] looked for those which met all of the following criteria: reported relevant endpoints (behaviour and/or treatment outcomes); scientifically acceptable designs; at least 80% follow-up; six months' follow-up in long-term treatments; statistical analyses; and protection against false negative results. They looked at studies of both short and long-term treatments. Only two studies satisfied all criteria, a main failing being the omission of evidence of patient health. They cited as one of the best studies that of Colcher and Bass [23] who investigated compliance with streptococcal pharyngitis medication. Patients in the study were assigned to three groups with the following conditions:

1. 10 day course of oral medication with the usual instruction;
2. 10 day course plus special instruction emphasizing the need to take the full course even if symptoms subsided;
3. Compliance obviated by administering treatment in a single parenteral dose.

Condition (2) was adequate in ensuring high compliance with significantly superior results on compliance and streptococcal recurrence when compared with condition (1). The clinical results achieved in (2) were equivalent to those with Condition (3).

Other studies reviewed showed that short-term compliance with medication could be marginally but reproducibly increased by reducing the frequency of dosage to once or twice a day [24] and by special packaging and calendars [25]. Specific instructions regarding a simple short-term regimen are generally seen to be sufficient to achieve compliance. Where long-term regimens are concerned Haynes *et al.* concluded that, to date, no single intervention of any sort was sufficient to improve long-term compliance. They reinforced Green's earlier comment that [21] in chronic degenerative disease no intervention by itself yielded immediate or sufficient impact on health indicators. For long-term regimens, therefore, multiple strategies are required including, from the studies reviewed: self monitoring, home visits, tangible rewards, peer group discussion, counselling by health educator or nurse, and special pill packaging. In the combinations studied most of the successful interventions involved cues and rewards. An example of the studies using a combination of interventions is that of Sackett *et al.* [26] with patients with hypertension who were non-compliant with medication. The intervention consisted of an interview to find out patients' daily habits which could be used to cue medicine taking; patients were also given instruction in blood pressure measurement. They were then seen twice a month by a non-professional assistant who reviewed their self-monitoring records of medicine taking and blood pressure and provided rewards for increased compliance and reduced blood pressure. A 21% increase in compliance was achieved. A much simpler study which could more easily be adopted in routine clinical situations was that of Takala *et al.* [27] also for hypertension patients, with the following elements:

1. Written instructions on medication;
2. A follow-up card which recorded at each visit the patient's blood pressure, current medication and date of next visit;
3. A contact made in cases of failure to attend for scheduled visits.

Significant reductions were found in the numbers who dropped out of treatment and a significant proportion had lowered blood pressure at the end of the study year. Haynes *et al.* [16] have produced a list of actions which have been shown to work in this area of compliance with medication (Table 5.6). Practitioners need to know what forms of intervention are effective and which achieve their results simply and cheaply. It is important also to know, particularly where long-term regimens are concerned, which strategies are viewed positively by patients.

The emphasis in much discussion of compliance is on the compliance of the patient. We might also refer to the 'compliance' of the professionals with strategies which have been shown to increase adherence to regimens. Haynes

Table 5.6 A short list of compliance improving actions that have been shown to work

For all regimens
Information:
    Keep the information as simple as possible
    Give clear instructions on the exact treatment regimen, preferably written

For long-term regimens
Reminders:
    Call if appointment missed
    Prescribe medication in concert with patient's daily schedule
    Stress importance of compliance at each visit
    Titrate frequency of visits to compliance need

Rewards:
    Recognize patient's efforts to comply at each visit
    Decrease visit frequency visit if compliance high

Social
    Involve the patient's spouse or other partner

also commented:

> Despite the knowledge that sound investigations have produced during the last two decades concerning the enhancement of compliance, many practitioners remain unaware of basic compliance management principles.

He emphasizes the need for training programmes to enable health care providers to apply proven techniques. In conclusion, there is a general view that the theoretical frameworks for compliance research need further development. At the same time compliance figures could be improved if knowledge already available was applied generally.

INFORMATION EXCHANGE BETWEEN DOCTORS AND PATIENTS

It has long been recognized that the informational needs of patients are not adequately met and the literature has been reviewed and discussed [28, 29, 30, 31]. Visser, for example, reports a survey of 754 patients from six hospitals in which the supply of information was rated an average of 7.3 on a scale from nought to ten [32]. The information supplied about department and hospital procedures was judged not sufficiently clear by 27% and not extensive enough by 34% of patients. Medical information was not clear to 24% and 28% did not consider the extent of information provided as sufficient. The findings were seen to confirm the conclusion of Dekkers [33] based on several investigations, that between 30% and 40% of hospital patients are not satisfied with the information they receive. The most consistent result in studies of patients' views was that more tended to be dissatisfied with the amount and nature of information they received than with any other aspect of treatment.

The failure to meet information needs satisfactorily can happen for reasons of omission: oversight, disruption by competing activities or poor professional communication; or commission: denying informational needs and withholding information. Korsch and Negrete's study of 800 separate mother–doctor interactions illustrated the failure to provide adequate information [34]. Almost half of the mothers left the consultation still unsure about what had caused their child's illness, and 20% felt the illness had not been properly explained. One explanation for findings of this kind is that patients did not ask for the information they needed, a frequent occurrence according to Visser. Professionals also report difficulties in assessing patient needs. In a study of informed consent with consultants in eight countries Taylor and Kilner [35] reported that 40% said that it was always difficult to assess patients' desire for information. A careful assessment of information needs is a necessary part of the communication process.

Information can be consciously withheld. Reasons for this have been suggested: the withholding of information as a means of maintaining control; the reluctance to convey uncertainty; and the difficulties associated with giving bad news. For example, Davis's study of parents of children with polio [36] reported that where the prognosis was fairly well established health professionals still maintained it was uncertain. Holding back the information served to delay the obligation to counsel and comfort. A further illustration was provided by Elian and Dean [37] who were allowed to work with a consultant's patients as long as these patients did not find out that they had multiple sclerosis. And yet, of 167 interviewed, 83% favoured knowing their diagnosis and 137 actually did know it – 40 had received the information from a doctor other than the consultant, 32 had diagnosed themselves and a large number had found out by accident. Only 45 had been informed by the consultant. Their view was that the consultant should provide the information. An editorial [38] in the edition of the *Lancet* which contained the study report said:

> ... It is indefensible on ethical and humanitarian grounds that patients should be left to make one of the most devastating discoveries in their lives by accident and without any professional support or explanation.

Providing for informed consent requires a full sharing of information. Professionals' attitudes to informed consent can act as a barrier to success. In Taylor and Kilner's study [35], 95% of respondents saw the informed consent requirement as an intrusion into the doctor–patient relationship. Fifty per cent felt that when it was associated with participation in a randomized controlled trial the doctor's dual role as scientist and caregiver was exposed. This created discomfort. No association was found between the legal requirements in specific countries on informed consent and the amount of information physicians reported giving to their patients. While some of their comments reflected a concern that the regulations for informed consent interfered with the sensitive sharing of information as and when patients were ready there was also evidence of physicians' claim to rights to control information. Only 37% believed that the best judge of the amount of information disclosed should be the patient. The variation in patients' needs should not, of course, be overlooked. Cassileth [39], for example, examined information preferences among cancer patients. People who sought detailed information tended to be younger as were those who wanted as much information as possible, whether good or bad news. Preferences were independent of sex. Of twelve types of information seven were perceived as absolutely necessary by at least half of the patients studied.

If the exchange of information between doctors and patients is to be more effective closer studies of these interactions are required. An important one is that of Tuckett and others [40] who studied 1302 consultations between doctors and patients. Their aim was to explore the extent to which ideas were shared in the medical consultation and they started from the view that the consultation was a meeting between experts: the doctor with scarce specialist knowledge and the patient, by dint of experience, immersion in a culture and past experience, with a set of ideas about the issue of concern. The researchers examined the information that doctors chose to give and seek from patients and the information patients volunteered to, and sought from, doctors. The ideas shared were linked to four predesignated topics: diagnostic–significance, treatment–action, preventive–action and implications. They reported that while doctors seemed to express a view about treatment–action and diagnostic–significance in all or nearly all consultations they were much less likely to indicate whether prevention was relevant and very unlikely indeed to indicate what they thought about implications – the social and emotional consequences of illness. Doctors spent a fair amount of time sharing what they thought but much less trying to share what patients thought. A main finding of the study was that the consultation was a one-sided affair: doctors and patients did not achieve a full dialogue and did not exchange ideas to any great degree. Doctors did little to encourage patients to present their views, often actually inhibited them, evaded what they did say, did not tailor instruction to the known details of the patients' lives, and the few efforts to establish patients' ideas and explanations were brief to the point of being absent. On the other hand, patients offered little which would have triggered dialogue – as they neither made clear nor were made to make clear their ideas – they could not receive explanations in reaction. Doctors could not know if the information they offered was understood correctly nor could patients know if their understanding was correct.

Only some aspects of information sharing between patients and professionals have been mentioned here, but from the evidence quoted and from other studies there is the need for the following activities if successful and satisfactory communication is to occur:

1. Helping patients to recognize and communicate their information needs;
2. Helping health professionals (especially doctors) to recognize fully that information needs exist and to elicit these needs;
3. Developing positive attitudes among health professionals towards the sharing of information and providing the institutional climate and resources to facilitate such sharing;
4. Increasing understanding about the ways that information sharing is constrained in health care contexts;
5. Identifying effective and efficient means of achieving satisfactory communication.

A few examples of patient education studies which have focused on information issues follow: Wallace [41], looking in more detail at the types of information patients wanted, examined the extent to which patients welcomed special preparatory communication in minor gynaecological surgery and also the types of information, timing and the format of presentation. Only 10% did not welcome special preparation and all patients welcomed some written preparation. The preferred type of information was procedural (when choosing between procedural, sensory, coping or reassuring information) but after exposure to sample materials and a booklet the preference was actually for a composite of all types of information. Most patients preferred to receive information from the surgeon. Wallace concluded that as most patients like information prior to hospitalization the provision of a booklet to back up the doctor is generally the most practical solution to providing cost-effective preparation for routine surgery with adults. Many studies have investigated the effectiveness of providing information, either alone or together with other methods, in preparation for surgery. Information can be procedural or sensory, or both and can be general or specific. Procedural information describes the nature of the medical procedure itself, when and where it takes place, by whom it will be provided and attendant risks. Sensory information describes the sensations the patient may expect to feel. Studies have been reviewed by Melamed [42] and Williams and Kendall [43]. According to the latter the research literature on the efficacy of information provision interventions for the reduction of adult distress and improvement of patient adjustment offers only equivocal evidence. They see some support for the efficacy of providing sensory information over procedural information.

One way of enhancing information exchange in primary care is to share the patient record. This has been advocated by Metcalfe who said [44]:

> The central idea is that sharing of the patient record symbolizes sharing the responsibility for health – an adult to adult relationship which protects or restores the patient's autonomy and dignity.

He recognizes the shift that this sharing can have on the power relationship: to have information about someone that he does not have himself is to be in a powerful controlling position which is inimical to the adult–adult relationship which should exist between doctors and patients. Fischbach *et al.* [45] have reported on a pilot project of the joint production of the patient record in which they found that patients participated actively regardless of socio-economic status. The additional information available to them had not made patients 'too directive' with providers, open disclosure had not led to malpractice or to improper self-care. They believed that co-authorship was an effective means of conveying complete, accurate and understandable information to both patient and provider. The patient's as well as the doctor's perspective was heard and appreciated. Positive outcomes from sharing problem cards developed from patient records in a group practice have been described by Tomson [46]. Records were shared with 100 patients. The sharing gave patients an opportunity to review their health needs and in some cases to correct inaccurate information: 80% were grateful for seeing the card, 88% felt cards should be shared and 51% thought seeing their cards would help them to manage their health better. Finally the last stage of the study by Tuckett *et al.* [40] discussed above was designed to communicate to doctors and some patients ideas and suggestions for improving communication. They used detailed case discussion, an intensive curriculum programme, a contribution to vocational training courses, small group discussions with GP trainers and a patient education pamphlet. Both doctors and patients valued the experience of the activities but they concluded:

> Attempts to articulate and exchange the doctors' models and ours led to a very considerable understanding of the potential role of patients' ideas but not necessarily or quickly to dramatic changes in behaviour.

PATIENT PARTICIPATION

Key outcomes of a self-empowerment approach to health education are active participation in health care and health decision-making. Greenfield *et al.* [47] have said that while there is evidence that patients can and wish to play a more active role in their care, studies leave unanswered questions of how to prepare patients for greater involvement in physician–patient interaction and whether greater involvement in care is related to better health outcomes. Evidence of the wishes for greater involvement in decision-making comes from consumers, women's and patients' rights groups and in more general comment. Writing in the *Lancet*, Slack has said [48]:

> It seems to me that communication between patients and doctors should not be used to persuade patients to do what physicians want them to do, rather it should be used to outline the possible plans of action, so that patients can decide clinical matters for themselves.

He acknowledges that some patients may not wish to assume this active role and they should not be forced to do so but he concludes with the suggestion that physicians stop thinking in terms of compliance and recognize the rights of patients to make their own decisions and help them to do so. The previous chapter provided some discussion of decision-making in school health education and outlined a 'vigilant' strategy of decision-making. This strategy is recommended for use in situations where the choice made has important consequences and when individuals want to make the best choice for themselves. For such decision-making to be possible in health care contexts the right of the patient to a role in decision-making has to be recognized and the process facilitated. This facilitation can involve some or all of the following: ensuring that patients are aware that choices are possible; specifying the alternatives; making information available on alternatives or helping patients acquire it; offering counselling support in the stages of weighing up alternatives and in the post-decision period, and ensuring that patients have the personal skills to use their decision-making competencies in the social situations of hospitals and primary care and when normal health is impaired.

A number of studies have looked at aspects of decision-making and active participation by patients. Greenfield *et al.* [47] carried out an intervention study with patients with peptic ulcer designed to alter the traditional patient role in physician–patient interaction. In a 20 minute session before a scheduled visit to the doctor patients were helped to read their medical record and to focus on the management of their own disease. In addition, an algorithm was used to clarify the logic of the medical process and to identify decisions relevant to the patient's own care. It was intended that this preparation would increase effective involvement in interaction with the physician. At follow-up six weeks later the intervention group had fewer limitations on physical and role-related activities, they preferred a more active role in decision-making and were as satisfied as the control group with their care. The intervention group were twice as effective as the controls in obtaining information from the physician. Although they did not ask more questions, other attempts to control conversation were more effective in eliciting information. Patients often actually avoided questions – as if they threatened the relationship and used more roundabout ways of gaining information. Joking and attributing topics to others were strategies used. It was suggested that these strategies may not be recognized by doctors as information seeking. The writers cautioned against applying their findings to other conditions and they did not go on to look at health outcomes, other than by self-report.

Although this study looked at the active participation of patients and aspects of information seeking in the consultation it did not actually measure decision-making competence. A study by Morris and Royle [49] has provided evidence that actually being offered a choice has positive outcomes. They investigated whether being offered a choice of surgery influenced levels of anxiety and depression pre- and post-operatively. A significantly higher percentage not offered the choice experienced clinical levels of anxiety and depression pre-operatively and up to two months post-operatively. By six months differences were not statistically significant although the trend was unaltered.

Efforts to increase patient participation do not always promote positive responses in patients. Roter's 1977 study [50] in a family and community centre was designed to increase patient question asking during the medical visit. The study group was low income, predominantly black and female and not typical of some of the groups who have urged active patient participation. The intervention group were each given 10 minutes with a health educator who worked with them through a protocol designed to enable patients to ask questions about their condition in the consultation. The control group had an interview about the centre facilities and were given an information sheet. The experimental group asked more direct questions and fewer indirect questions than the control group. The interactions of the experimental group women were characterized, however, by negative affect: anxiety and anger. The interactions for the control group patients, on the other hand, were described as mutually sympathetic. The experimental group was less satisfied with care received but did demonstrate better appointment keeping during the four month monitoring period and also showed significant increases in internal locus of control. Roter interpreted her data by drawing on Dissonance Theory. The experimental intervention focused patients on information seeking and gave them some skills and encouragement in asking questions in the consultation. In taking an active orientation the passive patient role was challenged and contributed to the negative mood of the interaction. The dissonance between the active decision-making and the usual passivity of their patient roles was resolved by changing self-image as exemplified in changed internality. Steele *et al.* [11] have pointed out that the follow-up period was short and the appointment keeping rates while statistically significant were small and called into question the implications drawn from the study. They feel Roter demonstrated that patients can be activated to ask more questions but that her evidence does not unambiguously point to strong positive effects and outcomes.

Speedling and Rose have focused directly on involving doctors and patients together in clinical decisions [51]. Using a method of quantitative analysis of the probabilities of events and the weighted importance of each event's outcome a decision tree is built up and patients attach a 'quality of life' assessment to each alternative. In the process of deriving utility values patients are empowered to act on their own behalf. No evaluation is yet reported. Speedling and Rose feel that the most immediate benefit from clinical decision analysis will be in giving legitimacy to the patient's point of view and encouraging a more active role in the doctor–patient relationship. They conclude:

> The approach we are recommending may well require more time by physicians with patients. This may entail increased opportunity costs, at least, to physicians. But the pay-off is that patients are enabled in the course of their participation in clinical decision-making to behave in ways that enhance their well being.

The analysis performed by Steele *et al.* [11] of the 'active patient' concept was noted earlier. Commenting in particular on the research studies they drew the following conclusions:

1. Because the active patient concept has been defined and operationalized in various ways it is difficult to know if apparent differences in the

participation preferences of patients are genuine or reflections of assessment procedures.

2. Sample sizes in studies have been small, non-representative and cross-sectional. Future research needs to focus on the 'natural history' of patient participation preferences. It also needs to focus on the various determinants of information needs and the preferences for active involvement;

3. There is no coherent theory guiding research and an orientating framework is essential.

In making recommendations to health professionals they suggest that a mechanical application of an activated approach that is not responsive to patients' varying needs may not produce the desirable outcomes attributed to this ideal model of patienthood. Professionals will need to actively elicit and try to understand patients' perspectives and formulate approaches with them, at the same time recognizing and responding to changes in those preferences.

Chapter three claimed that a sound theoretical framework will provide a substantial basis for practice. As we have seen, reviewers of both the compliance literature and that on the active participation of patients have criticized the current state of the theory which guides research. While a fuller development of theory is needed there is, nonetheless, a sound knowledge base to guide practice. The remainder of this chapter will examine some aspects of patient education in primary care and hospitals.

THE ORGANIZATION OF EDUCATION IN HEALTH CARE CONTEXTS

In the first place it is convenient to discuss primary care and hospital situations separately although later it will be argued that much better coordination is needed between the two sectors if education is to be a more coherent activity and, in the end, a more successful one. Although much patient education is hospital focused in terms of the proportion of patient contacts and the continuing relationships within it, primary care is arguably the more important sector for health education.

PRIMARY CARE

Primary care includes those services provided outside hospitals mainly by general practitioners, dentists, pharmacists, opticians, community nurses, midwives, practice nurses and health visitors. In the UK primary care services deal with nine out of ten contacts with the health service and most of the contacts are patient initiated. The services include management of illness and a variety of activities with the well population registered with the practice. Except in emergencies and some minor injuries patients normally enter hospital care by referral from primary care. In the UK 90% of family doctors work in practices employing some ancillary staff and over 75% practise in groups. The membership of primary health care teams varies but it is common to have in addition to general practitioners, health visitors, community nurses, midwives and district nurses.

In the last ten years a number of reports and official documents have addressed wholly, or in part, the subject of health education and prevention in primary care. These include the 1981 document *Care in Action* [52], a series of reports from the Royal College of General Practitioners [53, 54], consultative documents on primary care and the community nursing services [55, 56], Project 2000 [57] and a Government White Paper [58]. Like the earlier prevention document [59], Care in Action emphasized individual responsibility for prevention and it looked at ways that the National Health Service (NHS), in adopting a preventive role, could provide the information people needed to make sensible decisions about personal health. It said that health authorities should insist on commitment to policies of health promotion and preventive medicine, ensure resources are directed to these purposes and establish priorities for programmes which meet the health interests of local populations [60]. The Royal College of General Practitioners' report [53], using the term 'anticipatory care', noted existing preventive work in primary care and identified particular subjects for health education within the normal consultation: antenatal and postnatal care; smoking, assessment of coronary risk status, and family planning. Further activities which would involve cooperation with other members of the primary care team and identification of people not presenting for consultation included primary immunization, developmental surveillance, early detection and treatment of elevated blood pressure and preventive work with the elderly. Finally, suggestions were made for prevention through working with others in the community. The consultative document on primary care [55] identified as key objectives the promotion of health and the prevention of illness and the subsequent White Paper [58] stated that the Government wished to strengthen the GP's role in health promotion by:

1. Paying special fees to encourage doctors to provide health checks and necessary follow-up to patients registering for the first time with an NHS doctor;
2. Considering incentives to achieve specified target levels of vaccination, immunization and screening, as well as to meet the costs of call and recall;
3. Considering amendments to doctors' terms of service to clarify their role in the provision of health promotion services and the prevention of ill health.

The paper also included prevention recommendations for dentists, pharmacists and community nurses. These documents use the terms prevention, health education and health promotion but there is little which goes beyond a preventive model of health education. Project 2000 [57] which addressed the education and training needed for nursing, midwifery and health visiting is a more wide-ranging document and says that in exploring future needs it was concerned to examine trends in social life, health and disease. It called for a reorientation in initial training towards the community and says that health promotion should be given high priority as a topic in its own right as well as being considered separately for each care group.

The Royal College of General Practitioner's (RCGP) document identified three arenas for general practitioner health education activity: in the consultation, with the practice population as a whole and in the community. Although the third area of activity identified fits in well with WHO ideas of primary health care and some discussion of community focused health education has been provided [60], there has been little development of evaluated studies to report. There has been an emphasis in discussion on the role of the general practitioner rather than on the contribution of the primary health care team as a whole. Those concerned with the social control potential of the medical profession express reservation [62] at the expansion of the doctor's territory in taking on health education. There is evidence that doctors are interested in increasing their involvement in health education [61] and a small-scale study has explored some of the conceptions held of health education in the context of general practice. Calnan, Boulton and Williams [62] report a study carried out with 34 doctors with a responsibility for postgraduate and continuing education in general practice. All saw prevention and health education as important within general practice. Prevention and health education were seen as a new domain of medical expertise, largely practice based, and apparently few had any clear ideas of the roles they could play in health education in the community. The definitions of health education held seemed to reflect four views:

1. Health education as a technical service to build into practice routines including, for example, an effective screening programme. The role in promoting behaviour change in patients was emphasized;
2. Health education in terms of response to patients presenting problems, with an emphasis on explanation to promote understanding and to help patients cope and make choices; This group showed reservation about opportunistic health education and were more likely to see health education on lifestyle issues as intrusive and moralizing;
3. Integration of the first and second. This group had been influenced by the RCGP initiatives and had sought to develop policies for their own practices;
4. A restricted approach in which health education was part of daily work but defined mainly in terms of problem-related interventions on smoking, weight and sometimes alcohol.

Research which has examined actual patient education in the consultation has used both observational methods and surveys. The study by Tuckett *et al.*

[40] discussed earlier concluded that prevention was discussed in only 25% of consultations. In focusing on the lifestyle issues of smoking, diet and alcohol consumption the consultations were assessed in terms of the opportunities that were provided for health education, the discussions that occurred, and the advice given. A distinction was made between problem-related health education where topics were raised in connection with the presenting problem and non-problem-related health education when the doctor raised topics independent of the presenting problem. A large proportion of consultations provided opportunities for problem-related education, especially in smoking. The majority of opportunities were not used. The opportunities for non-problem-related education were virtually never explored. In a separate paper Boulton and Williams [63] commented that the way the doctors overlooked opportunities cannot be seen in neutral terms as just 'lost opportunities'. Patients may interpret and attach as much significance to comments not made as to those which are made. A more recent study has reported on the frequency with which health promotion topics occurred within the consultation and on patients' attitudes to such introductions. In a five doctor practice with 8300 patients [64], 100 consecutive adults consulting the doctors over a two day period were given a questionnaire at the close of the consultation. It contained a satisfaction scale and a checklist of 10 health promotion topics. Patients recorded if topics were raised, the person who raised them, whether they felt comfortable discussing the topics and the degree to which discussion was helpful. The results can be seen in Table 5.7. Health promotion was discussed

Table 5.7 Number of consultations at which 10 health promotion items were discussed and the patients' mean satisfaction scores

Topic discussed	Number of consultations	Mean satisfaction score
Smoking	19	4.37
Diet	19	4.32
Weight	19	4.30
Family planning	12	4.29
Blood pressure	31	4.28
Exercise	24	4.26
Cervical smear	13	4.23
Alcohol	11	3.92
Immunization*	4	–
Breast self-examination*	4	–

* Mean satisfaction score not calculated because number of consultations too small.

in 64 (74%) of the 86 consultations for which questionnaires were analysed. Blood pressure was mentioned in the largest number and breast self-examination in the least. Patient satisfaction was not significantly influenced by inclusion of the health promotion topics and most (84%) found the discussion helpful. The researchers noted the high proportion of consultations in which health promotion topics were raised. High satisfaction scores could be due to a reluctance to report true feelings about the service or because expectations were low. This study provides no evidence on the success of introducing health promotion topics other than in satisfaction terms. The most widely quoted study of the effectiveness of health education intervention within the consultation has been that of Russell *et al.* [65]. The study was carried out on 2138 cigarette smokers attending the surgeries of 28 general practitioners in London. Patients were randomly assigned to one of four groups with the following conditions:

1. Patients were asked if they smoked before their consultation but received no further information or advice;
2. Patients filled in a questionnaire on smoking habits before the consultation;
3. Patients received advice to stop smoking from the general practitioner;
4. Patients received advice as in (3) plus a leaflet and advised that they would be followed up.

Those who stopped smoking in the first month after the intervention and were still not smoking a year later were recorded. There were 0.3% in Group 1, 1.6% in Group 2, 3.3% in Group 3 and 5.1% in Group 4. The findings of the study have been discussed by Calnan and Johnson [66] who agree that it offers evidence to suggest that advice given by a general practitioner is effective in changing people's smoking habits. It is not clear, however, which aspect of the consultation process or routine makes the crucial impact. A more recent study by Russell, Stapleton, Hajek *et al.* [67] was an attempt to see if the measure shown to be effective in the earlier study could be incorporated into the daily routine with patients rather than as an intrusive element for the purposes of a short-term study. In this investigation, 101 general practitioners in 27 practices in London took part in a quasi-experimental study which was designed to examine whether a brief intervention applied to all smokers seen by practitioners and sustained on a continuous basis could in time have a cumulative effect and reduce prevalence of smoking. Of 21 practices in one health district, seven opted for a brief intervention with support from the smokers' clinic, four opted for the intervention without support and six acted as care controls. A further 10 practices in a second health district provided further controls. Six cross-sectional surveys were carried out over three years, each consisting of all adults attending a doctor during a defined two week period. The estimated decline in self-reported smoking prevalence over the first 30 months from the start of the intervention was 5.5% in the group receiving intervention plus support, but only 2.0% in the group receiving the intervention only and 2.1% and 3.0% in the control groups receiving usual care. At this stage in the study results suggest that intervention on a routine basis by a general practitioner is most effective when backed up by further support.

Most of the studies which have focused on health education occurring within the consultation have reflected preventive approaches. A general practice study which has addressed patient participation is that of Bird, Cobb and Walji [68]. It was carried out in a new general practice in an inner city multiracial and multicultural area of Birmingham with high mortality and morbidity rates. The aim of the new practice was to develop patient choice and responsibility and investigate methods of meeting patient needs. The practice encourages an open style of reception to give patients informal and ready access to receptionists. It piloted the first nurse practitioner project in the UK and the practice recognizes and encourages patients' rights of access to their medical records and each patient is handed his or her records on arrival in the waiting room. The project reported aimed to achieve a higher level of patient participation through adopting a three stage consultation. The extent of participation was assessed by questions put to patients and staff after the consultation. The 30 minute extended consultation included a session with a receptionist for assisted access to the medical record, a 15–20 minute session with a doctor or nurse and a self-help session with a receptionist. The extended consultation was welcomed by patients who showed, it was reported, a marked degree of participation and it also increased the satisfaction and cooperation of project staff. It had not been the aim to assess the project in terms of therapeutic outcome but it was believed that a consultation process which gives patients a more responsible role could be shown to result in benefits in health. Projects of this nature set a model for health promotion in general practice built around a more active model of the patient than that offered in the RCGP and some of the other documents on health education in primary care.

HOSPITALS

In the hospital sector in the UK there has been a gradual development of condition-specific health education along with the more general provision of anticipatory care for hospitalization and surgery. However, in the USA, there is a longer history of commitment to hospital wide education of patients. Although some of the influences which contributed to this development are general ones some were more specific to the form of organization of health care in the USA. In 1964 the American Hospital Association [69], at a conference, took the position that it should act as the nationwide agency for stimulating the development of patient education which was recommended as an integral part of patient care and thus a direct responsibility of hospital personnel. This conference has been noted as one impetus, together with the consumers rights' movement, for a Patient's Bill of Rights [70] approved by the House of Delegates in 1973 which stated that the patient has the right to obtain from his physicians complete and current information concerning his diagnosis and treatment in terms he can reasonably be expected to understand. This background of patients' rights has not featured as strongly in developments of patient education in the UK. By 1974 the President's Committee on Health Education emphasized the importance of reorientating the health care system to the maintenance of good health and prevention rather than primarily to treatment of acute illness [1]. Also in 1974 the Blue Cross Association [71] reflected on demands for health care systems to improve effectiveness and efficiency and, while assuring quality of health care services to contain rising health care costs. It saw patient education as one mechanism among many for responding to this need. A number of further statements have been made by the American Hospital Association (AHA) including in 1981 [72]:

> Patient education services should enable patients and their families, when appropriate, to make informed decisions about their health, to manage their illnesses and to implement follow up care at home.

It has been stated that every contact between a health professional and a patient is an opportunity for education. For this to become a reality the importance of health education would need to be recognized by all professional groups who would also need appropriate training for their educational role. While the new proposals for nursing training give health promotion a high profile the same cannot be said for medical training. Maryon Davis [73], in a discussion of the GP's role in health education, has observed:

> The RCGP reports highlighted the need for adequate training of doctors in interpersonal communication skills at medical student level and as vocational trainees. However, a recent survey of British Medical Schools has shown that only a few make any serious attempt at such training. Indeed, specific teaching on prevention and health education in the medical undergraduate curriculum is still far from universal.

To date, patient education in British hospitals has tended to be condition specific or addressed to particular stages in a hospital 'career'. Education to assist patients on entering hospital and in preparation for surgery has been extensively evaluated and there are a number of reviews [42, 43]. Interventions have compared various types of information with or without development of various coping skills and a number of outcome measures have been used: medication, length of hospital stay, anxiety measures and costs. The overall conclusion from reviews is that pre-operative education is of benefit in a wide variety of conditions although different combinations of information and coping strategies may work in different conditions and with particular individuals and groups. An example of a study which demonstrates the greater effectiveness of coping strategies over information alone is that of Ridgeway and Mathews [74]. Patients about to have a hysterectomy were randomized into three groups, each receiving a different booklet. The first group had one providing general information on the ward routine, the second a booklet on the operative procedure and the sensations to be expected and the third explained ways that concerns or worries could be reappraised more positively. The third group was able to employ this strategy for the anaesthetic procedure, for pain and recovery. This last group were more active three weeks later and suffered fewer symptoms after the operation.

The adoption of the nursing process with individualized care plans will allow assessment of patients' educational needs and should ensure that all patients with a particular condition are not seen to have identical learning and counselling needs. Much early patient education was planned around predesigned protocols. Although it was intended that they be modified in relation to specific need, education was essentially professionally determined rather than patient led. If we accept the idea of active patient participation in care it is axiomatic that patients are actively involved in the assessment of needs. When programmes are professionally determined they may fail to address areas of particular significance to patients or when needs have been recognized the education provided may be inappropriate. Webb has studied the needs of women who have had a hysterectomy [75]. Instead of the detailed information they wanted about the recovery period they were given imprecise information, much of it of a prohibitory type. Leaflets provided, when attempting to be more precise, often assumed stereotypical ideas of women's activities. Webb notes particularly the needs for advice on sexual activity and counselling on sexuality. In a small survey of trained nurses she reported that the importance of sexuality and the giving of support and counselling was endorsed. However, when asked what advice to give to a woman going home after hysterectomy none mentioned general issues of sexuality or emotional issues.

CO-ORDINATION

The co-ordination of patient education activities is an important issue. Although schools are encouraged to have specialist co-ordinators and patient education co-ordinators exist in America the role is not an established one in the UK National Health Service. In any episode of hospital care patients can encounter a number of different professionals, ancillary staff, other patients and their own families and friends. All can provide contributions to their education, formally or informally. If these varied inputs go uncoordinated it is highly unlikely that a coherent programme results. Co-ordination for each individual patient could be enhanced if educational inputs were all carefully recorded in the patient's record. If the 'educational' record formed part of the discharge information sent back to the general practitioner, continuity of education could be achieved. While co-ordination of condition specific education can, and does occur, the presence of a co-ordinator with institution wide responsibilities for the development and support of patient education can monitor the development of education as part of care in all conditions. Currently there is considerable variation in the degree to which the educational needs of specific groups of patients are recognized and efforts made to meet them. The co-ordinator could be a nurse with further training or a special health education officer.

Evidence of the effectiveness of co-ordination comes from a study in Michigan in the USA. Eighteen criteria for patient education were incorporated into a survey of subject based programmes. Of 281 programmes reported, 219 (78%) had either a full-time or part-time co-ordinator. The mean number of criteria met by these programmes was 13.8 with a full-time co-ordinator and 12.7 with a part-time co-ordinator but only 8.3 where there was no co-ordinator [76]. There was some variation in the number of criteria met according to the type of co-ordinator. Where the co-ordinator considered education to be his or her prime responsibility more criteria were likely to be met than where responsibilities were diverse. If the co-ordinator had received further training, programmes tended to be more comprehensive and meet more criteria.

METHODS AND RESOURCES

The usual need to select teaching methods and resources in line with educational objectives and the characteristics of learners and situations applies equally to health care contexts. Evaluations of various methods and resources have been carried out. A few points only will be raised.

First, we need to consider how far teaching methods and resources should be tailored to individual preferences. If we promote individualized care plans and active participation by patients it seems to follow that teaching approaches should be selected through dialogue with patients. Wilson-Barnett [6] has observed that the earlier didactic emphasis of patient education is being questioned and there is a shift towards a more patient-centred involvement. She cites a study by Ozbolt and Goodwin which evaluated [77] a programmed learning booklet which could be used by patients following pulmonary surgery according to their individual abilities and recovery rates. Adherence to the programmed approach was shown to have a significantly positive effect, patients suffering fewer infections and periods of hospitalization than others in this situation. Illness places restrictions on what patients are ready and able to learn and this must be clearly recognized. Considerable counselling may be needed before the readiness to learn new capabilities is reached.

Secondly, the question of whether people other than professionals should be involved in education needs to be addressed. As in other areas of health education, peer education has come in for discussion. Peer educators are defined by Bartlett [78] as persons who currently or formerly have experienced the illness or condition and have been specially recruited to assist in educational activities. They have been used for such conditions as cancer, asthma, renal transplants, ostomies and other conditions. The American Reach to Recovery programme for mastectomy patients is a specific example. Van den Borne *et al.* [79] reviewed studies of the effects of contacts between cancer patients. They reported that of the 18 identified most did not satisfy methodological conditions necessary to draw conclusions. Four out of six studies with sound methodological design showed positive effects of contacts with fellow sufferers. Positive effects were: more knowledge about (breast) cancer; better movement of arm after mastectomy and more use of breast prostheses; stronger improvement in general health perception; less disturbance of body image; and more reduction in negative feelings. In none of the studies were results found indicating a negative effect from fellow patient contacts. Bartlett, in his review [78], said that early experience with the use of peer educators was encouraging but limited empirical research had been undertaken. Based on findings from existing programmes he suggested that peer educators could be used most effectively when: the illness was chronic; the illness was socially stigmatizing due to physical handicaps; and/or impairment of self-concept or body image existed.

Finally, the effective use of mass media in health education will be examined in Chapter Six but a brief observation can be made here. The informational needs of patients were highlighted earlier in this chapter. Notwithstanding the limitations of leaflets patients generally appreciate receiving them. Timing of such provision needs, however, to be carefully addressed. In Wallace's study [41] discussed earlier, patients expressed a consistent preference for preparation (including booklets) prior to hospitalization. She pointed out that early preparation may have the advantage of facilitating emotional adjustment over a longer period and also, perhaps, to stimulate the patient to seek information and emotional support which could in turn reduce anticipatory anxiety. Parrinello [80], who reported on an evaluation of an arterial bypass booklet, said that over 90% of respondents found the booklet helpful but those who had an opportunity to discuss it with a health care worker found it of greater value. Timing of delivery and an opportunity to discuss the content of written materials should be relatively easy to organize.

COSTS AND BENEFITS OF PATIENT EDUCATION

The importance of exercising caution in using cost-benefit measures to evaluate health education has already been discussed in Chapter Three. It is, therefore, interesting to note here that the evidence that patient education reduced the costs of care was an early trigger to its development and has been a continuing influence in the USA. This effectiveness in economic terms has been recognized by Health Maintenance Organizations which provide care for nine million people [81]. In the guidelines for health promotion and education services in HMOs it says:

> When the HMOs act was passed in 1973 the case for the advantages of health education and health promotion was largely theoretical. Because medical technology was still seen by most people as the primary path to health improvement most health care professionals did not support education programmes. Now, less than 10 years later, much has changed. Modestly increased expenditures in health education and health promotion have led to more sophisticated program development and rigorous evaluation and these are beginning to provide documentation of efficacy and cost effectiveness of 'health education programmes'.

Bartlett [78] has recently reviewed patient education strategies to identify those that will pay off under prospective pricing imposed in 1983 for the hospital care of Medicare patients under which hospitals are reimbursed at a present rate for each patient admission, according to the patient's diagnosis-related group. Among the cost containment strategies patient education was advocated as a means of reducing medical costs and improving quality of care. He examined pre-admission education, medication self-administration programmes, out-patient education, discharge planning education, family education, peer education, cooperative care units, early discharge and home health programmes and identified for seven of them diagnosis-related groups for which they could be recommended. In an earlier editorial Bartlett [82] discussed some of the issues pertaining to seeing patient education as a cost saver:

> In this cost conscious environment, it is very tempting for patient educators to advocate the need for patient education primarily as a cost savings tool. In economics jargon, patient education is being justified less as a consumable service which is valuable in its own right, and more as a social investment which will reduce net costs.

Bartlett sees this strategy as perilous on two grounds. First, it undermines aspects of patient education which do not save money and which may well increase costs. Providing more education to facilitate informed consent is one example. He believes that it would, in fact, be difficult to demonstrate a direct relationship between most informal educational activity in hospitals and subsequent cost savings. Secondly, it condones a double standard. Newly proposed medical treatments and procedures may be routinely approved on the basis of medical necessity while patient education must demonstrate both its effectiveness and capacity to cut costs. As many patient education activities are associated with savings it is worth saying so but education as an integral part of every patient's care is not necessarily likely to save money overall.

PROFESSIONAL TRAINING

Although the evidence exists from intervention studies for successful outcomes from health education, that knowledge needs to be put into practice in health care contexts as a whole. This requires commitment to education and appropriate training. Wilson-Barnett and Close [83] have both examined the nurse's role in patient education and considered some of the reasons for their being less effective than they might be. Factors mentioned include: lack of assessment skill, lack of teaching skills, inadequate preparation at basic and post-basic level, and low priority given to patient education.

CONCLUSIONS

This chapter has reviewed selectively some aspects of the evaluation of education in health care contexts. Such education has developed at varying paces in different countries and in many remains underemphasized and underfunded. There is no uniform commitment to a particular philosophical approach and the earlier domination by advocates of the preventive approach has been extensively challenged by the general movement to promote greater active participation by patients in all aspects of health care. The accumulated evidence that patient education can contribute to reductions in health care costs has been particularly telling in developing a commitment to patient education. Caution has been expressed, however, at using economic benefits as the main or even sole criteria of judging the success of education. Many elements of patient education may involve increases in expenditure. Focusing on economic benefits can distort educational activity towards achieving specific outcomes, often those more associated with a preventive model than models of the self-empowerment type. In a climate in which there is a growing emphasis on the active involvement of people in their own health care there needs to be a commitment to the idea that education in health care contexts is valuable in its own right.

While there is a demand from patients for more comprehensive and more appropriate education this demand is not yet fulfilled, even if relatively straightforward outcomes such as information sharing are considered. Official reports and other documents have argued for increased education. In the area of primary health care in the UK criticism can be made of the largely individualistic focus of health education which is recommended although some initiatives may be more in tune with education for self-empowerment [68] ideas. A greater commitment to health education in basic and continuing education is required. While nurses, the professional group with the largest role in the education of patients, recognize their role, a number of barriers to fulfilling it adequately have been identified. A study [5] is currently exploring the ways that nurses are prepared for their health promotion roles as part of basic training. Health education requires inter-professional collaboration and this could be enhanced if more inter-professional training took place at basic and continuing levels. To overcome the tendency for some health conditions to receive a fuller component of education than others (even where objective need can be judged as equivalent) and to provide a more effective service overall, the appointment of patient education co-ordinators on the USA model is recommended where they do not already exist. They would have similar roles to health education specialists in the community: catalyst, co-ordinator, curriculum development, continuing education, resource provision, management, etc.

Hospital stays are being progressively shortened in length. Some health conditions require extended programmes of education to support return to health. These cannot be put into practice effectively during the hospital stay especially when people may have considerable adjustments to major life changes before contemplating new learning. Illness puts variable constraints on people's learning competencies and it could be argued that the hospital should be used only for education related to the most immediate needs. Even where the hospital period can be used fully there is still the need for continuation of education after discharge. For a condition requiring a spell in hospital, education should begin in primary care, be continued at the initial visit to the consultant, through the admission period and after discharge to primary care. A record of education could be kept by the patient (with copies held in primary care).

Finally, eight principles of patient education [84] have been drawn by Bartlett from a series of articles reviewing 450 empirical studies, literature reviews and other reports. These, he says, could enlighten and guide future patient education and research:

1. Planners of patient education programmes need to thoroughly specify the patient behaviours desired and identify the obstacles to performing those behaviours;
2. A combination of educational and behavioural strategies is more effective than one method. However, planners must balance effectiveness gains with the increased resource consumption such methods entail;
3. The quality of education may be more important than the methods used. In particular, individualization appears to be specially important;
4. Personalized approaches are more effective than mediated approaches and patient education requires effective interpersonal skills on the part of the caregiver;

150

5. Knowledge is necessary but generally not sufficient for behaviour change;
6. Patient education should be oriented towards what the patient should do, not just what the patient should know;
7. Patient educators need to direct more attention to the long-term performance of desired behaviours, enhancing the patient's social support and co-ordinating patient education with community based health promotion efforts;
8. Patient education programmes need to be co-ordinated with sources of regular medical care although the actual educators do not necessarily need to be direct caregivers.

He concludes by saying:

> The answers to many research questions remain cloudy, and other questions remain to be formulated. Yet, a considerable body of knowledge now exists upon which effective, practical and acceptable patient education programs can be developed. More research attention now needs to be directed to the question: why aren't we applying the knowledge we already have?

REFERENCES

1. President's Committee on Health Education (1974) *Report of the President's Committee on Health Education*, Department of Health Education and Welfare, New York City.
2. Green, L., Squyres, W. D., D'Altroy, L. H. and Hebert, B. (1980) What do recent evaluations of patient education tell us? in: *Patient Education: An Enquiry Into the State of the Art*, (ed. W. D. Squyres), Springer Publishing Company, New York.
3. Mullen, P. D., Green, L. W. and Persinger, M. S. (1985) Clinical trials of patient education for chronic conditions: a comparative analysis of intervention types. *Preventive Medicine*, **14**, 753–81.
4. Rimer, B., Keitz, M. K. and Glassman, M. A. (1985) Cancer patient education reality and potential. *Preventive Medicine*, **14**, 801–18.
5. Bartlett, E. E. (1985) Editorial: At last, a definition. *Patient Education and Counseling*, **7**, 323–4.
6. Wilson-Barnett, J. (1988) Patient teaching or patient counselling? *Journal of Advanced Nursing*, **13**, 215–22.
7. Fahrenport, M. (1987) Patient emancipation by health education: an impossible goal. *Patient Education and Counseling*, **10**, 26–37.
8. Savage, W. (1986) *A Savage Enquiry: Who Controls Childbirth?* Virago, London.
9. Holohan, A. (1977) Diagnosis: the end of transition, in: *Medical Encounters: The Experience of Illness and Treatment* (eds A. Davis and G. Horobin) Croom Helm, London.
10. Szasz, T. S. and Hollender, M. H. (1956) The basic models of the doctor–patient relationship. *Archives of Internal Medicine*, **97**, 587–92.

11. Steele, D. J., Blackwell, B., Guttman, M. C. and Jackson, J. C. (1987) Beyond advocacy: a review of the Active Patient Concept. *Patient Education and Counseling*, **10**, 3–23.

12. Roter, D. (1987) An exploration of health education's responsibility for a partnership model of client–provider relations. *Patient Education and Counseling*, **9**, 25–31.

13. Bartlett, E. E. (1988) *Preparing for strategic planning Patient Education and Counseling*, **11**, 1–2.

14. Becker, M. H. and Maiman, L. A. (1980) Strategies for enhancing patient compliance. *Journal of Community Health*, **6**, 113–35.

15. Leventhal, H. and Cameron, L. (1987) Behavioural theories and the problem of compliance. *Patient Education and Counseling*, **10**, 117–38.

16. Haynes, B. R. (1987) Guest Editorial: Patient compliance then and now. *Patient Education and Counseling*, **10**, 103–5.

17. Apostolides, A. Y., Hebel, J. R. and McDill, M. S. (1974) High blood pressure: its care and consequences, in urban centres. *International Journal of Epidemiology*, **3**, 105–18.

18. Birket, N. J., Evans, E., Taylor, D. W. *et al.* (1986) Hypertension control in two Canadian communities: evidence for better treatment and overlabelling. *Journal of Hypertension*, **4**, 369–74.

19. Cameron, R. and Best, A. J. (1987) Promoting aherence to health behaviour change interventions: recent findings from behavioural research. *Patient Education and Counseling*, **10**, 139–54.

20. Haynes, B. R., Wang, E. and Mota Gomes, M. (1987) A critical review to improve compliance with prescribed medications. *Patient Education and Counseling*, **10**, 155–66.

21. Green, C. A. (1987) What can patient educators learn from 10 years of compliance research? *Patient Education and Counseling*, **10**, 167–74.

22. Epstein, L. H. and Class, P. A. (1982) A behavioural medicine perspective on adherence to long term medical regimes. *J. Consult. Clin. Psychol.*, **50**, 950–71.

23. Colcher, D. S. and Bass, J. W. (1972) Penicillin treatment of streptococcal pharyngitis, a comparison of schedules and the role of specific counselling. *JAMA*, **222**, 657–9.

24. Tinkelman, D. G., Vanderpool, G. E. and Carroell, M. S. (1980) Compliance differences following administration of theophylline at 6 and 12 hour intervals. *Am. Allergy*, **44**, 283–6.

25. Linkewich, J. A., Catalano, R. B. and Flack, H. L. (1974) The effect of packaging and instruction on outpatient compliance with medication regimes. *Drug Intell. Clin. Pharm.*, **8**, 10–15.

26. Sackett, D. L. *et al.* (1975) Randomised trial of strategies for improving medication compliance in primary hypertension. *Lancet*, **i**, 1205–7.

27. Takala, J., Niemela, N., Rosti, J. and Sivers, K. (1979) Improving compliance with therapeutic regimes in hypertension patients in a community health centre. *Circulation*, **59**, 540–3.

28. Ley, P. (1977) Psychological studies of doctor–patient communication, in: *Contributions to Medical Psychology*, (ed. S. Richman) Pergamon Press, Oxford.

152

References

29. Byrne, P. S. and Long, B. E. L. (1976) *Doctors Talking to Patients*, HMSO, London.
30. Pendleton, D. and Hasler, J. (eds) (1983) *Doctor–Patient Communication*, Academic Press, London.
31. Di Matteo, M. R. and Di Nicola, D. A. (1982) *Achieving Patient Compliance*, Pergamon Press, Oxford.
32. Visser, A. Ph. (1984) Patient education in Dutch hospitals. *Patient Education and Counseling*, **6**, 178–89.
33. Dekkers, F. (1980) Patient education between right and practice, (I, II, III and IV). *Med. Contact*, **35**, 640–3, 674–7, 709–12, 737–40.
34. Korsch, B. M. and Negrete, V. F. (1972) Doctor-patient communication. *Scientific American*, **227**, 66–73.
35. Taylor, K. M. and Kilner, M. (1987) Informed consent: the physician's perspective. *Social Science and Medicine*, **24**, 135–43.
36. Davis, F. (1963) *Passage Through Crisis: Polio Victims and Their Families*, Bobbs, Merrill, New York.
37. Elian, M. and Dean, G. (1985) To tell or not to tell the diagnosis of multiple sclerosis, *Lancet*, **ii**, 27–8.
38. Editorial (1985) Telling patients with multiple sclerosis, *Lancet*, **ii**, 26.
39. Cassileth, B. R., Zupkis, R. V., Sutton Smith, K. and March, V. (1980) Information and participation preferences among cancer patients. *Annals of Internal Medicine*, **92**, 832–6.
40. Tuckett, D., Boulton, M., Olson, C. and Williams, A. (1985) *Meetings Between Experts; An Approach to Sharing Ideas in Medical Consultations*, Tavistock Publications, London.
41. Wallace, L. M. *Psychological Studies of the Development and Evaluation of Preparatory Procedures for Women undergoing Minor Gynaecological Surgery*, PhD thesis, University of Birmingham, England.
42. Melamed, B. (1977) Psychological preparation for hospitalisation, in: *Contributions to Medical Psychology*, (ed. S. Rachman) Volume 1, Pergamon Press, Oxford.
43. Williams, C. L. and Kendall, P. C. (1985) Psychological Aspects of Patient Education for Stressful Medical Procedures, *Health Education Quarterly*, **12**, 135–50.
44. Metcalfe, D. (1980) Why not let patients keep their own records? *Journal of the Royal College of General Practitioners*, **30**, 420.
45. Fischbach, R., Sionolo-Bayog, A., Needle, A. *et al.* (1980) The patient and practitioners as co-authors of the medical record, *Patient Education and Counseling*, **2** (1), 1–5.
46. Tomson, P. (1985) Sharing problem cards with patients. *Journal of the Royal College of Practitioners*, **35**, 534–5.
47. Greenfield, S., Kaplan, S. and Ware, J. (1985) Expanding patient involvement in care. *Annals of Internal Medicine*, **102**, 520–8.
48. Slack, W. (1977) The patients' right to decide. *Lancet*, **ii**, 240.
49. Morris, J. and Royle, G. T. (1988) Offering patients a choice of surgery for early breast cancer: a reduction in anxiety and depression in patients and their husbands. *Social Science and Medicine*, **6**, 583–5.
50. Roter, D. (1977) Patient participation in the patient–provider interaction. The

effects of patient question asking on the quality of interaction satisfaction and compliance. *Health Education Monographs*, Winter, 281–315.

51. Speedling, E. J. and Rose, D. N. (1985) Building an effective doctor–patient relationship: from patient satisfaction to patient participation. *Social Science and Medicine*, **21**, 115–20.

52. Department of Education and Science (1981) *Care in Action: A Handbook of Policies and Priorities for the Health and Personal Social Services in England*, HMSO, London.

53. Royal College of General Practitioners (1981a) *Health and Prevention in Primary Care: Reports from General Practice*, RCGP, London.

54. Royal College of General Practitioners (1981b) *Prevention of Psychiatric Disorders in General Practice*, **20**, RCGP, London.

55. DHSS (1986) *Primary Health Care: An Agenda for Discussion*, HMSO, London.

56. DHSS (1987) *Neighbourhood Nursing – a Focus for Care: Report of the Community Nursing Review*, HMSO, London.

57. United Kingdom Central Council for Nursing, Midwifery and Health Visiting (1986) *Project 2000: A New Preparation for Practice*, UICC, London.

58. Government White Paper (1987) *Promoting Better Health; Government Programme for Improving Primary Health Care*, HMSO, London.

59. Department of Health and Social Security (1976a) *Prevention and Health: Everybody's Business*, HMSO, London.

60. Watt, A. (1986) Community Health Initiatives and their relationship to General Practice, *Journal of the Royal College of General Practitioners*, **36**, 72–3.

61. Bluck, M. E. (1975) *Public and Professional Opinions on Preventive Medicine* (unpublished), Tenovus Cancer Education Centre, Cardiff.

62. Calnan, M., Boulton, M. and Williams, A. (1986) Health education and General Practitioners: a critical appraisal, in: *The Politics of Health Education* (eds S. Rodmell and A. Watt) Routledge and Kegan Paul, London.

63. Boulton, M. and Williams, A. (1983) Health education in the general practice consultation: doctor's advice on diet, alcohol and smoking. *Health Education Journal*, **42**, 57–63.

64. Sullivan, D. (1988) Opportunistic health promotion: do patients like it? *Journal of the Royal College of General Practitioners*, **38**, 24–5.

65. Russell, M. A. H., Wilson, C., Taylor, C. and Baker, C. D. (1979) Effect of general practitioners' advice against smoking, *British Medical Journal*, **2**, 231–5.

66. Calnan, M. W. and Johnson, B. M. (1983) Influencing health behaviour: how significant is the general practitioner? *Health Education Journal*, **42**, 39–45.

67. Russell, M. A. H., Stapleton, J. A., Hajek, P. *et al.* (1988) District programme to reduce smoking: can sustained intervention by general practitioners affect prevalence? *Journal of Epidemiology and Community Health*, **42**, 111–15.

68. Bird, A., Cobb, J. and Walji, M. T. I. (1988) Increasing patient participation using an extended consultation: an inner city study. *Journal of the Royal College of General Practitioners*, **38**, 212–14.

69. American Hospital Association (1964) *Health Education: Role and Responsibilities of Health Care Institutions*, AHA, Chicago.

70. American Hospital Association (1972) *A Patients' Bill of Rights*, American Hospital Association, Chicago.

71. Blue Cross (1974) *White Paper on Patient Health Education*, Blue Cross Association, Chicago.
72. American Hospital Association (1981) *The Hospital's Responsibility for Patient Education Services*, AHA, Chicago.
73. Maryon Davis, A. (1984) Health Education in the Surgery. *Health Education Journal*, **43**, 4.
74. Ridgeway, V. and Mathews, A. (1982) Psychological preparation for surgery: a comparison of methods. *British Journal of Clinical Psychology*, **21**, 271–80.
75. Webb, C. (1985) *Sexuality, Nursing and Health*, John Wiley and Sons, Chichester.
76. Pack, B. E., Hendrick, R. M., Murdock, R. B. and Palma, L. M. (1983) Factors affecting criteria met by hospital based patient education programs, *Patient Education and Counseling*, **5**, 76–84.
77. Ozbolt Goodwin, J. (1979) Programmed instruction for self care following pulmonary surgery, *Int. J. Nurs. Stud.*, **16**, 29–40.
78. Bartlett, E. E. (1988) Which patient education strategies will pay off under prospective pricing? *Patient Education and Counseling*, **12**, 51–91.
79. Van den Borne, H. W., Pruyn, J. F. A. and Van den Heuvel, W. J. A. (1987) Effects of contacts between cancer patients on their psychosocial problems, *Patient Education and Counseling*, **9**, 33–51.
80. Parrinello, K. (1984) Patients' evaluation of a teaching booklet for arterial bypass surgery. *Patient Education and Counseling*, **4**, 183–9.
81. Mullen, P. D. and Zapka, J. G. (1981) *Health promotion and education*, in: *Services in HMO's*, US Public Health Service, Washington, DC.
82. Bartlett, E. E. (1985) Social consumption or social investment? *Patient Education and Counseling*, **7**, 223–5.
83. Close, A. (1988) Patient education: a literature review. *Journal of Advanced Nursing*, **13**, 203–13.
84. Bartlett, E. E. (1985) Forum: patient education: eight principles from patient education research. *Preventive Medicine*, **14**, 667–9.

6

THE MASS MEDIA
IN HEALTH PROMOTION

Nothing is easier than leading the people on a lesh. I just hold up a
dazzling campaign poster and they jump through it.

Joseph Goebbels, Director, Ministry for Popular
Enlightenment and Propaganda [1]

In this chapter, the mass media are viewed in the same strategic way as, for
instance, community development, patient education or the schools. Just as
the schools have particular characteristics and may thus make a qualitatively
different impact from, say, informal education in the community, mass media
have their peculiar strengths and weaknesses. Ideally they would be used as
part of a comprehensive programme which employs the range of strategies and
agencies described earlier in this book. All too frequently they have been used
in far from splendid isolation – either because the prospect of a fully
co-ordinated programme has been too daunting, or more likely because they
have been assumed to possess a power akin to that of a kind of educational
'magic bullet'. The view expressed at the head of this page is not unique to Dr
Goebbels!

It should by now be clear that to ask whether health education works is to ask
a meaningless question. This tenet certainly applies to the analysis of mass
communication campaigns – which, over the years, have been the cause of
much heated debate about effectiveness and efficiency. Rather than asking
whether mass media work, we should be asking what kind of effect we might
expect from different kinds of media used in different situations and contexts
to present different sorts of message about different subjects to different target
groups. We must also ask questions about both the intended and unintended
or incidental effects of mass media – and examine the extent to which such
effects should be taken into consideration or even deliberately manoeuvred as
a tool of health promotion.

We are faced with a complex picture and yet it is possible to provide valid
generalizations – both at the level of communication theory and at the more
pragmatic level of guidance for users. This chapter will, then, seek to
illuminate certain key issues in the use of mass media. It will examine the
peculiar features of the media and their different forms; it will consider the
incidental and unplanned effects of media; it will discuss the essential elements

of theories of mass communication and their pragmatic application in social marketing; it will ask what lessons might be learned about marketing health and will place particular emphasis on pre-testing. It will conclude with a sampler of health education programmes having a major mass media component, reinforcing the general – and perhaps stunningly obvious – point that a successful community programme incorporates mass media as a subsidiary but important element within the programme as a whole.

THE MEANING OF MASS MEDIA

As the words suggest, the two key features of mass media are their mass audience and the fact that there is no interpersonal communication between the originator of the message and the mass audience: the message is mediated. It is the mass audience which is so enticing to the communicator: it offers the seductive but illusory prospect of instant influence. As de Tocqueville [2] observed: '... nothing but a newspaper can drop the same thought into a thousand minds at the same moment'. Goebbels experienced a similar but more ambitious optimism for his propaganda ministry. With the advent of radio and television the possibility of wholesale change at national or even international level created joy in the minds of those seeking to manipulate population behaviours and alarm in the minds of those who wished to preserve the integrity of individual freedom to think and decide. However, although it is certainly possible to contact a mass audience, the second major characteristic of mass media makes it extremely unlikely that the population might be manipulated at the whim of the propagandist. In other words the fact that the message is mediated makes it impossible to gain immediate feedback of the results of the communication and thus provide a tailor-made communication which is responsive to the needs, personality and moods of the audience. As has so often been noted, the blunderbuss attributes of mass media are inconsistent with offering the 'different strokes for different folks' which are a component of an efficient influence process. Figure 6.1 makes this important point about feedback and reminds us of the difference between communication and education.

In interpersonal communication the communicator effectively codes a message for transmission to an audience (typically one person or a small group of people). The format of the message will most often be symbolic (e.g. written or spoken speech) but may be iconic – in which case pictures may be used to clarify the message. Alternatively, because it is considered likely to produce certain learned outcomes, an enactive format could be employed. This would require some form of audience participation to communicate the message and achieve the communicator's purpose. For example role play might be used to increase awareness of a social issue or to change audience attitudes. Non-verbal

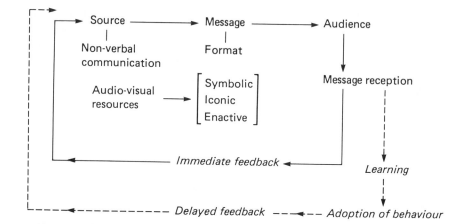

Figure 6.1 The communication process (derived from Tones [3]).

communication is an important component of the whole communication package.

It is of course apparent that mass media may simulate some of the features of this communication process – the presenter of a television programme may be specially chosen to be credible to the audience and may seek to ensure that his or her non-verbal communication is consonant with the programme goals. Again a variety of iconic messages may be used on television or other visual media. Some attempt may be made to achieve audience participation. However there is no way of knowing whether or not the audience has participated, has responded to the pictures or the charm of the presenter or whether, indeed, the audience has even understood the various messages let alone acted upon them. Although feedback may be provided for media producers – in the form of audience research, return of newspaper coupons, measures of population behaviour before and after programmes – there is no instant and observable response from the individuals comprising the audience. Audience phone-ins during radio programmes probably provide the closest approximation but the encounter is typically very short and excludes the majority of the listeners. Delayed feedback is no substitute for immediate feedback if anything other than the communication of relatively simple messages is to be achieved comprehensively and efficiently. Moreover immediate feedback not only allows the communicator to repeat, clarify and vary the message, it enables him or her to look for unwanted side-effects such as the arousal of excessive anxiety – a point of some ethical importance.

Most communication attempts are concerned to do more than ensure that the message has been correctly interpreted and understood. In reality their purpose is to generate some learned outcome – the acquisition of new information or understanding; a change in belief and attitude; the learning of a new skill and even the adoption of a new practice or change in lifestyle. It is usually acknowledged by media workers that there is a 'hierarchy of effects': it is relatively easy to 'agenda set' and communicate simple information; it is increasingly difficult to change attitudes, teach complex skills and persuade people to adopt new behaviours – especially where these involve exertion, discomfort or the abandoning of pleasure! The various intermediate indicators of programme success which were described in Chapter Three and the model underlying these relate to this communication dilemma for the mass media. In order to achieve the more difficult and often long-term outcomes, the requirements of immediate feedback and the personalizing of approaches make it difficult for mass media to compete with interpersonal education.

Before proceeding to clarify further the capabilities of different forms of media, we should note the distinction between mass media and the various media devices used as adjuncts to interpersonal communication and education. The film used as an audio-visual aid to a lecture or as a trigger for group discussion may appear superficially similar to a mass media television programme. In effect the film is a learning resource which is part of the iconic and enactive format of the communication; it is directly controlled by the communicator without loss of the important feedback principle. A good example of such use is provided by the work of Evans and McAlister based on McGuire's inoculation theory [4, 5, 6]. These studies utilized film or video as part of a programme designed to inoculate young people against social pressures to smoke. By and large, film was effective in producing behavioural outcomes only when accompanied by other techniques such as peer-led teaching and structured role play. McAlister *et al.* [7] were able to claim that students receiving this media-aided interpersonal teaching were recruited to smoking at less than half the rate of controls not receiving the programme. Similar results using lifeskills training in the field of substance misuse provide evidence of the importance of interpersonal education in the problematic arena of persuading the young '... to eschew deeply satisfying activities which are validated by peer and other social pressures'. The effectiveness of mass media-based smoking programmes should be judged against this alternative – or rather complementary – approach [8].

It is interesting in this general context to consider the special case of programmed learning. At first glance a programmed text or programme designed for use in audio-visual form would appear to have characteristics of both a resource to be used as part of interpersonal education and at the same time share some of the features of mass media. A programme could, for instance, be used totally outside the interpersonal encounter – either on a self-access, student-centred basis or through mass distribution as a book. Since properly validated programmes are highly efficient teaching devices, this would appear to give the lie to earlier assertions about the limitations of mass media. The fact is, of course, that a programmed text or related device has (i) been designed for a specific audience (cf. the notion of market segmentation below) and (ii), through the proper process of validation and standardization, it incorporates the principle of immediate feedback in its construction (providing the student with 'IKR' – immediate knowledge of results). The dissemination of such programmes with their intrinsic capacity to interact with the audience might well combine the advantages of interpersonal education with the attractions of reaching a mass audience. The implications for open learning and distance learning are self-evident although a discussion of these is beyond the scope of this book. Reference to this tactic does, however, remind us of the heterogeneous nature of mass media – a fact we must consider before seeking to make generalizations.

MEDIA VARIETIES

It is apparent that mass media vary considerably in their potential and capabilities – despite the common characteristics discussed above. They differ in form and format: leaflets and posters are substantially different from the electronic media of television and radio. They differ in their potential for reaching audiences and in the nature of the audience they reach: local radio listeners have different characteristics from readers of quality national press; in the UK Open University and Channel Four documentaries will appeal to viewers who may not be addicted to soap opera. They differ in their credibility and trustworthiness. Fuglesang [9] offered a salutory reminder that modern media technology is relevant only to about 20% of the world population who can read and write and have access to electronic media. Folk media using, for example, puppets and the oral tradition of proverb and storytelling, replace the technology and mass audience of western society. However the focus of this book is on developed countries and three examples will illustrate the different potential of various forms of media.

The first example illustrates the superiority of cinema advertising compared with what many would regard as the most powerful medium – television. Douglas [10], in a guide to advertising, reminds us that cinema not only offers higher quality sound and image definition than television but also differs in audience composition and involvement (in addition to the fact that it is possible to advertise 'illicit' products in the cinema which it is not possible to present on television – at least in many countries.) Douglas cites Marplan research which compared recall of a hitherto unknown product after exposure to cinema and television advertising. Young women who had seen the commercials were interviewed on the following day. Recall of the main point of the commercial by the cinema audience was 26% compared with 9% by the television audience. In the context of discussion about what we might expect from media exposure, it is interesting to note that spontaneous recall was only 2% for the television audience (but 8% for the cinema audience). Recall after prompting went up a further 36% for television audiences compared with 56% for cinema audiences. Douglas ascribed this superiority to the greater impact produced by screen size, better sound and image quality and absence of distractions.

The second example offers evidence of the kind of result which might be expected from one of the trusty stock-in-trade media devices of the health promoter – the exhibition. Research carried out by the Transport and Road Research Laboratory (TRRL) in 1970 [11] recorded numbers of people attending road safety exhibitions, audience characteristics and their source of information about the exhibition, their progress round the exhibition and the time spent at each exhibit or display. The TRRL adduced the following principles:

1. Attendance at even the best road safety exhibitions is unlikely to exceed 1000 per day. It is often much less than this. The prospects of getting at... (major target group)... are therefore extremely poor.
2. Local press publicity can increase the attendance by at least 50%.
3. The audience at exhibitions appears to be a broad cross section of the population ... it has not been possible to find whether they ... are in most need of propaganda.
4. When going round exhibitions visitors tend to spend very short times at exhibits. The average time spent at many exhibits is less than one minute. None of the visitors see all the exhibits, many see less than half. Animated exhibits attract a lot of attention, but often distract visitors from the static displays.

The third example concerns credibility. It is an axiom of attitude theory that beliefs and attitudes are unlikely to change if the source of the communication is perceived to be untrustworthy, lack expertise or other forms of authority. A similar point is made in Communication of Innovations Theory by the principle of homophily. It is therefore interesting to ask whether different forms of mass media are more acceptable than others and whether these are more or less credible than alternative forms of interpersonal communication. Budd and McCron [12] interviewed 692 adults from Central England and, among other things, invited them to indicate how far they would trust information about changing one's life for the sake of one's health derived from each of 12 sources. These sources included medical personnel, lay people and media. The family doctor received the highest rating (an average score of 3.51 on a four point scale). The four lowest ratings (1.8, 1.72, 1.69 and 1.68 respectively) were accorded to a magazine article, television advert, newspaper article and, last of all, a friend or neighbour. Radio and television documentaries scored at an intermediate level (2.43; 2.39) but were boosted by having doctor involvement! Even the humble poster was rated third most credible when displayed in a GP's surgery or waiting room.

A more recent study [13] makes a related point. However, while television advertising – especially about health – was treated with scepticism and mistrust, women's magazines and certain television personalities were often considered more credible than some health professionals – at any rate on the subject of feeding a family.

INCIDENTAL AND PLANNED EFFECTS OF MEDIA

Before considering what the generalizations from Mass Communication Theory have to offer for health education practice, we must note a further dimension to the classification of mass media effects. Whereas the main concern of health education is the development of programmes deliberately designed to influence audience characteristics, it is important to recognize that mass media may well have incidental and often unpredicted effects. Rather like the hidden curriculum in the school setting, these incidental effects may have to be taken into account as possibly unhealthy pressures or canalized in the interests of health promotion.

The fact that mass media can have a dramatic and unforseen impact has been fully recognized since Cantril [14] documented the sizeable panic produced among the citizenry by Orson Welles' production of H. G. Wells' *War of the Worlds* in the 1930s. Less dramatic but more insidious is the way in which press and television report health issues. Even the recording of cancer cure is likely to be couched in terms which reinforce the general alarm and pessimism conjured up by the very term. Wellings [15] makes a similar point about the public's processing of media reporting of the 1983 'pill scare'. Draper and his colleagues made related points about the ways in which the very grammar of television reporting tends to introduce bias which, for example, favours the supremacy of high technology medicine at the expense of the less glamorous but potentially more beneficial preventive and health promotion measures [16].

Again the incidental presentation of health issues in entertainment programmes and soap opera may foster misleading images and attitudes. Characterization may serve to validate images of unhealthy lifestyles as part of a norm-sending process. The portrayal of alcohol on television conveys a norm of heavy drinking and associates comsumption of alcohol with benefits rather than costs [17, 18].

The impact of advertising unhealthy products is a highly contentious political issue. Advocates of advertising, not unsurprisingly, stress its social benefits and minimize the negative effect on recruitment [19]. The effect of cigarette promotions on children has been the subject of recent research [20, 21, 22, 23]. Although it is not yet possible to demonstrate unequivocally that there is a causal relationship between advertising, sponsorship and smoking recruitment, it seems likely that children who smoke are generally more aware of cigarette advertising and sponsorship than non-smokers and more favourably disposed to the brands. What is clear is that such advertising and sponsorship establishes a hidden curriculum which legitimizes smoking and denotes its continuing acceptability.

We will now, however, turn to the deliberate use of mass media to produce desired learning outcomes – focusing particularly on their potential for producing behaviour change and the adoption of approved practices.

MASS COMMUNICATION THEORY

An analysis of research and theory into the effects of mass media suggests a shift in opinion over the years from an apparently magical belief in their omnipotence (fostered perhaps by a mixture of Dr Goebbels and Vance Packard) to an almost totally opposite assertion that mass media will not produce any significant changes in actual behaviour – especially in the difficult domain of health. A more cautiously optimistic view is currently prevalent. Day in a foreword to Douglas [10] describes colourfully the emotion generated by the debate about the effectiveness of media advertising:

> Advertising has always been wreathed in metaphysical mists. From the time of the first medicine-man selling snake oil from the back of the stagecoach, to the self-induced hypnosis created by so-called 'subliminal' advertising, to the about-to-be wonders of global commercials via satellite, there has always been a need on the part of some people, at least, to believe in the talismanic properties of advertising and its supposed power to 'manipulate' its audience.

Day adds, 'I have yet to see the evidence that advertising unsupported by product performance has ever had more than a temporary effect in persuading anyone to do anything against their own best interests'.

This view is consistent with the orthodoxy which came to replace the early 'direct effects' or 'hypodermic' models of media influence. According to the latter the community presented itself as a compliant patient for its injection. If the injection did not work either a different medicine was called for or a larger dose! The influence of Katz and Lazarsfeld [24] and Lazarsfeld and Merton [25] led to a kind of 'null effects' model in which mass media were considered to have a minimal impact. Katz and Lazarsfeld proposed their two-step hypothesis of influence according to which of the adoption of behaviours by a social group or community resulted from interpersonal interaction with opinion leaders who were (i) more receptive of media information than the mass of people, and (ii) were sought out for advice by the community and were thus relatively influential. Lazarsfeld and Merton further argued that mass media would not induce change unless one or more conditions were met: 'monopolization', i.e. where there are no contrary influences and messages;

'canalization', i.e. where a particular message or recommendation for action plugs into existing motivations and preferences; and 'supplementation', i.e. where interpersonal efforts supplement media-based messages. Klapper's influential [26] review consolidated this general view of media limitations. Reinforcement rather than conversion was the prime role of the media:

> Within a given audience exposed to particular communications, reinforcement, or at least constancy of opinion, is typically found to be the dominant effect (of mass media), minor change as in intensity of opinion is found to be the next most common; and conversion is typically found to be the most rare (p. 15). (Cited by Wallach [27]).

Mendelsohn's [28] conceptualization of mass media replaces the image of the hypodermic with that of an aerosol:

> Rather than being a hypodermic needle, we now begin to look at mass communication as a sort of aerosol spray. As you spray it on the surface, some of it hits the target: most of it drifts away; and very little of it penetrates.

It is worth noting in passing that Mendelsohn does acknowledge the possibility that at least some of the message hits the target even though presumably very little actually results in desired behaviour change.

The audience has, so far, been represented as a relatively passive entity which is more or less difficult to influence – depending on whether it is the hypodermic or the aerosol which is wielded. It is however misleading to consider the recipients of the message as either undifferentiated or passive. As was noted in an earlier chapter, Communication of Innovations Theory classifies the community into categories in accordance with their relative openness to change. This analysis is useful in that it not only views the audience as a heterogeneous group but also relates readiness to adopt innovations to the perceived characteristics of the new idea or practice – and the likely costs or benefits which might result from adoption. In other words the recipients of mass media messages neither passively accept nor reject the influence but rather analyse and interpret it in an active fashion – typically in the context of interpersonal interactions with family or friends. Mendelsohn [29] makes a distinction between 'Homo mechanicus' and 'Homo volens', the latter being an '... active organism who often seeks out useable information – the dynamic individual who uses only that information he or she needs from the media while disregarding the useless stuff'.

This latter approach has elsewhere been referred to as a uses and gratifications model, suggesting as it does that the active recipient of media messages selects from those messages what (s)he needs to gratify current motivation. As Dorn and South [30] have pointed out, this interpretation is very acceptable to the promoters of unhealthy products since it denies accusations of manipulation of a naïve and gullible public! They also note how this conflicts with both right and left wing theories of media manipulating the populace. Right wing mass manipulative models view people as being often naïve and feckless and therefore corruptible by unhealthy media influences. Left wing theories view the mass of people as being subjected to control by a capitalist elite which uses its ownership of media to exploit its audience.

Budd and McCron [12] emphasize that mass media influences cannot and should not be isolated from a social context in which they '... interact and sometimes compete with, other sources of information and influences in complex ways, and that the individual selects, and compares from these diverse sources to construe a meaningful explanation for himself about particular issues which may, or may not, be in line with the intention behind any or all of the sources of information available to him'. The social context can also be interpreted in terms of what Dorn and South [30] refer to as a 'consensual paradigm', i.e. media collude with and encapsulate, in cliché and stereotype, social norms – exemplified earlier by reference to the norm-sending role of soap opera and news reporting. Dorn [31] further draws our attention to his preferred class–cultural model which urges health educators to take account of the subcultural constructions of meaning of, for example, different social classes and ethnic groups. Ball-Rokeach and De Fleur [32] propose a dependency model involving a tri-partite relationship between media, audience and society. An interesting implication of this theory is that '... when people's social realities are entirely adequate ... media messages may have little or no alteration effects... In contrast, when people do not have social realities that provide adequate frameworks for understanding, acting and escaping, and when audiences are dependent in these ways on media information received, such messages may have a number of alteration effects'.

It should by now be clear that it is not enough to say that mass media can or cannot readily influence audience behaviour. It is also apparent that the media influence process is a complex one. One simple fact can however be stated: in normal circumstances, mass media will not easily change people's behaviour unless individual motivation and normative influences are favourable. McKinlay's lament [33] on the failure of mass media to promote health is eminently explicable when this simple fact is taken into account.

How embarrassingly ineffective are our mass media efforts in the health field (e.g. alcoholism, obesity, drug abuse, safe driving, pollution, etc.) when compared with many of the tax-exempt promotional efforts on behalf of the illness generating activities of large-scale corporations. It is a fact that we are demonstrably more effective in persuading people to purchase items they never dreamed they would need, or to pursue at risk courses of action, than we are in preventing or halting such behaviour.

The comparison which McKinlay makes between commercial advertising and health marketing is particularly apposite at a time when health educators are urged to learn from the superior expertise of commerce and adopt the social marketing approach. The relevance of social marketing will therefore now be considered. In particular it should be possible to see how recommended approaches articulate with communication theory as discussed above. Moreover if we are to make sound judgements about the evaluation of mass media in health promotion, we should understand the kinds of expectations of success inherent in social marketing as well as noting the rules pertaining to efficient management of educational interventions using media.

HEALTH EDUCATION AS SOCIAL MARKETING

Marsden and Peterfreund [34] argued that adoption of marketing principles would provide public health departments with a guide and incentive to help them '... shed a bureaucratic tradition and a lacklustre image which compromises their ability to provide services and to function as authoritative sources of health information'. Others, who have perhaps interpreted health promotion rather narrowly as a profile-raising excursion into energetic media-backed publicity, look to commerce for tips on how to sell health (see for instance Docherty [35]; Player [36]). However, Bonaguro and Miaoulis [37] outlined a marketing approach to Green's well-known PRECEDE* model asserting that the goals of marketing and health promotion are similar. Since one of the major aims of this chapter is to examine what kinds of success we might realistically expect from mass media-based health education, it is clearly important to look critically at these claims for the social marketing approach. Do we have a new panacea – or, more modestly, what insights can we gain from the best commercial practice for the marketing of health?

First of all, we should note that the notion of health marketing is not that recent a discovery. In 1977 Lovelock [38] commented on the value of marketing concepts and strategies for health marketers. He also referred the reader to earlier work by Kotler [39] and Zaltman *et al.* [40]. More recently, Solomon [41] identified ten key marketing concepts having relevance for health promotion through public communication campaigns:

1. The marketing philosophy;
2. The 'four Ps' of marketing;
3. Hierarchies of communication effects;
4. Audience segmentation;
5. Understanding all the relevant markets;

* For details of this, the reader is referred to Green, L. W., Kreuter, M. W., Deeds, S. G. and Partridge, K. B. (1980) *Health Education Planning: A diagnostic approach.* Mayfield, Palo Alto, California.

6. Information and rapid feedback systems;
7. Interpersonal amd mass communication interactions;
8. Utilization of commercial resources;
9. Understanding the competition;
10. Expectations of success.

These ten concepts will serve as a basis for discussing what we might learn from commercial approaches to marketing but in order to assess their relevance we should be in no doubt about the fundamental differences between the selling of commercial products and the selling of health.

As McCron and Budd [42] have pointed out, the question of advertising effectiveness is shrouded in myth yet the popular view is not only that advertising is powerful but it must work because businesses spend so much money on it. It is, in fact, salutory to note the difference in expectations of success between businesses and those who look for quick results from health education! This is, however, only one of the distinctions between the commercial and public domains. These differences may be summarized as follows:

1. There is clearly a considerable difference in the size of budgets typically available to commercial and public domain communicators.
2. Commercial advertisers would normally set much lower standards for success than those commissioning health education programmes. Whereas the latter would often expect evidence of behaviour change – preferably dramatic – the former would have much lower ambitions and might not expect any change in, for example, sales at all. During the late 1970s a well known chain of bakers spent some £300 000 on ten television commercials. These were thought to have been a great triumph even though there had been no increase in volume sales. The firm was content to maintain their market in the context of a general rise in bread consumption! (Reported in *Daily Mail*, 13 February, 1980).
3. A more important distinction between the marketing of health and commercial products is the fundamental difference in the nature of the products on offer. The commercial product offers the customer gratification of some existing need; if the customer does not like the product, the manufacturer will produce something he or she does like – or will change its image. The highly successful campaign to sell the chocolate bar 'Yorkie' was in the last analysis based on people's liking for chocolate. The campaign's success lay in appropriate manipulation of brand image to appeal to psychological needs other than the taste gratification. By contrast health education is frequently trying to sell a product which commercial advertisers would consider no-one in their right mind would buy! Potential customers are not uncommonly urged to stop doing something they find enjoyable and start doing something unpleasant or difficult. Playing with

brand imagery is of course possible (as we will note in the section on pre-testing) but this involves the adding of 'psychographic icing' to an often rather unpalatable cake.

What is more, the product which is being promoted by health education is frequently intangible and offers gratification at some indeterminate time in the (often distant) future. This almost exactly reverses the pattern of commercial sales technique which promises immediate gratification – often on credit.

4. A further important distinction concerns ethical considerations. While commercial advertising is now constrained to avoid blatant lying, it is by its very nature economical with the truth. Education, by definition, should be concerned with helping people make informed decisions (although there are proponents of a persuasive prevention model who are eager to use advertising techniques to manipulate and coerce). Again health education should be concerned with avoiding unwanted side-effects – such as anxiety or unresolved dissonance. Commercial advertising is also concerned to avoid negative images and connotations which are likely to have an immediate impact on sales figures. However it is much easier to do this since the basic message is invariably positive: our product will meet your needs and make you feel good. Again, health education cannot, ethically, make a decision to ignore or abandon the equivalent of an unprofitable market. Indeed disadvantaged groups and other resistants to the sales talk often form the main market.

5. Finally, because commercial advertising can rely on the pre-existence of audience motivation, the change in the audience which it seeks to produce is often limited to brand awareness and the creation of a positive attitude to the particular product. The behavioural response is relatively simple – the purchase of a product which in all probability differs from previously purchased products only in its packaging – physical or psychological. Health education seeks to change deeply seated attitudes and even values and sometimes to produce the adoption of often complex behaviours.

The very real differences between the marketing of health and commerical products should, however, not blind us to the lessons to be learned from good commercial marketing practice. Indeed perhaps the most important lesson is that the products on sale are very different! We will use Solomon's ten-point analysis as a basis for the discussion.

1. Market Philosophy

The first point worthy of note has to do with the concept of 'market philosophy' which is based on the idea of 'exchange', i.e. that there should be equity between marketer and consumer: the prime goal is to meet consumer needs (real or imagined); the customer is always right! As Marsden and

Peterfreund [34] reminded us, the cavalier presentation of health services would make the commercial marketer blush. Apart from the obvious need (in the words of the Ottawa Conference) to re-orient health services, the way in which some health educators patronize their clients can be counter-productive. Mendelsohn [29] makes the point very forcibly:

> Among the 'needs' we all have is not to be bombarded with information we already have or do not have any use for (e.g. information asserting that excessive drinking may be bad for us); not to be commanded to do something that is vague and unachievable without explicit simple instructions regarding its achievement (e.g. 'drive carefully'); not to be unreasonably frightened (e.g. any drinking during pregnancy, no matter how moderate, will surely result in the birth of a monster); and not to be insulted by the health communicator who implies that every one the communicator is trying to address is (1) ignorant... (2)... sinfully 'irresponsible' in that they don't give a damn about their own lives/or the lives of others; and (3) they are slothfully 'apathetic' in not immediately doing without question what the communicator commands them to do.

An important question concerns the definition of consumer 'needs'. As we will see, community development urges us to base our programmes on 'felt needs'; frequently these needs do not match the epidemiological reality and require a complex negotiation with the client group which is beyond the scope of mass media.

2. Four P's – Product, Price, Place, Promotion

Solomon's second point was concerned with the four P's, namely product, price, place and promotion – what others have called the 'marketing mix'. There are clear messages for the health educator: the (health) product should be tangible, attractive and accessible. While some health promotions meet all three of these criteria, many others are unnecessarily vague. For example, the sale of condoms or wholemeal bread involves tangible products which are relatively accessible and which may be attractively packaged, but general messages to 'take more exercise' or 'look after yourself' are less tangible and, for a majority of people, inaccessible and downright unattractive. The relative lack of attractiveness of the product has already been noted but the notion of accessibility is of interest. While there may be an element of physical accessibility in health promotions (e.g. access to clinic; availability of healthy food) the question of psychological accessibility may be overlooked. It is clear that many people wish to adopt a healthier lifestyle but lack skills and support to do so. The lack of these facilities effectively renders the desired change inaccessible (see Health Action Model, Chapter Three).

The matter of price is self-evident. In health promotion the cost is more likely to be psycho–social than financial. It is only necessary to remind the reader of the central part which the notion of costs and barriers plays in the Health Belief Model (discussed in Chapter Three).

Place and promotion may be considered together. Place emphasizes the importance of distribution of the goods and retail outlets. Promotion reminds us that advertising is only one element of the marketing mix. The relevance of both of these will be taken up later when we consider the seventh of the ten points.

3. Hierarchy of Communication Effects

The third concept refers to the 'hierarchy of communication effects'. This describes the importance of recognizing what was called in Chapter Three the causal chain between input and output. Commercial marketing acknowledges that success becomes increasingly difficult to achieve as we move from measures of simple market penetration to behaviour change. McGuire (43) comments on this 'distal measure fallacy' and points out nicely the different criteria of success used by the public and commercial sectors:

> All too often the communicator evaluates the campaign or its component parts in terms of a response step early in the chain, quite distant from the later step (no. 10) that actually constitutes the criterion of success. The public communication campaigner should look with horror upon the practice in the commercial advertising industry of buying 50 billion dollars' worth of time and space each year solely on the Step 1 (exposure) criterion of Neilsen ratings or circulation figures as if all that counts is reaching the public.

Despite McGuire's objection and for reasons stated earlier, because of pre-existing motivations of the public, market penetration may be all that is necessary to sell products.

4. Audience Segmentation

The fourth concept is that of audience segmentation. It is concerned with the idea of market aggregation and argues that media campaigns will be more effective insofar as they can move towards disaggregation. In other words if messages and channels can be devised which appeal to different homogeneous sub-sets of the population, more effective and efficient results will be achieved. It is worth observing in passing that interpersonal communication is based on what would be called total market disaggregation, i.e. the condition achieved by interpersonal approaches which supply 'different strokes for different folks'.

The criteria for segmentation range from the cruder geographic and demographic variables – e.g. targeting lower social class groups via popular press – to more sophisticated measures of personality (sometimes referred to in advertising parlance as 'psychographics'). Stein [44] ascribed part of the success of a cancer information service to its targeting of four groups: smokers who want to quit, persons over 50, cancer patients and their families, and blacks. Mendelsohn [45] described an effective crime prevention campaign which found it impossible to refine its message delivery to reach specific groups. Nonetheless the blunderbuss approach adopted appeared to work but produced different effects in different segments of the audience. For instance in relation to demographic variables, affluent people (at proportionately lower risk) made greater gains in intention to engage in neighbourhood crime prevention activity than did the higher risk less affluent groups. On the other hand lower income groups showed a greater readiness to report suspicious looking people to the police. In respect of psychographic criteria, the campaign appeared to have resulted in greater overall levels of preventive competence among those who initially believed themselves to be relatively less able to safeguard themselves and their property. The attitudes of those perceiving themselves initially to be less at risk of crime were more likely to have been influenced by the campaign that those perceiving themselves to be more vulnerable. The latter group, however, were more likely to act and follow the specific crime reduction recommendations made by the programme. Lavigne *et al.* [46] viewed market segmentation as a central feature of their APPLAUSE Project (Appropriate public presentations for learning about alcohol and other drugs using segmentation effects). This illustrates particularly well how pre-testing of population groups and individuals forms an integral part of programme planning. Lavigne *et al.* subdivided their market segment of parents into two further high and low risk groups and listed demographic and psychographic characteristics. For instance, the high risk group were more likely to be blue collar and male, having negative attitudes to legal and social controls over alcohol use and being less likely to believe that parents influence their children's behaviour. They were also more likely to engage in risky drinking behaviours and to have experienced health and social consequences of drinking. This segmentation allowed the project team to develop strategies designed to take account of these inter-group differences. Apart from the self-evident value of identifying and pre-testing key market segments, perhaps the main principle to be extracted from the points made above is the difficulty faced by mass media in achieving precisely tailored programmes; such fine tuning must be left to interpersonal interactions.

5. Market Understanding

The fifth of Solomon's recommendations is to understand the market. In effect this is an injunction to recognize the existence of secondary markets which might facilitate or inhibit access to and the success of programmes in influencing the primary target groups. On a simple level we might invite media workers to 'look for the gatekeeper'. If a programme depends on the display of posters in clinics and the nurse or doctor in charge is upset by the poster presentation no amount of pre-testing on the target group will prevent disappointment. The poster will not be displayed!

6. Feedback

Solomon's sixth recommendation concerns the evaluation process. In short he urges that each programme, in addition to summative evaluation, should incorporate formative/process evaluation to allow the programme to be modified through the provision of rapid feedback of results.

7. Interpersonal and Mass Communication Interaction

His seventh point centres on the interaction of interpersonal and mass communication. It is virtually axiomatic that mass communication may be enhanced by interpersonal education. Commercial practice has recognized this guiding principle in its firm separation of advertising from the broader promotion/marketing function and, more specifically, in its recognition of the importance of the retail outlet in influencing customer purchasing patterns.

8. Commercial Resources

Here, Solomon makes the point that those marketing health should utilize commercial resources where possible. There is readily available commercial expertise (e.g. market research firms) which may have greater expertise than, say, a small health education department. The firm (suggests Solomon) may even provide their services at discount rate or even for nothing – in order to improve their own brand image!

9. Competition

When marketing health, it is essential to understand the competition – and produce a better product! The competition for health education consists primarily of the anti-health lobby and its political supporters. One of the most interesting recent attempts to learn from this maxim is described by Chesterfield-Evans and O'Connor [47] who report on the Australian BUGAP campaign (Billboard utilizing graffitists against unhealthy promotions). Chapman's [48] 'Lung Goodbye' offers the would-be subversive a handy set of tactics to combat the powerful Goliath of the tobacco industry.

10. Expectations

In planning a campaign, it is necessary to formulate realistic targets, and not be cajoled into colluding with unrealistic expectations of success.

THE LESSONS OF SOCIAL MARKETING
AND MASS COMMUNICATION THEORY

Having reviewed social marketing theory's recommendations for success and noted the extent to which this is compatible with the different orientation of health education, we should now be in a position to relate this review to general mass communication theory and ask what we might legitimately expect from mass media in health promotion. We should, therefore, note the complexity of interpersonal communication and the learning process and limit our expectations. We should note the particularly difficult task of selling health and curtail our expectation of success even further. Mass media will not normally be able to achieve certain health education goals:

1. They will not convey complex messages and create understanding of the often complicated issues related to health and disease – such as the interplay of risk factors in coronary heart disease.
2. They will not readily teach complex motor or social interaction skills – such as breast self-examination or the capacity to deal assertively with interpersonal pressures.
3. They will not produce attitude change in resistants nor will they provide the support necessary for motivated individuals who wish to change their behaviour in adverse physical and social circumstances.

On the other hand mass media will deliver simple messages and, where people are already motivated, this may trigger often dramatic changes in behaviour. Provided that audience penetration can be achieved (the simplest measure of media effectiveness), mass media can be stunningly successful in their agenda-setting function. As has been frequently noted, it is difficult to tell people what to think but very much easier to tell them what to think about. Unfortunately this powerful agenda-setting function which is so very relevant to the radical, critical consciousness raising role described in Chapter One cannot be used on the powerful medium of television because of its political unpalatability.

Mass media will, clearly, only achieve their potential if programmes are constructed in accordance with good communication practice – many of which have been discussed in the context of social marketing. It is worth adding that good communication practice will also take account of the models described in Chapter Three and utilize the well accepted principles of attitude theory. The communication model at the beginning of this chapter provides a framework which has been fully elaborated by McGuire [4], Albert [49] and Flay [50] – all of whom provide analyses based on the Hovland-Yale model which emphasizes *inter alia* the importance of source and message factors in achieving attitude change.

Two other broad recommendations may be made. The first of these has to do with Solomon's observations (point seven in his list) about the interaction of media communication and interpersonal communication. This offers the generalization that mass media will be more effective in achieving goals other than agenda-setting the more they manage to enlist interpersonal support (and thus lose their media-like characteristics). This is of course integral to the use of educational media – such as Open University – which attempt to create viewing groups to offer mutual support and to enlist the interpersonal and pedagogical skills of local tutors.

This generalization, as we have seen, is a major tenet of Communication of Innovations Theory and the two-step hypothesis discussed earlier in this chapter. Chaffee [51], in an interesting analysis of political campaigns, makes a similar point. He argues that about one fifth of a community pay little attention to politics; one third are politically active communicators but about one half of the total population follow politics in a relatively passive fashion via the media and '.. are moved to interpersonal discussion only on the occasion of a highly salient, unanticipated, or ambiguous political event'. It is this interpersonal discussion which influences political attitudes. Chaffee supports this view with the observation that watching the Watergate hearings on television was less important than discussing them in accounting for any changes in political attitude. He goes on to make a point of especial relevance for our understanding of the potential of mass media for influencing attitude and behaviour. Media are most effective on their own when there is (i) low audience involvement in the matter under discussion, (ii) there is little difference in available choices and (iii) the message is unopposed.

Liu [52] provides an intriguing examination of mass campaigns in communist China and reminds us that the Chinese have always stressed the importance of training activists to support their mass media campaigns. Flay *et al.* [53,54] discusses the synergy of media and interpersonal education from the opposite perspective and shows how media in the form of television programmes can boost the effect of school-based education – and trigger further interpersonal influence in the form of parental involvement.

The second recommendation for effective media practice seeks to underline the importance of pre-testing of health education programmes. Although this is related to the notion of audience segmentation, pre-testing received little prominence in Solomon's discussion. It will receive much greater emphasis here not merely because of its importance as part of effective practice but because of the way in which it illuminates the process of evaluation generally and the importance of the various intermediate indicators discussed in Chapter Three.

PRE-TESTING THE PROGRAMME

Pre-testing must form part of any well-designed health education programme. It is also an integral part of the process of evaluation. Two main pre-testing goals may be distinguished: the first is to pre-test relevant characteristics of the target population, the second is to pre-test the programme and its component parts.

The first form of pre-testing has already been mentioned in the discussion of audience segmentation. Its purpose is two-fold. Relevant population or target group measures indicate those group and individual characteristics which the programme designers must take into consideration if they are to meet consumer needs and foster effective learning. They also serve as a baseline or yardstick against which the programme's success may be judged through the application of post-tests as part of the normal function of summative evaluation. The data provided can then be fed back into the system to enhance future similar activities. Formative process evaluation is, as indicated in Chapter Two, an integral part of effective programme development and such formative research is also central to the pre-testing of messages and general programme content.

Palmer [55] provides an excellent example of audience pre-testing in formative research in his description of the development of the Children's Television Workshop Health Minutes programme – a series of minute-long presentations on health topics. Pre-testing focused on 10 measures: (i) individual needs and values (to which programmes could appeal as part of the 'canalization' process), (ii) barriers to health behaviours, (iii) family members' involvement in health decisions, (iv) prior improvements in lifestyle (seeking to associate new health behaviours with prior health promoting decisions), (v) subject matter explorations (previous relevant knowledge or ignorance), (vi) knowledge of symptoms, (vii) health lexicon (in order to devise an appropriate vocabulary for hispanic speakers), (viii) prior influence of television and radio (impact of earlier programmes on health behaviours), (ix) inventory of household medications, and (x) parents' perceptions of themselves as child trainers.

Clearly the measures of individual characteristics and their immediate socio-environmental situations will depend on programme purposes and may be defined in various ways – technical or non-technical. Romano [56] describes research into smoker characteristics using focus group interviews which resulted in the development of four psychographic profiles. These were 'The Fatalists; the Diligent; the Avoiders; and the Oblivious'! Subsequently programme materials were developed to take account of these different personality types.

Turning now to the pre-testing of programmes rather than potential audiences, Romano [57], in one of the most useful guides available on the subject, has identified two major stages: concept development and message execution. The first of these is concerned with the evolution of potential messages and associated rough artwork – often in the form of animatics. These are devised initially as a result of a priori decisions about their likelihood of achieving programme goals. The tentative messages are then pre-tested on a representative sample of the target group [58]. Leathar [59] provides a classic example of the way in which a message had to be modified in response to evidence of misperception after pre-testing. He describes the reactions to an anti-smoking poster developed to remind people of the link between smoking and ill health. The setting was a graveyard; the cigarette was represented symbolically as a tombstone. A line of copy at the bottom of the picture asked the rhetorical question 'Why do you think every packet carries a government health warning?'. Although the original version received several awards from professional advertisers, it was misperceived by the primary target group, smokers. This example of selective perception and defensive avoidance is described by Leathar as follows:

> Smokers, on the other hand, saw things somewhat differently. In general, they showed a high level of psychological defensiveness towards the entire advert. Initially, they claimed to see the cigarette as a variety of unrelated objects: a stick of rock, lipstick, even a telegraph pole. Furthermore, they superficially assumed the bottom line simply to be the conventional Government Health Warning itself, thus failing to see it as a statement relating the visual material to the warning. They thus not only misperceived the symbolic visual presentation of the cigarette tombstone, but saw little, if any, relationship between this and the factual copy line which was intended to be the main theme of the advertisement. This confusion was further compounded by the image presented. Like non-smokers, smokers attributed a certain 'lightness' to the impression created, but this was attractive and pleasant and in no way symbolic of ill-health. It reminded them of pleasant and rather idyllic country scenes, of bluebells and daffodils and pretty girls; of sunshine and ploughmen's lunches in 'nice' country pubs.

The scene was subsequently restructured as a result of the pre-testing in order to provide a rather more funereal impression and the line 'Ashes to ashes' was introduced as a symbolic link.

One of pre-testing's major functions is to develop messages and programmes tailored to a given market segment. In commenting on the irrelevance of many messages for lower social class groups, Player and Leathar [60] underlined the importance of providing socially sensitive advertising. They challenged the advice given to those requiring support in coping with the withdrawal symptoms following attempts to give up smoking – advice such as 'suck a clove', 'doodle with a paper clip' or 'start a new social activity'! In order to avoid such middle-class bias at the concept development stage, Leathar [59] used a projective technique to determine target group reactions to the packaging of two alternative forms of booklet offering advice on how to stop smoking. Working-class respondents showed a clear preference for one of the two covers when asked to describe the 'personality' which each of the covers conveyed to them. The preferred cover was associated with a person who drank in typical pubs, was open and friendly and could be relied upon to lend money and help you out. In the words of Communication of Innovations Theory, the most attractive cover was more homophilous. In advertising parlance the preferred booklet had a better brand image.

The techniques and instruments used in pre-testing are, of course, not fundamentally different from those used in evaluating health education programmes generally. The various indicators of success listed in Table 3.2 could equally be applied to pre-testing and it is not difficult, for instance, to relate these to the standard pre-testing questions developed by the US Office of Cancer Communications Health Message Testing Service [58]. Table 6.1 is

Table 6.1 Guidelines for interpreting responses to standard pre-testing questions (from Romano, 1984 [58])

	High score range (%)	*Average* score range (%)	*Low* score range (%)
Attention/recall (Percent remembering seeing message after one exposure)	41 or higher	30–40	29 or lower
Main idea (Percent remembering main idea of message after one exposure)	36 or higher	25–35	24 or lower
Worth remembering (Percent indicating 'yes')	76 or higher	60–75	59 or lower
Personally relevant (Percent indicating message is talking to someone like themselves)	66 or higher	50–65	49 or lower
Anything confusing (Percent indicating 'yes')	9 or lower	10–20	21 or higher
Believable	91 or higher	75–90	74 or lower
Well done	66 or higher	50–65	49 or lower
Convincing	71 or higher	55–70	54 or lower
Informative	76 or higher	60–75	59 or lower
Made its point	91 or higher	75–90	74 or lower
Interesting	66 or higher	50–65	49 or lower
Pleasant	66 or higher	50–65	49 or lower

particularly interesting because it not only provides a pragmatic list of measures related to the pre-testing of television public service advertisements (PSAs) but also provides guidelines for interpreting the results. It will be recalled that establishing meaningful and realistic standards of success is a fundamentally important task for health education programming.

Standard pre-testing techniques comprise: individual in-depth interviews, central location intercept interviews, self-administered questionnaires, focus group interviews, gatekeeper review and readability testing. As may be imagined these are based on standard quantitative and qualitative research approaches as discussed in Chapter Two. One or two further comments will serve to illustrate the particular flavour of pre-testing approaches.

The focus group interview or panel testing seeks to gain insight into the characteristics of given communications and programmes by recording the discussion of a panel consisting of representatives of the target group and noting their reactions to the pilot materials. Conversation, questioning or more specialized tactics – such as the projective technique mentioned above – may be used in this context.

The central location intercept interview may also be called a 'hall test' since interviewees, typically identified by quota sampling, will be invited to a hall or other convenient central location for panel testing – or indeed any other kind of research into audience reactions. Romano [57] also describes a more expensive version of the hall test – 'theatre testing' – which allows larger numbers to respond to visual and electronic communications.

The technique of gatekeeper review acknowledges the importance of researching the reaction of key individuals who will control the target audience's access to given health education programmes.

One of the more important and specialist applications of pre-testing involves the analysis of written materials. A detailed discussion of this area is beyond the scope of this chapter but requires some brief review. Since the majority of communication and learning materials in health education are in written form, it is clearly important that the target group responses are properly tested. It is of course possible to use any of the techniques discussed above to judge the suitability of written materials. For instance a 'copy editing' technique could be used in conjunction with individual or group interviews. This involves the respondents actually writing on, say, a pamphlet or leaflet and scoring out offensive items, underlining confusing phrases and writing in alterations or additions. However, the testing of written materials normally comprises three broad approaches: content analysis, typographical analysis, and measuring readability. Content analysis has its own technology but in its simpler form consists of systematically sampling written passages or books and categorizing content in whatever way is most likely to illuminate the particular research and its goals. For instance Davison [61] analysed the questions asked at a series of public cancer education sessions and examined their implications for the content of cancer education. The study of mass media programming by Best *et al.* [16], which was referred to earlier, was based on a content analysis of news reporting just as Hansen's observations on the incidental portrayal of alcohol on mass media documented references to and depiction of alcohol in advertising, documentaries and entertainment programmes such as soap opera. Redman [62] in a useful chapter on printed and non-print materials in patient education, reports a content analysis of 27 mental health pamphlets which demonstrated that:

> ... approximately 60% of the content was in the middle-class cultural mould and that another 30% consisted of ambiguous platitudes... The conclusion of this analysis was that the mental health movement was unwittingly propagating a middle-class ethic under the guise of science...

Research into the design of print has received rather less attention in health education and tends to focus on the relative legibility of different type-faces, use of upper case compared with lower case letters and the general aesthetic presentation (see for instance Stewart [63]). On the other hand the assessment of readability is or should be part of the routine process of developing written communications.

Three main strategies tend to be used in measuring reading ease. The first of these uses a frequency count principle arguing that people will be more likely to comprehend commonly used words. And so vocabulary is checked to see if it forms part of an agreed core of basic, i.e. frequently used, language. Perhaps the best known of these approaches is the Dale-Chall list which includes the 3000 most commonly occurring words in the American language [64]. A second procedure is based on calculations of the redundancy inherent in particular written passages, i.e. the amount of repetition, overt or covert. The Cloze Procedure [65] removes every fifth word from a passage and invites respondents to estimate the meaning of the missing word. The higher the success rate, the greater the comprehensibility of the passage.

However, the most commonly used approach to assessing readability is based on the empirical finding that the comprehensibility of written material is correlated with sentence length and number of polysyllabic words within the sentence. Short sentences containing words having few syllables tend to be easier to read than long sentences containing a high proportion of long words. Although the most popular of these various formulae internationally is undoubtedly the Flesch formula [66], a simpler version is the FOG (Frequency of Gobbledegook) formula [67]. The Office of Cancer Communications on the other hand uses the SMOG (Subjective Measures of Gobbledegook) Formula [68].

It is important to be aware that all of the reading ease measures referred to above do not pre-test a representative sample of the actual target group and are thus not as reliable nor as valid as genuine pre-testing. For instance the popular Dale-Chall, Flesch, FOG and SMOG formulae were all indirectly derived from results of the McCall-Crabbs Standard Test Lessons in Reading and thus relate to average developmental stages of reading competence in American children. As Pichert and Elam [69] point out, 'Readability formulas may mislead you'! Nonetheless there are real correlations between these formulae and the intelligibility of written data and they provide valuable pre-testing tools when used with caution. In any case, once we move beyond the realm of checking comprehension and recall into the realm of attitudes and intentions, we would be advised to take the results of all pre-testing with the proverbial pinch of salt. Attempts to discover how people will actually react to communications and programmes on the basis of their comments about acceptability, interest, personal preference or stated intention, should always be guided by a degree of scepticism. This of course applies even more so when observations are made about other people's likely responses!

A SELECTIVE REVIEW OF MEDIA STUDIES: GENERAL OBSERVATIONS

The mass media strategy is in one important respect different from the remaining delivery strategies discussed in this book. Although each of these has its own idiosyncracies and flavour, mass media differ fundamentally in the lack of personal contact between educator and audience. The media strategy is therefore of particular interest – especially since it promises so much but, in many people's view, delivers relatively little. This latter part of the chapter will therefore present evidence which should help us decide what we might realistically expect from mass media. In judging this evidence, we must of course bear in mind the general principles, stated in the first part of the book, that the quality of evidence will depend on (i) the definition of success employed therein, (ii) the extent to which appropriate research designs have been used, and (iii) the choice of particular methods based on intelligent use of learning and communication theory. The latter point will not, of course, apply to the mass media strategy except insofar as media are used to represent particular tactics such as face-to-face interaction (e.g. a video of a counselling session) or group work (e.g. a film of a smoking cessation clinic). In such instances learning tactics are being employed at second hand. The only other situation where choice of appropriate teaching methods is important in the context of mass media use is when the latter are supplemented by auxiliary interpersonal methods.

Particular varieties of media do of course have different capabilities and characteristics – as we have seen above – and the review which follows will provide separate evidence of the potential of some of these for achieving different kinds of outcome. More particularly we will consider the use of posters and leaflets and compare these, implicitly or explicitly, with the arguably more powerful electronic media – radio and television. In addition, we will examine the capabilities of mass media for dealing with some specific health problems including a particularly problematic issue – that of substance misuse.

What then might we say about mass media efficiency? Can we generalize or must we again say it depends on the type of media, subject matter and target group? As indicated in the introduction to this book, Gatherer *et al.* [70] have provided one of the most recent attempts to provide a comprehensive answer to the question, 'Is health education effective?'. As a result of analysing 49 reported evaluations of mass media programmes, they concluded that mass media were in fact inferior to individual instruction and groups. Seven out of eleven of their cases demonstrated some changes in knowledge (of the order of 6% and typically short-lasting); two out of two studies demonstrated some attitude-shift (of between 3 and 6% – though four studies recorded an attitude change in the wrong direction); 20 out of 30 studies showed some behaviour change. As regards this latter category, Gatherer *et al.* note that behaviour change is most likely where a single action is required (e.g. clinic attendance or use of a phone-in service); it tends to be relatively short lived; and change is less likely to occur when general changes in behaviour pattern are required.

Atkin [71] also provides a review of campaign effectiveness; his analysis was not intended to be the kind of comprehensive catalogue which Gatherer *et al.* compiled but provides a rather more thorough and sophisticated analysis of the reasons why certain campaigns were or were not effective. He commented, for instance, on the failure of a campaign to teach Cincinnati residents about the United Nations. Neither knowledge gain nor affective change resulted from a '… heavy flow of multi-media messages'. According to Atkin, lack of success was due to excessive quantity of information at the expense of quality. He ascribed other failures to the use of unpopular media channels and lack of audience penetration; use of vague messages rather than making specific recommendations; poor audience segmentation; generating audience reaction through hard-sell techniques, and failure to take account of the audience's latitude of acceptance.

On the other hand when learning theory and the principles of effective media communication were taken into account, programmes have been demonstrably successful. Atkin cites a programme on sexually transmitted diseases called 'VD Blues' (Greenberg and Gantz, [72]) which attracted a wide audience, increased their perception of the seriousness of the problem, enhanced knowledge levels – especially about mode of transmission and cure – and apparently resulted in thousands of people visiting VD clinics after the programme. He also referred to a successful programme described by Mendelsohn [73] which utilized a quiz format to communicate information about a National Driver Test Program. This had an estimated audience of 30 million viewers, generated over a million letters and '... stimulated thousands to enrol in driver improvement courses'.

There are other well documented examples of successful media programmes which should satisfy critics. For instance, Farhar-Pilgrim and Shoemaker [74] described a series of campaigns designed to influence Americans' extravagant use of energy. Applying Communication of Innovations Theory, they concluded that proper design which took account of audience motivation could produce very acceptable results. They demonstrated, for example, a good level of penetration – their messages reached 83% of city adults an average of 14 times. The target group seemed to be more willing to pay for energy saving devices (the percentage varied between 5% and 17%). Moreover, an increase in sales of such devices was recorded and a higher proportion of the target group undertook various energy saving practices such as installing shower flow control devices than a comparison group: the adoption rate was between 16% and 27% higher than the comparison – depending on the device in question. While this example might not appear to be directly relevant to health education practice, it does illustrate that campaigns which ask people to take action for the collective good can be effective provided that appropriate appeals are made to self-interest (in this case, financial gain).

Bell *et al.* [75], in their review of research in health education (1948–1983) also report examples of effectiveness. For instance, an assessment of the Glasgow rickets campaign claimed an eight-fold increase in demand for vitamin D supplements for older Asian children together with a 33% increase in requests for paediatric drops [76]. The review also included England and Oxley's study [77] which reported a halving of the rate of head infestation among a population of 147 385 children after a regional campaign. Again, Bell *et al.* record the success of a programme in increasing the level of rubella vaccination which involved general practitioner support of a national publicity campaign directed at women in the practice population. Within the study population, 1187 women responded to a request to attend for screening and 106 of the 133 who were eligible for immunization accepted this [78].

Turning now to the use of educational broadcasting, it is clear that properly constructed programmes can have a wide range of desirable effects. Rogers [79] showed how the BBC 'Merry-Go-Round' sex education programme (when used in the context of classroom teaching) could change beliefs and attitudes. Children who experienced the programmes not only increased their knowledge of sexual vocabulary but also developed different attitudes to nudity, reproduction and toilet habits: in other words they acquired a greater and more healthy openness in relation to sexuality.

Again McCron and Dean's [80] thorough evaluation of a series of programmes produced by Channel 4 Television on health matters ('Well

Being') revealed a wide range of beneficial outcomes. They summarized some of these effective outcomes as follows:

> ... in television terms, a relatively successful programme attracting a considerable audience, which showed a relatively high appreciation of the programmes... follow-up activities ...were useful in ... promoting a degree of audience feedback and participation ... programmes promoted thinking and encouraged the development of new understandings.

A review by Gordon [81] of a traditional mass media-centred campaign also reveals how a mix of radio, TV, posters and pamphlets can have a behavioural outcome. A mix of 800 posters, 50 000 leaflets, mass mailing of letters to groups and clubs, press releases, press advertising, 11 radio spots and the involvement of three TV stations generated attendance at a Baltimore diabetes clinic on the three following days in the following proportions: day one, n = 512; day two, n = 790; day three, n = 1350. Interviews with those attending the clinic seemed to confirm that attendance had been primarily due to media information (64% press; 14% radio; 8% TV; remainder interpersonal contact). As the author notes, '... large groups of individuals stand ready to take action on any given issue and merely lack the information or cue to make the action possible'. Certainly in this case, media triggered action. It would, however, be patently wrong to say this would happen for any given issue. Indeed, analysis of the examples of the media programmes above will in all cases indicate the presence of a key condition: pre-existing audience motivation; time and professional presentation necessary for communication of complex information; adjunct of interpersonal pressure, etc. However, it is rather difficult to find an easy explanation of the apparent success of a media-based intervention by the Indian Cancer Society which claimed to have doubled attendances at its six Bombay clinics specializing in the early detection of cancers. This would have been expected, a priori, to have been a difficult task. The journal article provides insufficient detail from which to determine which important pre-conditions seem responsible for overcoming the important affective barriers which often militate against successful cancer education [82]. Following the 10 points of social marketing, the charitable involvement of an advertising agency might indeed, as claimed, have provided the skills and expertise necessary for a sensitive campaign! On the other hand, it may be the case that developing countries are more susceptible generally to mass media interventions and/or that it is easier to utilize community networks to enhance the impact of mass media. Alternatively, it may be that in western, urbanized society health education is more concerned with requiring the abandoning of pleasures and addictions associated with affluence whereas the major barriers in developing countries have to do with cultural misconceptions and associated issues. Whatever the reason, there seems to be consistent evidence of successful media interventions in these countries. For instance, Jenkins [83] reviews 17 projects: most reveal some significant changes and many of these are behavioural. These include a 3% decline in population growth rate (Costa Rica); an improvement in breastfeeding from 25% to over 50% (Micronesia, Yap Islands); 75% of all under-fives vaccinated on one day (Nicaragua); an increase from 0% to 24% adding oil to meals to enhance the energy content after a radio campaign (Phillipines); an increase from 20% to 59% having latrines (Tanzania).

Evidence of the effectiveness of family planning campaigns have normally come from developing countries. Taplin [84] reported that six projects 'improved contraceptive availability, increased sales of products, spread knowledge and stimulated wider use of methods promoted...'. A campaign in Esfahan increased pill accepters by 54% and total contraceptive use by 64% over a six-month period. Again, the impact of China's family planning programme is legendary and, as Liu [52] indicated, this combined a blend of media and interpersonal persuasion. By 1972, 79% of China's population was using contraception; the rate of population increase was reduced from 23 per 1000 in 1963 to 4.7 per 1000 in 1974.

The *International Quarterly of Community Health Education* (Vol. 5, pp. 149–166, 1985) included a study by Cernada and Lu [85] in a list of articles, selected by health educators, of the most worthwhile publications of the 1970s. This described a mass media demonstration project which provided evidence of successful penetration, knowledge and attitude change and an increase in low cost contraceptive practice. It could, of course, be argued that it is relatively easy to sell at least some varieties of family planning practice: health educators are offering a tangible product together with real benefits in terms of reduction of anxiety and economic pressures while minimizing loss of gratification. Relatively few thoroughly evaluated studies of family planning education are available for western countries – possibly because the service does not really need promoting! Those that are available seem to indicate reasonable levels of success. For instance a study of a press/poster/leaflet campaign in Lambeth in 1972–3 increased numbers of new patients at clinics by 68%, total attendances by 26% and clinic sessions by 46%. A similar programme in Holland aimed at young people under the age of 18 succeeded in trebling numbers of clinic visitors at a time of year when attendance figures normally dropped – both studies are reported by Smith [86].

One final point will be made about the use of mass media in developing countries. It will be recalled that the major single benefit – perhaps the sole benefit – of mass media is their capacity to reach a mass audience – and to do so relatively cheaply. As Leslie [87] indicates in her review of mass media and nutrition education, '... the most firm conclusion suggested by the evaluations is that mass media health and nutrition education projects can reach large numbers of people (up to several million) in a relatively short period of time. The evaluations also indicate that, although there is a considerable range in costs among projects it is possible to achieve this outreach at a cost as low as $0.01 per person'. She goes on to point out that between 10% and 50% of the audience remember the main nutrition message and that when a specific nutrition message has been designed, there is '... a reasonable expectation that the target audience could modify their behaviour accordingly and ... a reasonable expectation that this modified behavior could bring about an improvement in health or nutrition status...'.

This chapter will be concluded by considering three situations where particular aspects of mass media or the kind of message they convey will determine the likelihood of success. In this way a major theme of this book will be reiterated: it is of relatively little value making generalizations about effectiveness without a careful analysis of goals, strategies and methodology. First, we will consider the influence of media characteristics by considering and comparing the use of leaflets and posters. Secondly, we will look at a functionally different kind of health education problem – persuading individuals to use seat-belts. Thirdly, we will consider goals and content by reviewing particularly problematical issues for health education – the misuse of substances. This will include comments about drugs generally and alcohol and smoking in particular.

POSTERS AND LEAFLETS

Before considering the potential of these two popular devices, we should reiterate the distinction made earlier between the use of media as mass media and the use of media as audio-visual aids or learning resources. It is almost a truism to say that the appropriate use of an audio-visual aid will enhance any given teaching method. For instance Burt *et al.* [88] described a successful piece of patient education in which interpersonal education by medical and nursing staff delivered to survivors of acute myocardial infarction was supplemented by written advice and pamphlets. Sixty two per cent of the smokers in the experimental group had remained non-smokers for between one and three years compared with 27.5% in a control group. This study did not quantify separately the relative contribution of the written materials. However, Russel *et al.* [132] were able to show that leaflets added a couple of percentage points to the effectiveness of the verbal advice provided by a doctor.

The use of leaflets as mass media – i.e. without interpersonal support – is more problematical. Tapper-Jones and Davis [89] documented a detailed and comprehensive survey of a sample of Welsh general practitioners' use of leaflets. The study demonstrated clearly that leaflet use was widespread in primary medical care: the vast majority of doctors used leaflets and/or other teaching aids. Of the sample of 176 GPs, 91% used diet sheets, 85.5% a variety of hand-drawn diagrams, 58.5% various leaflets, 39% pre-printed diagrams, 26% plastic models, 19% a patient counselling compendium, 15.5% 'Family Doctor' booklets and 3.5% 'some other aid'. The major suppliers of the leaflets were, first of all, various pharmaceutical companies and, second, Health Education Council. Interestingly, GPs rated television as the most effective means of communication followed by 'personal advice from doctors' – the reverse of Budd and McCron's [12] observation of patients' rating of credibility!

The study by Russel *et al.* which was cited above, led to the development of a specially tailored booklet containing advice on giving up smoking. This was despatched to all GP's in England and Wales. Its fate serves to illustrate some of the limitations of the leaflet – and will now be considered in the context of social marketing's notion of a 'hierarchy of effects'. We should first note that a leaflet must often be delivered to a 'gatekeeper' who will make it available to the prime user. The leaflet must be acceptable to the prime user and its message must then impinge on the consciousness of the target population: people must pick up the leaflets, read them, pay attention to the messages contained therein and, if they have been properly pre-tested, they should understand their content. Hopefully, they may also believe the message and this belief may in turn contribute towards the development of a favourable attitude to a healthy outcome which may then predispose the learner to adopt some behaviour or, possibly, to change some unhealthy practice – assuming of course that the social and physical environment will support and not inhibit such a course of action!

Spencer [90] attempted to track the GUS ('Give Up Smoking') leaflets mentioned above. His survey revealed that 57% of the sample did not remember having received the booklets. Of those who did recall having received them, 72% found them acceptable and 39% had used them. However, only one in three of this user group appeared to have used the booklets in the prescribed fashion, i.e. as a consultation aid requiring the GP to provide a personalized message for the patient in the context of interpersonal advice and exhortation about stopping smoking. Posters accompanied the booklets and 69% of the 43% of doctors who had any recollection of receiving the kit claimed to have displayed the poster in the practice premises.

The ubiquitous and frequently maligned poster has been subjected to many appraisals – most of which demonstrate very low effectiveness when used without interpersonal support. Posters are, almost by definition, designed to convey persuasive messages without such adjuvant support (by contrast with a chart which is meant to be used as a teaching aid). Grant [91] studied the impact of two differently styled posters urging women to have a cervical smear. These were prominently displayed in a number of clinics and women were interviewed in order to determine what they recalled of the posters. Relatively few could recall the posters (although one designed in a question-and-answer format was superior to the other). Significantly the women who were most aware of the posters had already had a smear test; their recall doubtless reflected self-congratulatory selective attention! A similar study by Cole and Holland [92] reported that only 16 out of 198 women could remember accurately two posters displayed in a health centre waiting room. Over 90% did not read available leaflets or take one home.

A particularly optimistic attempt to use posters was described by Auger *et al.* [93]. Both posters and mobiles were used in a hospital setting to influence smoking behaviour. While the researchers did not imagine that a poster could influence the smoking habit, they thought that smokers in canteen areas might be persuaded not to smoke in that given situation or perhaps to extinguish their cigarettes. An ingenious form of indicator of success was employed: base line 'debris indices' were developed by counting and measuring cigarette butts before and after the poster/mobile display. The results? No change! It should be noted, in passing, that this study pre-dates the substantial normative shift away from smoking and the prevalence of non-smoking policies in hospitals, restaurants and the like. It might well be the case that posters would have some trigger effect if used today in a similar context.

The Transport and Road Research Laboratory has carried out several experimental studies of media impact. One study demonstrated that by taking learning theory into account and sequencing the information presented in a poster, a significant improvement in correct interpretations of safe road crossing practices could be produced in children of various ages. While 36% of all children aged five to seven misinterpreted all messages on a draft poster, only 9% got the messages wrong on the revised 'sequenced' poster. Clearly, as the designers noted, understanding is only weakly related to road-crossing behaviour; nonetheless, the same organization demonstrated that posters used by the roadside could actually influence driving practices. After displaying double crown size posters for a week in six sites, the number of overtaking actions fell from 1866 to 1355 and the proportion of risky overtaking declined from 9% to 4.5%. However, posters used in a similar way had no effect on more complex driving behaviours – such as keeping an adequate distance between cars on the M4 at Slough! (TRRL [94, 95]).

The final example to be discussed in this section on posters and leaflets is a well designed and extensively monitored campaign to prevent children's accidents. It is particularly interesting in that it: (i) used booklets in conjunction with a series of television programmes, (ii) its measure of effectiveness encompassed most of the kinds of indicator examined in Chapter Three and (iii), because it appealed to caretakers of young children, motivation to take action must have been relatively high – certainly by comparison with programmes which required the audience to undertake uncomfortable activities or forego gratification. The campaign consisted of three components;

a ten programme television series lasting ten minutes per programme and employing a popular television personality as presenter; a 36 page booklet; a community initiative which sought to establish local 'Play it Safe' groups consisting of a variety of lay and professional people concerned with safety. The impact of the programme has been thoroughly documented [95, 96]. The effectiveness of the TV programme will be summarized before analysing the separate effect of the booklets. Results will be described in accordance with the 'chain of indicators' ranging from awareness through to behaviour change.

First, audience penetration was good. Some 8 million people on average watched each programme (15.5% of the viewing population over the age of four). By the end of the series 59% of adults and 40% of children had seen at least one programme. The viewing figures indicated a representative social class distribution; as it was hoped to reach lower socio-economic groups, audience segmentation was thus satisfactory. Secondly, viewers had a positive attitude to the programmes: 96% of viewers found them interesting; 47% found them 'very helpful' and a further 37% considered them 'quite helpful'. More important, however, for the achievement of campaign goals is the audience attitude to the preventive measures which the programmes attempted to promote. In seeking to gain insight into these outcome measures – and the intermediate variables which influenced them – some 2000 people were interviewed before and after the campaign. A sample of viewers was also compared with a matched group of non-viewers and their beliefs, attitudes and reported changes in practice were compared. The results can be summarized as follows:

1. Viewers tended to have more favourable reactions on four measures of six general attitudes to child safety;
2. Viewers were more likely than non-viewers to accept the probability of specific accidents occurring in eight out of 11 test situations;
3. Viewers were also more likely than non-viewers to believe that parents could do something to prevent the 11 accident situations described in the booklets. Whereas neither of the differences in (1) and (2) were statistically significant, two of these efficacy beliefs did meet the criterion of statistical success.

Thirdly, in respect of actions taken, viewers were on average more likely to have translated positive attitude into practice. Of a possible list of 15 specific safety actions, viewers took 5.97 actions compared with non-viewers' 5.44. Again, this difference was not significant statistically. However, when a separate analysis of viewers who were 'responsible for children every day' was carried out, the differences in this category and in the categories listed above did reach a level of significance. In other words, the section of the target group which perceived the direct relevance of the recommendations was influenced significantly to a greater or lesser extent. Whether a difference of 0.9 safety actions taken is considered a success clearly depends on expectations of a mass media campaign!

Turning next to the contribution of the booklet, the following information was provided by the BBC's research department. Between December 1981 and the end of March, 1982, a total of 1.5 million copies had been distributed – a figure which included 45 000 individual requests. Research into the population reached by the booklet indicated that some 11% of a total of 1926 adults interviewed had seen the publication and 4% claimed to have read it. By comparison, 15% of a sample of 1080 programme viewers had seen the booklet and 6% claimed to have read it. Predictably the proportion of lower socio-economic groups having written for the booklet, seen it or read it was smaller than middle-class groups. Some 75% of the 1080 viewers claimed to have read all of the booklet and 71% of these claimed to have read it thoroughly. Ninety seven per cent were pleased with the publication and found it useful. Fifty nine per cent considered it taught them 'a lot of things I didn't know' but 76% believed that 'sensible parents would already follow most of the advice in the booklet'. What of actions taken? Although there may well be over-claiming, it does seem to be the case that the booklet had prompted actions among at least some readers. For example 16% of booklet readers (which, remember, is 16% of the 4% of the population who claimed to have read it) stated that they now took more precautions in the kitchen; 15% were more careful with medicines and dangerous liquids; 10% took safety action concerning glass; 6% took more fire precautions and checked electrical safety; 4% secured windows, made stairs safer and secured cupboards.

A further interesting observation may be made about the impact of the total campaign. Some 15 local groups had been formed before the TV series was actually shown – as a result of advance publicity and liaison work. This additional source of interpersonal support might be expected to maximize the impact of the campaign proper. In fact a study in an inner city area by Colver *et al.* [97] showed that 55% of the working class families interviewed did not watch any of the TV programmes and only 9% of a group specially encouraged to watch the series took any of the 15 safety actions. However when a comparable group received a home visit and were given specific advice, some 60% actually took some kind of action.

The evaluations of posters and leaflets discussed above clearly make the point that the peculiar features of given media will influence the likelihood of a successful outcome. However, these intrinsic factors will compete with other components of the whole influence process making prediction difficult if not impossible: for instance the success of the 'Play it Safe' booklets was affected by the context of the TV programmes, by the audience's beliefs about children's vulnerability to accident and, above all, by the addition of interpersonal education in Colver's study. Sometimes the anticipated benefits of given media may not materialize. For example, Harris [98] reported on the failure of a local radio-based campaign to persuade the community to take on responsibility for preventing hypothermia in elderly relatives and neighbours. One of the key indicators – whether or not elderly people living alone had been visited in the previous seven days – seemed to show that there had been a 9% decline in visits after the programmes! At first glance, the 'folksy' nature and community orientation of local radio might have made it particularly suitable for this kind of campaign. Although hypothermia might not seem to be a particularly problematical health topic – most people would not be expected to be hostile to helping old people – the subject matter of many programmes offer an almost desperate challenge to the ingenuity of those seeking to produce change through mass media.

In the next section of this chapter, the results of a particularly rigorous study will be presented which seems to the author to indicate just what unsupported mass media can achieve under difficult but not impossible circumstances – promoting the wearing of seat-belts. The concluding section of this chapter will review an acknowledged problem area – that of substance abuse in general. It will comment on drug education, identifying the prevention of alcohol misuse as especially difficult compared with tobacco smoking.

SEAT-BELTS

In 1973, Levens and Rodnight [99] assembled evidence of the effectiveness of a series of controlled area experiments in the use of mass media to promote seat-belt wearing in Britain. The value of the study rests on the following facts: (i) evidence of important driver/front seat passenger characteristics is presented, (ii) precise details of media input and their cost are provided, (iii) objective evidence of specific behaviours is described, and (iv) we can be as confident as anyone can that the results of media programmes can be ascribed to the input rather than other 'contaminating' events.

First, the pre-testing of driver characteristics revealed the following useful data: drivers appeared to already be motivated to wear seat-belts. Some 85% of those interviewed claimed to have a positive attitude to seat-belt wearing, believing that this would cut down injuries. It seemed that despite this attitude many drivers did not 'belt up' – and it was not possible to rely on reported use of belts since drivers consistently over-estimated it. The number claiming to wear seat-belts more than half the time was 57% but observed levels of wearing were only 17%. Any measure of programme effectiveness must therefore try to use observation rather than self-report.

Further research into the failure of drivers to use seat-belts, despite their generally favourable attitude, suggested that this might be due to beliefs that although belts would reduce accidents, drivers were not susceptible to such accidents in a variety of situations (despite objective evidence to the contrary).

In Health Belief Model (HBM) terms, the target group clearly believed in the effectiveness of seat-belts but were ambivalent about susceptibility and seriousness. At all events a programme was devised which used three appeals: 'appeal to the head', 'appeal to the heart' and 'appeal to the nervous system'. In other words a logical/factual approach compared with an emotional approach and an approach which tried to instil a habit so that seat belt wearing became routinized. Qualitative research indicated that this latter was probably the most effective and the slogan, presented by someone having high source credibility, 'Klunk, Klick After Every Trip' was considered to have provided a mnemonic. The implication of this being that in HBM terms, the main perceived cost was merely the effort involved in establishing a routine (apart, of course, from the 15% who were implacably opposed on ideological grounds!).

The programmes were then launched in different regions in Britain utilizing different levels of expenditure – mostly on television advertising but supported by poster display. The results were carefully monitored by observing levels of seat-belt wearing at a variety of sampling points. The rate of wearing increased in each of the regions sampled and to some extent reflected the level of media expenditure. There did seem, however, to be a decay effect with the exception of the final area where the trend seemed to be upward – perhaps indicating the start of a normative shift. The extent of the effect is summarized by Levens and Rodnight as follows: 'It is possible, within a media expenditure range corresponding to a national equivalent of from £235 000 to £720 000 (1972 prices) to raise the level of seat-belt wearing by a percentage ranging from 3% to 16% (from a basic 14%–15% start point) and to do so within a period of three weeks'. They concluded that a burst of advertising over three weeks followed by supportive posters for a further three weeks would be the most cost-effective way of proceeding. If we return to our earlier comment about the expectations of commercial advertisers, the changes produced would represent a very high level of success. However, the researchers do observe that having reached such a level any further effects could not be achieved by more mass media work. Using the level of seat-belt wearing prevalent in Australian states (where, at the time, legislation had been introduced) as a yardstick (i.e. 75% wearing), they concluded, 'The probable cost of bridging the gap between 32% and 75% wearing by persuasive advertising alone ... could never be justified in benefit terms'.

In Britain, the need for such media-based health education has disappeared with the advent of legal compulsion. It is worth noting, as an aside, that although education failed to increase the level of wearing much above 30%, its agenda setting function facilitated the enactment of health policy as described in Chapter One. In other parts of the world, health education is still needed to protect vehicle occupants. In this context it is interesting to note how a broad-based media plus community programme in North Carolina followed good commercial practice and offered various incentives to drivers wearing seat-belts (in the form of prizes and the opportunity to draw a winning lottery ticket). The programme was successful in raising the level of wearing from 24% to 41% in six months and sustaining it at 36% after a further six months [100]. Let us compare this level of success with programmes which seek to modify substance abuse and influence levels of drug and alcohol use and smoking.

SUBSTANCE ABUSE

By comparison with safety education, family planning and many of the other topics receiving consideration above, attempts to deal with the problems of substance abuse seem to be doomed to failure – especially if the sole mode of attack is mass media campaigns. In short, the task would seem to involve persuading individuals to forsake habits which give them pleasure and to which they may be addicted – in one sense or another – or which meet some important psychological or social need. The significance of these motivational barriers will be apparent when we consider examples of campaigns designed to promote smoking cessation and foster sensible drinking. First, however, we will consider a recent attempt to use mass media to influence illegal drug use.

Expert Opinion

Despite expert opinion and Home Office policy, the UK government made a decision to launch a mass media campaign costing some £2 million directed at heroin misuse. The amount of money involved may be put into some kind of perspective by noting that the major national health education agency's total budget at the time amounted to some £10 million. It is highly probable that the hidden goals of the campaign were to be seen to be doing something to deal with a problem of doubtful magnitude but which created a good deal of moral outrage and indignation. At any rate, an evaluation was commissioned by government. In assessing the results of this evaluation, four questions have to be asked: (i) should £2 million have been spent on the programme? (ii) Were any real changes detectable in the target audience at the end of the campaign? (iii) If there were any such changes, could they reasonably be attributed to the campaign? (iv) In the event of real changes being observed, were these really significant rather than merely statistically significant – i.e. might they make any contribution to the reduction of drug misuse?

Of course, a priori, the money should not have been spent in that way. First, epidemiologically the problem of heroin use did not justify such an expenditure. Secondly, the accepted wisdom of drug education asserted that programmes should not use unsupported mass media nor should they focus on one specific drug. However, to many people's surprise, the evaluation appeared to indicate that against all the odds there was a significant and relevant change in beliefs and attitudes (since heroin use was so unusual there was no possibility of measuring any actual behaviour change). It is not possible here to provide a detailed and critical analysis of the research (for fuller discussion see Tones [101]) but several valuable conclusions for media use generally may be drawn. First, it was apparent that the campaign had been very successful in penetrating the market (which comprised young people aged 13–20) and in achieving levels of awareness which ranged from 80% to 98% – depending on the assessment criteria used. It thus supported the general axiom that properly constructed programmes can indeed raise awareness successfully. The second point which can be made is that it is increasingly difficult to find adequate control groups for national media programmes and therefore any observed results cannot be unequivocally ascribed to the programme itself. This was unfortunate since there did appear to be statistically significant changes in a series of measures of belief, attitude and intention which appeared to indicate a general hardening of attitude towards heroin use. However, because a control group was lacking and because the perfectly acceptable practice of using randomly selected but separate population sub-samples to measure attitudes, etc. before and after the campaign had been used, it was possible to argue that the observed changes might have been due to pre-existing differences in the samples – even though these should have been removed by the process of random selection. Such an argument would have looked suspiciously like rationalization on the part of opponents of mass media drug education had it not been for several anomalies in the results. For instance there seemed to be a tendency for the pre-campaign sample to have a generally less cautious approach to life than the post-campaign samples: the pre-campaign group appeared more likely to argue with parents and a higher proportion claimed that they would, 'stand by their friends whatever they did'. These general attitudes could hardly have been influenced by a campaign dealing with a specific drug and the apparent hardening of attitudes could be ascribed to the fact that the post-campaign samples were generally more cautious, god-fearing – and already opposed to hard drugs!

However, a much more important point can be made about the heroin campaign. Let us assume that the claimed shift in attitudes and beliefs was genuine. What impact could this be expected to have on the likelihood of a group of young people resisting the offer of hard drugs? Apart from the fact that beliefs about the effect of heroin on the body would probably be challenged when the young people in question actually engaged with a heroin-using subculture, such beliefs and associated attitudes would be insignificant in real terms in the context of the various other alleged influences on drug misuse – such as unemployment, social deprivation, home background and socialization, personality factors, self-esteem, machismo, rebelliousness, curiosity, social interaction skills, peer pressure, cultural norms, availability of drugs and beliefs about the gratifications provided. In the face of these factors, the potential of mass media for influencing drug-related behaviour must be small. An alternative government strategy which allocated a similar amount of money to provide for about 100 drug co-ordinators for education authorities for a year, would appear to be much more cost-effective – even if it did not cater for the sense of moral outrage of the populace! However, let us move on to consider our most popular drug – alcohol.

Alcohol

At first blush – and under the influence of a stereotyped view of desperate junkies unable to 'kick their habit' – we might expect alcohol education to offer greater opportunities for effective intervention than the heroin campaign discussed above. In fact one of the biggest challenges to health promotion is posed by alcohol. The reasons are perhaps self-evident: unlike smoking, the health education message is relatively complex. It seeks to promote 'moderate' or 'sensible' drinking – and requires the individual to calculate relative strengths of different liquor; it requires judgement and decision-making. Moreover the use of alcohol is strongly supported by social norms while smoking is becoming an increasingly deviant behaviour. The vast majority of smokers acknowledge the negative aspects of their habit and claim that they would like to give up – seeking only a magic formula and appropriate support to help them do so. The tobacco manufacturers are under constant attack while the brewing industry has a much more positive image. On the other hand, like smoking, alcohol consumption provides considerable gratification – both physical and social. It is, thus, hardly surprising that examples of effective alcohol education are almost non-existent – particularly in the context of media campaigns and community wide programmes.

The effectiveness and efficiency of alcohol education programmes have been comprehensively reviewed. In addition to the general reviews of Gatherer *et al.* [70] and Bell *et al.* [75], Kinder [102] analysed some 66 studies on drug and alcohol education published between 1963 and 1973. Blane and Hewitt [103, 104] also produced state-of-the-art reviews in 1977 and 1980 of mass media. More recently Dorn and South [30] provided a critical appraisal of 404 publications. The conclusions to be derived from all of these reviews may be summarized as follows:

1. There have been relatively few methodologically sound evaluations (perhaps with the exception of a few studies of drink-driving).
2. Expenditure on health education has been completely insignificant compared with the promotion of alcohol. Such campaigns as there have been have tended to have limited geographical coverage and to have been broadcast at inappropriate times. As Dorn and South [30] observe, 'For every £1000 which is paid in liquor duty and tax in the UK, 43 pence is

spent on education about alcohol and its effects. In 1980 over £76 million was spent on drink advertising.'

The pro-alcohol messages conveyed directly and indirectly by media indicate both its social acceptability and its high level of prevalence.

3. A social marketing approach incorporating thorough pre-testing should be used by health educators.
4. There is a need for locally oriented community programmes having a strong interpersonal education component.
5. Alcohol education programmes frequently produce a change in knowledge and occasionally attitude but rarely influence drinking behaviour.

To some extent these observations might be made about most health education issues; it just happens that influencing alcohol consumption is especially difficult. We will now illustrate the points above – and other mass media issues discussed earlier – by reviewing selectively a few of the plethora of studies in this area. The first of these are concerned with the incidental effects of mass media.

The incidental, 'norm-sending' aspects of mass media were mentioned earlier in this chapter and reference was made to Hansen's [17] work on media images of alcohol. Several published studies underline the importance of this norm-sending role of media in relation to alcohol. The following are cited by Dorn and South [30]. Block [105] described the ways in which press reporting stereotyped and stigmatized the alcoholic. A series of investigations by Breed and Defoe [106–111] examined not only the portrayal of alcohol in magazine advertising but also in press reports, prime time television sitcoms, comic books and campus magazines. Gerbner [112] pointed out the higher prevalence of alcohol images in top-rated programmes. King [113] pre-dated Hansen's [17] observations by demonstrating similar types of presentation in British 'soaps'. Finn [114] reminded us of the wide variety of mass media by reporting a content analysis of greeting cards which again perpetuated the negative stereotyped images of the alcohol abuser.

One of the possible mechanisms whereby these incidental effects may be produced is that of modelling. Both Caudill and Marlatt and Garlington and Dericco [115, 116] have argued that media models may influence the drinking rates of male students.

The norms conveyed through media presentations are essentially unrealistic. These mythical messages suggest that:

1. Everyone drinks heavily (i.e. at a rate per unit time far in excess of real life drinking).
2. Drinking is associated with sexual prowess, romance, enjoyable social occasions, power and commercial success – and generally occurs in up-market situations.

3. Few negative consequences are shown. Drinkers remain clear-headed, do not have accidents, stay slim and healthy – or, alternatively, may be seen as anti-heroes. These latter provide a celebration of cosy self-gratification and folksy moderation in the face of attempts by fanatical zealots who try to impose unattainable ideals of health and fitness on the populace at large.
4. 'Problem drinkers' are presented only in the caricatured form of skid row down-and-outs.

Following the theoretical discussion at the start of this chapter, it is not, of course, intended to suggest that this background of 'normative noise' will necessarily have any direct effect on people's drinking. It does, however, following the principles of 'uses and gratifications', provide people with the 'evidence' to justify their current practices and resist the pressures of health education. In the face of this background 'noise' conveying the normality and desirability of heavy alcohol consumption, it is perhaps some consolation that media credibility is relatively low (at any rate when it can be seen to attempt to influence). As indicated earlier, Budd and McCron [12] demonstrated a low level of trust in health messages generally when delivered by mass media. This situation, not surprisingly, appears to apply to drugs and alcohol also. For instance Dembo *et al*. [117] reported that high school students perceived television and radio as having low credibility compared with other media and with interpersonal sources of information. It is not, however, clear whether the incidental presentation of health-related information is subject to the same degree of sceptical appraisal. It is probably wise to assume that it is not.

The implications of the work described above for health promotion are clear but not necessarily easy to achieve. At the level of policy, the controllers of broadcast media must be prevailed upon to ensure that the consequences of alcohol consumption are more realistically portrayed. At the level of individual health education, the natural scepticism of the viewing public must be nurtured by increasing awareness of media conventions and developing critical appraisal skills. Given the relative ineffectiveness of mass media in fostering 'sensible drinking' this aspect of health promotion merits increasing emphasis.

Turning now to these more deliberate attempts to influence people's knowledge, attitudes and practices with regard to alcohol, we might first ask about the trade's success in persuading individuals to start drinking and increase their level of consumption. As indicated earlier, (Henry and Waterson, [19]) the advertisers of alcohol modestly deny having any effects on recruitment, asserting that they offer a public service by allowing the existing drinker to select from available beverages: i.e. the goal is brand-switching. Several attempts have been made to give the lie to this assertion and demonstrate that advertising does have an effect on consumption. While it does seem likely that preferences for different kinds of alcohol (e.g. beer versus spirits) may be influenced (Brown [118]), it is difficult to find sound evidence that restrictions on advertising will reduce consumption (Ogbourne [119]) or show anything other than weak econometric associations. In the absence of such evidence, it becomes more difficult to urge governmental action. If there is an effect, it is clearly of a much lower order than the impact of such structural factors as fiscal, economic and legislative measures (Bourgeois [120]). However, even if advertising does not in fact increase total consumption, the norm-sending function should be sufficient to justify pressure for controls.

Again, if it is indeed true that advertisers with their vast advertising budget really cannot influence consumption, the chances for health education of reducing total consumption would, a priori, appear to be slight. Published research supports this view but also demonstrates the anticipated 'hierarchy of effects', i.e. that it is relatively easy to create awareness but increasingly difficult to influence recall, attitudes and behaviour. Some indication of this is provided by Maloney and Hersey's [121] detailed account of an intensive marketing strategy to transmit alcohol public service advertisements (PSAs) nationwide (in the USA). Messages were aimed principally at women and youth. Assessment of the campaign reach (penetration) as measured by the proportion of the target audience likely to be watching television at a given time of day multiplied by the market share of a particular television station indicated that the PSAs reached on average 31.8% of all adults, 22% of the female target group and 19% of young people. However, according to the authors, commercial practice suggests that product purchase requires at least three exposures to an advertisement – which in turn means a level of campaign reach of 42% of an audience. Although the average penetration was 22%, there were in fact 13 markets where more than 42% of the primary targets were exposed to the PSAs and three where the exposure was 60% or more.

And so, given a sufficient level of media expenditure, the first goal of awareness can clearly be attained. Two case studies will now be considered in order to illustrate what might be expected from media campaigns which try to surpass this relatively limited goal. The first was launched in the North-east of England and the second in California.

The Tyne-Tees Alcohol Campaign was piloted in 1974 (HEC [222]) and, in the view of many people, had unrealistic objectives of producing changes in consumption in a region noted for its heavy drinking. After a series of changes and developments the campaign continued into the 1980s. At a meeting to assess its effects (HEC [123]) eight key findings were listed. These illustrate what might realistically be expected from such a campaign:

1. People in the North-east were aware of their regional attitudes to alcohol being 'different'.
2. People in the North-east were more inclined to believe alcohol was a problem, though they were inclined to think of it as caused by other problems.

3. People in the North-east were more aware of sources of help.
4. More than 70% recalled the campaign and there were significant levels of recall of specific messages.
5. One in eight people claimed that it had some influence on their thinking about alcohol.
6. Safe drinking levels were believed to be lower in the North-east than in Leicester (a comparison region).
7. There was more awareness of 'equivalents' in the North-east than in Leicester.
8. There might be some antagonism building up towards health education messages.

The programme in California which we will now consider, is of special interest because it was designed particularly to take account of known limitations of mass media. It was called the 'Winners' programme (indicating its attempt to promote a positive image) and is described by Wallack and Barrows [124]. It ran for three years at a total cost of some $2.5 million. It was located in three sites: one acted as a control; one received a media-only programme and the third received media plus an additional community based effort (thus seeking to emulate the Stanford Heart Disease Prevention Programme (q.v.). Programme goals were as follows: awareness raising and provision of information; attitude-change and subsequently changes in actual drinking behaviours; medical indicators – viz. cirrhosis rates (after an appropriate time lapse) and social indicators in the form of drunk driving rates, arrests for disorderly conduct, etc. It was considered that success would lead to cost-benefits and an overall reduction in per capita consumption.

The target was adults aged 18–35 and after the first year it was hoped that other groups might be influenced.

The media programme included: three 30 second television commercials, three 60 second radio slots; press advertisements; 110 billboard displays. The media mix was calculated to reach 90% of the target group on an average of 35 occasions. The message content emphasized positive advantages of lower consumption, presenting images of the moderate drinker as happy, in control, sociable and macho. Women were depicted as self-assured and in control.

It is interesting to note how political factors almost immediately affected the programme planning. The Wine Institute exerted pressure which delayed the programme to the extent that there was a 40% lower exposure than had been originally planned.

The community programme was designed to incorporate an interpersonal element. Some 14 453 people attended meetings; 67 000 pieces of programme material (balloons, badges, etc.) were distributed; various publicity events were arranged; teacher training programmes were developed. According to the authors, however, the community programme did not meet expectations in that there was little integration with media inputs and a planned recruitment of volunteers who might hold home meetings did not materialize.

The results follow the now expected pattern: good levels of awareness, some attitude change and no behaviour change. For detailed results, readers are referred to the original article. However, the following will serve to indicate the nature and scale of the changes achieved.

1. There was a high level of slogan recognition (79% in adult group, 86% in youth group). As with many other results these tended to be more pronounced in the media plus community area and greater than in the control community.
2. There was a generally high level of correct interpretation of the messages (e.g. 70% adult; 84% youth) and 20% of adults and 30% of youth scored at least 8 out of 12 on a scale of overall comprehension. The problem of lack of feedback potential of media was, however, to be observed in that some 25% believed that one of the PSAs was promoting alcohol – even after pre-testing and subsequent change!
3. Recall was generally good (50% adults; 72% youth).
4. In general there was a disappointing level of change in the affective area. For example awareness of alcohol problems and concern about these problems showed relatively slight increases as did concern about own level of drinking (e.g. 8% adults and 2% youth). On an attitude scale containing 13 statements relating to advertising of alcohol, drunkenness etc., there was only one significant change (and that was in the adult group).
5. As for behavioural outcome, 15% of those who recognized the 'Winners' slogans reported a reduction in drinking or claimed they intended to do so, but there was no supporting evidence of this. There was no change in other items which attempted to measure quantity and frequency of drinking nor was there any change in a seven category drinking problem scale.

In short, it is clear that even in a very well constructed and evaluated programme which takes account of the dictates of social marketing, there is no evidence of behaviour change. It could, of course, happen that the campaign's impact on knowledge and awareness might, in the context of future developments, make the success of such hypothetical developments more likely. Wallack and Barrows [124] described the situation thus:

> The California Prevention Demonstration was unique in many ways, but in terms of the types of outcomes that were produced it was quite typical. The major evaluation findings of increased awareness, some gain in knowledge and no attitude or behaviour change is consistent with a myriad of other mass media programs and prevention efforts in general.

The authors argued that Lazarsfeld and Merton's views [25] were even more applicable to the current scenario than they were 40 years ago. They strongly assert the points made in the first chapter of this book, that mass media programmes in difficult areas like alcohol use will only be effective when complemented by significant public policy measures. As it is:

> Mass media campaigns and other kinds of individual-oriented interventions are safe because they virtually never challenge any powerful vested interests. Such interventions implicitly state that the problem is in the person and not in the system. Yet as we have suggested above, the person and the system are inseparable; you cannot address one without also addressing the other.

The results of workplace interventions, to be discussed in the next chapter, would bear out these views. However, research on mass media work in smoking yields much more impressive results – particularly when combined with interpersonal efforts and based on sound learning theory. The reasons for any such success compared with alcohol interventions were suggested earlier. For the moment, we will briefly consider some of the results of evaluations of programmes designed to foster smoking cessation.

Smoking

Before commenting on the effectiveness of mass media in combating smoking, we must note that just as alcohol use and misuse has its own peculiarities as a public health problem, the special characteristics of smoking must be taken into account before judgements are made. First of all, there are two qualitatively different smoking prevention tasks: the prevention of recruitment differs from the promotion of smoking cessation. The motives which underlie young people's adoption of the habit are not at all similar to the motivation which may prevent adult (or even young people) quitting. For young people tobacco and its pharmacology are largely irrelevant; smoking serves a symbolic purpose and meets instrumental needs – gratifying the values associated with machismo, toughness, precocity and the like. It also provides a valuable adjunct to self-presentation and social interaction. While some of these aspects may also be important to the adult smoker, the cigarette's role in affect control becomes much more prominent.

The educational tasks demanded by these two different prevention goals are thus distinct. In simple terms, the aims of preventing the onset of smoking involve the creation of a negative attitude to the habit and, more importantly, providing substitute gratification in the form of lifeskills, etc. On the other hand, since the majority of smokers already appear to have a negative attitude to their habit, the major preventive goal is to provide a trigger to cessation followed by support to minimize the chance of relapse. The very nature of these different educational objectives means that the mass media have been seen as more appropriate to the smoking cessation exercise rather than to preventing recruitment (although, as we have seen, television may be a useful supplement to school-based programmes which seek to prevent recruitment to smoking). As we will see, the effectiveness of mass media in stimulating cessation (the only justifiable goal) has depended on the extent to which support can be provided or mobilized – and this in turn has meant borrowing interpersonal techniques.

Two kinds of intervention will be described below. The first of these involves mere consciousness raising about the importance of stopping smoking – with or without the provision of more detailed information and mailed supporting literature. The second involves a more thorough television presentation incorporating several sessions and based on social learning theory. Typical of the former situation is the UK National No Smoking Day.

Reid [125] describes the relative effectiveness of two successive no smoking days – in 1984 and 1985. Apart from providing results which reveal the anti-smoking potential of this sort of publicity tactic, the hierarchy of effects is nicely illustrated. For instance, after pre-publicity designed to co-ordinate national health education efforts, on the day itself some 716 press reports were recorded together with 424 mentions on television or radio. Over a 14 day period there were 13 national radio or television slots and an estimated 134 hours of broadcasting (including in 1985 mentions on the popular 'soaps' 'Brookside' and 'Coronation Street').

Public awareness was high and amounted to some 79% of the population. There was local support from over 100 health education units as well as other organizations such as schools, hospitals, etc. In terms of acceptability, 70% of an interview sample agreed that the day was a good idea and only 7% were firmly opposed.

In order to determine the impact on smoking, a survey of 2000 adults was carried out in 130 sampling points throughout the country. The results were as follows: of 2000 adults, 735 were smokers; 95 (13%) reported trying to give up; and five succeeded in giving up for the day. A further study of 4000 adults three months later provided corroboration of the first survey. Eleven per cent reported they had tried to give up smoking on National No Smoking Day; 9% claimed to have been successful for two months before relapsing. However only three out of the 4000 were still non-smokers after three months (and only one of these claimed that this was due to the day itself!).

Was this a success or a failure? The cost incurred was £50 000 – and included expenditure on 250 000 posters and 300 000 smokers' contracts. At any rate, it was decided to repeat the day in 1985 with an increased budget (£100 000). Although no information was presented on cessation rates, it was clear that awareness was again high: some 76% had heard of the programme on television and 6.5% of smokers claimed to have given up for the day. An interesting indicator is provided of the booster effect of local involvement: some 22 000 people used a telephone to 'Dial a Tip' but 14 000 of these were from Plymouth where two local television personalities committed themselves to stop smoking during the week. It is clearly unwise to set unrealistic behavioural standards for a publicity venture such as National No Smoking Day. Rather it should be viewed as an agenda-setting exercise which might to some degree counteract the norm-sending messages transmitted by the tobacco advertisers and may even act as an ultimate trigger to a small number of individuals who have been screwing up their courage to abandon their habit!

A more extensive – but to some extent more abortive – media venture was reported by Raw and de Plight [126]. A 15 minute programme was presented at prime-time in a regular documentary slot. It had a 'hard-hitting evangelical style' ('... we want to make a frontal attack on smoking ... we're going to send you every known device to make you give it up and stop killing yourself.') That section of the public who were already motivated to quit and were waiting for the 'magic bullet' responded eagerly. Four thousand calls were received in thirty minutes and eventually some 600 000 people wrote in for the kit which was to help them stop smoking. Unfortunately only 20 000 kits were available. The public was not impressed!

Eventually a more limited kit was sent out to a sample of 20 000 applicants together with a questionnaire. The response rate was 12%. Of the 1752 who returned useable questionnaires: 1602 said they intended to stop smoking; 747 tried to stop; 57 succeeded for between two and three months; 41 were still not smoking after six months and 14 were abstinent at one year. The success rate among those who returned the questionnaires was thus 0.79%.

It should however be noted that 46% had found the kit unhelpful. Other studies of similar ventures have met with greater success: for instance Cuckle and Vunakis [127] studied a random sample of 4492 subjects out of half a million who requested a postal smoking cessation kit after a television programme on the hazards of smoking. Compared with a control group, cessation after one year was superior in the experimental group (11% versus 16%). Interestingly but not surprisingly validation via salivary cotinine measurement revealed lower results but there was still a statistically significant difference (7% versus 9%). These results are not dissimilar to those found by O'Byrne and Crawley [128] after an Irish programme. Some 5% of kit recipients claimed to have stopped smoking between three and five months after the campaign. The superiority of the American figures presumably reflects the greater normative 'push' to non-smoking in the USA compared with Eire. Normative factors would have to be considered also in the comprehensive and well-documented study by Puska *et al.* [129] in Finland.

In the general context of the North Karelian Heart Disease Prevention Project (q.v.) a smoking cessation course was presented on television in 1978. It was launched at a national press conference and was supported by extensive press reporting. The major voluntary organizations also informed their members about the programme and a serious attempt was made to encourage smokers to follow the programme in organized groups. Lay leaders of these groups were provided with support materials. The programme lasted four weeks; there were seven sessions broadcast during the evening and lasting 45 minutes each. The programmes were designed to incorporate interpersonal methods in that a group of ten smokers were featured in the studio and sessions were led by two experts. The techniques used by smoking cessation clinics were employed. In other words the mass media strategy was about as thorough as it could be: there was intensive and comprehensive coverage on the one available television channel; it was supported by additional publicity in the context of a regional programme which had raised awareness of the national heart disease problem; it employed interpersonal methods on screen and encouraged group support in local neighbourhoods. How well did it do? The results showed that 39.5% of men saw between one and three of the broadcast sessions (figures for women were 38.7%); 4.2% of men and 7.3% of women saw all seven. As for the impact on smoking, a survey carried out one year after the final programme revealed that 17% of smokers followed the programme but did not try to stop, and 1.4% stopped smoking but started again. Only 0.8% of those who were smoking at the start of the series were non-smokers after one year. Analysis of those who followed the programmes in a support group yielded the following results. In North Karelia 404 people were in these organized groups; 320 completed the course. Of those who completed the course, 21% succeeded in stopping smoking for a period of at least six months.

One of the most thorough and effective programmes employing mass media to promote smoking cessation is described by Best [130]. This used not only mass media but employed the principles of behaviour modification in the form of 'self-management' components previously used in face-to-face clinics. Six programmes were broadcast on consecutive weeks between 7.00–7.30 p.m. The potential audience was some 20 000 adults (in Washington DC). Viewers were invited to write in for the self-help guide mentioned above and each television programme was linked to a chapter in the booklet. Those who applied for the booklet served as the subjects of the evaluation.

At the end of the series, 86.5% of the survey group returned a completed questionnaire; 64.2% returned a second questionnaire at three months and 71.4% returned a questionnaire at six months. Cessation rates at these times were: 11.5%; 14.7% and 17.6% respectively.

How should we assess the results of both the Finnish exercise and the intervention described by Best? Puska *et al.* made the observation that although the programme achieved a rate of success which was small percentage-wise, some 10 000 smokers countrywide might have stopped smoking with the aid of the programme – and that is a lot of smokers in absolute terms. Best commented that the spontaneous quit rate (in the USA) was probably 5%; long-term success rates for smoking cessation clinics are of the order of 15–20% (perhaps higher if supplemented by prescription of nicotine chewing gum); face-to-face behaviour modification methods utilized by Best achieved 50% at six months. By these criteria the 17.6% achieved by his television programmes are good. In terms of cost-effectiveness, he calculated that the face-to-face method cost $200 per success; smoking clinics cost $250 or more while, because of the large audience reached by media, the television series cost some $48 per documented abstinence (at six months).

One final point will be made about the use of mass media and smoking prevention. While it is clear that education about smoking generally and education delivered by mass media in particular are undoubtedly more effective than alcohol education, we should bear in mind Wallack's observations about the importance of structural–social change in supporting education. Engleman [131] describes this synergism between publicity, education and legal/fiscal measures in influencing smoking rates. He argues that not only has education itself had an impact on smoking, but it has also been responsible for such increases in taxation on cigarettes as have been imposed in recent years. He refers to the USA and argues that had it not been for the first Surgeon General's Report in 1964 and the subsequent education and publicity, smoking would have been 22% greater than it was in 1975. Since that time the reductions have continued – although it seems likely that as we move into the asymptote, further progress will be increasingly difficult and mass media will have an increasing role to play in stimulating policy change rather than persuading individuals to quit. At the same time the main thrust of smoking education must be targetted on young people – mainly in the schools and utilizing appropriate interpersonal educational strategies.

Because of the controversial nature of mass media, this chapter has looked in some depth at the issues involved and the requirements of effective media work. The conclusion to be drawn is that mass media can serve a very useful purpose in health education when properly designed and when their inherent limitations are recognized. In general, greater success will be achieved when mass media are used in support of community-wide programmes – a point which will receive reinforcement when we consider the various heart health programmes in the final chapter. Before doing this we will give a rather less extensive review of a strategy which is increasing in popularity and which has peculiar features of interest. This strategy concerns the delivery of health education in the workplace.

REFERENCES

1. Rhodes, A. (1976) *Propaganda: the Art of Persuasion, World War II*, Angus and Robertson, London.
2. De Tocqueville, A. (1961) *Democracy in America*, Schocken Books, New York, (p. 134), cited by Paisley, W. J. (1981) Public communications campaigns: the

American experience, in: *Public Communication Campaigns*, (eds R. E. Rice and W. J. Paisley), Sage Publications, Beverley Hills.

3. Tones, B. K. (1981) The use and abuse of mass media in health promotion, in: *Health Education and The Media*, (eds D. S. Leathar, G. B. Hastings and J. K. Davies) Pergamon, London.

4. McGuire, W. J. (1973) Persuasion, resistance and attitude change, in: *Handbook of Communication*, (eds I. De Sola Pool *et al.* Rand McNally, Skokie, Ill.

5. Evans, R. I., Rozelle, R. M. and Mittlemark, M. B. (1978) Deterring the onset of smoking in children. *Journal of Applied Social Psychology*, **8**, 126–35.

6. McAlister, A. and Hughes, M. (1979) Playing the (role) part, *Audio-Visual Communications*, **22**, 650–8.

7. McAlister, A. *et al.* (1980) Pilot study of smoking, alcohol and drug abuse prevention. *American Journal of Public Health*, **70**, 719–21.

8. Botvin, G. J. *et al.* (1984) A cognitive-behavioural approach to substance abuse prevention. *Addictive Behaviors*, **9**, 134–47.

9. Fuglesang, A. (1981) Folk media and folk messages, in: *Health Education by Television and Radio*, (ed. M. Meyer) KG Saur, München.

10. Douglas, T. (1984) *The Complete Guide to Advertising*, MacMillan, London.

11. Transport and Road Research Laboratory (1970) *Design of Road Safety Exhibitions*, Leaflet SRU 6, May, 1970.

12. Budd, J. and McCron, R. (1979) *Communication and Health Education, A Preliminary Study*, Health Education Council, London.

13. Kerr, M. and Charles, N. (1983) *Attitudes to the Feeding and Nutrition of Young Children*, Health Education Council, London.

14. Cantril, H. (1958) The invasion from Mars, in: *Readings in Social Psychology*, (eds E. E. Maccoby, T. M. Newcomb and E. L. Hartley) Henry Holt, New York, pp. 291–300.

15. Wellings, K. (1986) Help or hype: an analysis of media coverage of the 1983 'pill scare', in: *Health Education and the Media II*, (eds D. S. Leathar *et al.*) Pergamon, London.

16. Best, G., Dennis, J. and Draper, P. (1977) *Health, the Mass Media and the National Health Service*, Unit for the Study of Health Policy, London.

17. Hansen, A. (1986) The portrayal of alcohol on television, *Health Education Journal*, **45**, 127–31.

18. Institute for Alcohol Studies (1985) *The Presentation of Alcohol in the Mass Media*, Report of a Seminar, January 1985. Institute for Alcohol Studies, 12 Caxton Street, London.

19. Henry, H. W. and Waterson, M. J. (1981) The case for advertising alcohol and tobacco products, in: *Health Education and the Media*, (eds D. S. Leathar *et al.*) Pergamon, London.

20. Piepe, A. *et al.* (1986) Does sponsored sport lead to smoking among children? *Health Education Journal*, **45**, 145–8.

21. Chapman, S. and Fitzgerald, B. (1982) Brand preference and advertising recall in adolescent smokers: some implications for health promotion. *American Journal of Public Heath*, **72**, 491–4.

22. Charlton, A. (1986) Children's advertisement-awareness related to their views on smoking. *Health Education Journal*, **45**, 75–8.

23. Aitken, P. P., Leathar, D. S., O'Hagan, F. J. and Squair, S. I. (1987) Children's awareness of cigarette advertisements and brand imagery, *British Journal of Addiction*, **82**, 615–22.

24. Katz, E. and Lazarsfeld, P. (1955) *Personal Influence: the Part Played by People in the Flow of Mass Communication*, Free Press, Glencoe, Ill.

25. Lazarsfeld, P. F. and Merton, R. K. (1975) Mass communication, popular taste and organised social action, in: *Mass Communications*, (ed. W. Schramm) University of Illinois Press, Urbana, Ill.

26. Klapper, J. T. (1960) *The Effects of Mass Communication*, Free Press, Glencoe, Ill.

27. Wallach, L. M. (1980) *Mass Media Campaigns: the Odds Against Finding Behavior Change*, University of California Social Research Group, School of Public Health, Berkeley, Ca.

28. Mendelsohn, H. (1968) Which shall it be: mass education or mass persuasion for health? *American Journal of Public Health*, **58**, 131–7.

29. Mendelsohn, H. (1980) *Comments on the Relevance of Empirical Research as a Basis for Public Education Strategies in the Area of Alcohol Consumption*, Dept. of Mass Communication, University of Denver.

30. Dorn, N. and South, N. (1983) *Message in a Bottle*, Gower, Aldershot, Hants.

31. Dorn, N. (1981) Communication with the working class requires recognition of a working class: a materialist approach, in: *Health Education and the Media*, (eds D. S. Leathar *et al.*), Pergamon, London.

32. Ball-Rokeach, S. J. and De Fleur, M. L. (1976) A dependency model of mass media effects. *Communication Research*, **3**, 3–21.

33. McKinlay, J. B. (1979) A case for refocussing upsteam: the political economy of illness, in: *Patients, Physicians and Illness*, (ed. E. G. Jaco), Free Press, New York, p. 12.

34. Marsden, G. and Peterfreund, N. (1984) Marketing Public Health Services. *International Quarterly of Community Health Education*, **5**, 53–71.

35. Docherty, S. C. (1981) Sports sponsorship – a first step in marketing health? in: *Health Education and the Media*, (eds D. S. Leathar, *et al.*) Pergamon, London.

36. Player, D. A. (1986) Health promotion through sponsorship: the state of the art, in: *Health Education and the Media II*, (eds D. S. Leathar *et al.*), Pergamon, London.

37. Bonaguro, J. A. and Miaoulis, G. (1983) Marketing – a tool for health education planning, *Health Education*, January/February, 1983, 6–11.

38. Lovelock, C. H. (1977) Concepts and strategies for health marketers. *Hospital and Health Services Administration*, Fall, 1977, 50–63.

39. Kotler, P. (1975) *Marketing for Non-Profit Organizations*, Prentice Hall, New York.

40. Zaltman, G., Kotler, P. and Kaufman, I. (eds) (1972) *Creating Social Change*, Holt Rinehart and Winston, New York.

41. Solomon, D. S. (1981) A social marketing perspective on campaigns, in: *Public Communication Campaigns*, (eds R. E. Rice and W. J. Paisley), Sage, Beverly Hills.

42. McCron, R. and Budd, J. (1987) Mass communication and health education, in: *Health Education: Perspectives and Choices* (2nd ed.), (ed. I. Sutherland), National Extension College, Cambridge.

43. McGuire, W. J. (1981) Theoretical foundations of campaigns, in: *Public*

Communication Campaigns (eds R. E. Rice and W. J. Paisley), Sage Publications, Beverly Hills, California.

44. Stein, J. A. (1986) The cancer information service: marketing a large-scale national information program through media, in: *Media in Health Education II*, (eds D. S. Leathar *et al.*) Pergamon, London.

45. Mendelsohn, H. (1986) Lessons from a national media prevention campaign, in: *Health Education and the Media* (eds D. S. Leathar, G. B. Hastings and J. K. Davies), Pergamon, London.

46. Lavigne, A. S., Albert, W. and Simmons, M. (1986) The Application of Market Segmentation in Alcohol and Drug Education: the APPLAUSE project, in: *Health Education and the Media* (eds D. S. Leathar, G. B. Hastings and J. K. Davies), Pergamon, London.

47. Chesterfield-Evans, A. and O'Connor, G. (1986) Billboard utilizing graffitists against unhealthy promotions (BUGAP) – its philosophy and rationale and their application in health promotion, in: *Health Education and the Media* (eds D. S. Leathar, G. B. Hastings and J. K. Davies), Pergamon, London.

48. Chapman, S. (1986) *The lung goodbye: a manual of tactics for counteracting the tobacco industry in the 1980s* (2nd ed.), International Organization of Consumers' Unions, The Hague, Netherlands.

49. Albert, W. H. (1981) General models of persuasive influence for health education, in: *Health Education and the Media* (eds D. S. Leathar, G. B. Hastings and J. K. Davies), Pergamon, London.

50. Flay, B. R. (1981) On improving the chances of mass media health promotion programs causing meaningful changes in behavior, in: *Health Education by Television and Radio* (ed. M. Meyer), K. G. Saur, München.

51. Chaffee, S. (1981) Mass media in political campaigns: an expanding role, in: *Public Communication Campaigns* (eds. R. E. Rice and W. J. Paisley), Sage Publications, Beverley Hills, California.

52. Liu, A. P. (1981) Mass campaigns in the People's Republic of China, in: *Public Communication Campaigns* (eds R. E. Rice and W. J. Paisley), Sage Publications, Beverley Hills, California.

53. Flay, B. R. *et al.* (1986) Reaching children with mass media health promotion programs: the relative effectiveness of an advertising campaign in a community-based program and a school-based program, in: *Health Education and the Media* (eds D. S. Leathar, G. B. Hastings and J. K. Davies), Pergamon, London.

54. Flay, B. R. *et al.* (1987) Implementation effectiveness trial of a social influences smoking prevention programme using schools and television, *Health Education Research*, 2, 385–400.

55. Palmer, E. (1981) Shaping persuasive messages with formative research, in: *Public Communication Campaigns* (eds R. E. Rice and W. J. Paisley), Sage Publications, Beverley Hills, California.

56. Romano, R. (1985) Pre-testing smoking messages, in: *Smoking Control*, (eds J. Crofton and M. Wood), Health Education Council, London.

57. Romano, R. (1984) *Pre-testing in Health Communications*, National Cancer Institute, Bethesda, Maryland.

58. Romano, R. (1984) *Making PSAs Work*, National Cancer Institute, Bethesda, Maryland.

59. Leathar, D. S. (1980) Defence inducing advertising, in: *Taking Stock: What Have*

We Learned and Where Are We Going? Procedings of the ESOMAR Conference, Monte Carlo, September, 1980, pp. 153–73.

60. Player, D. A. and Leathar, D. S. (1981) Developing socially sensitive advertising, in: *Health Education and the Media* (eds D. S. Leathar, G. B. Hastings and J. K. Davies), Pergamon, London.

61. Davison, R. L. (1983) Questions about cancer: the public's demand for information. *Journal of the Institute of Health Education*, **21**, 5–16.

62. Redman, B. K. (1984) *The Process of Patient Education*, (Chapter 7), CV Mosby, St Louis, Toronto.

63. Hartley, J. (ed) (1980) *The Psychology of Written Communication*, (Part 3), Kogan Page, London.

64. Dale, E. and Chall, J. A. (1948) A formula for predicting readability: instructions. *Education Research Bulletin*, **27**, No. 37.

65. Holcomb, C. and Ellis, J. (1978) Measuring the readability of selected patient education materials: the Cloze Procedure. *Health Education*, **9**, 8.

66. Flesch, R. (1948) A new readability yardstick. *Journal of Applied Psychology*, **32**, 221.

67. Harrison, C. (1980) *Readability in Classrooms*, University Press, Cambridge.

68. McLaughlin, G. (1969) SMOG grading: a new readability formula. *Journal of Reading*, **12**, 639.

69. Pichert, J. W. and Elam, P. (1985) Readability formulas may mislead you. *Patient Education and Counselling*, **7**, 181–91.

70. Gatherer, A., Parfit, J., Porter, E. and Vessey, M. (1979) *Is Health Education Effective?* Health Education Council, London.

71. Atkin, C. K. (1981) Mass media information campaign effectiveness, in: *Public Communication Campaigns* (eds R. E. Rice and W. J. Paisley), Sage Publications, Beverley Hills, California.

72. Greenberg, B. S. and Gantz, W. (1976) Public television and taboo topics: the impact of 'VD Blues'. *Public Telecommunications Review*, **4**, 59–64.

73. Mendelsohn, H. (1973) Some reasons why information campaigns can succeed. *Public Information Quarterly*, **37**, 50–61.

74. Farhar-Pilgrim, B. and Shoemaker, F. F. (1981) Campaigns to affect energy behavior, in: *Public Communication Campaigns* (eds R. E. Rice and W. J. Paisley), Sage Publications, Beverley Hills, California.

75. Bell, J. *et al.* (1985) *Annotated Bibliography of Health Education Research Completed in Britain from 1948–1978 and 1979–1983*, Scottish Health Education Group, Edinburgh.

76. Dunnigan, M. G. *et al.* (1981) Policy for the prevention of asian rickets in Britain: a preliminary assessment of the Glasgow rickets campaign. *British Medical Journal*, **282**, 357–60.

77. England, P. M. and Oxley, D. E. (1980) Head infestation in Humberside: a health control exercise. *Health Education Journal*, **39**, 23–5.

78. Hutchinson, A. and Thompson, J. (1982) Rubella prevention: two methods compared. *British Medical Journal*, **284**, 1087–9.

79. Rogers, R. S. (1973) The effects of televised sex education at the primary school level. *Health Education Journal*, **32**, 87–93.

80. McCron, R. and Dean, E. (1983) *Well Being – An Evaluation*, Channel 4 Television Broadcast Support Services, London.

81. Gordon, E. (1967) Evaluation of communications media in two health projects in Baltimore. *Public Health Reports*, **82**, 651–5.
82. Ajit, T. C. (1982) A life worth living. *Public Relations*, Winter, 1982, 3–5.
83. Jenkins, J. (1983) *Mass Media for Health Education*, International Extension College, Cambridge.
84. Taplin, S. (1981) Family planning campaigns, in: *Public Communication Campaign*, (eds R. E. Rice and W. J. Paisley), Sage Publications, Beverley Hills, California.
85. Cernada, G. P. and Lu, L. P. (1982) The *Kaohsiung Study, Studies in Family Planning*, **3**, 198–203.
86. Smith, W. (1978) *Campaigning for Choice; Family Planning Association Project Report No. 1*, Family Planning Association, London.
87. Leslie, J. (1981) Evaluation of mass media for health and nutrition education, in: *Health Education by Television and Radio* (ed. M. Meyer), K. G. Sauer, München.
88. Burt, A. *et al.* (1974) Stopping smoking after myocardial infarction, *Lancet*, i, 304–6.
89. Tapper-Jones, L. and Harvard Davis, R. (1985) *A Project to Develop Publications to Support Health Education Within the General Practice Consultation*, Health Education Council, London.
90. Spencer, J. (1984) *General Practitioners' Views of the 'Give Up Smoking (GUS) Kit'*, Health Education Council, London.
91. Grant, A. S. (1972) What's the use of posters? *Journal of the Institute of Health Education*, **10**, 7–11.
92. Cole, R. and Holland, S. (1980) Recall of health education display materials. *Health Education Journal*, **39**, 74–9.
93. Auger, T. J., Wright, T. J. and Simpson, R. H. (1972) Posters as smoking deterrents. *Journal of Applied Psychology*, **56**, 169–71.
94. Transport and Road Research Laboratory (1967 and 1972) *Testing a Children's Poster* (Report SRU 2), and *Improving Driving by the Use of Posters Beside Roads* (Report SRU 28), TRRL, Crowthorne, Berkshire.
95. British Broadcasting Corporation (1982) *'Play It Safe': Child Accident Prevention Campaign*, BBC Broadcasting Research Special Report, November, 1982, BBC London.
96. Jackson, R. H. (1983) 'Play It Safe': a campaign for the prevention of children's accidents, *Community Development Journal*, **18**, 172–6.
97. Colver, A. P., Hutchinson, P. J. and Judson, E. C. (1982) Promoting children's home safety, *British Medical Journal*, **285**, 1177–80.
98. Harris, J. (1983) *Interpretive Summary of Hypothermia Campaign Evaluations, Winter of 1982/3*, Health Education Council, London.
99. Levens, G. E. and Rodnight, E. (1973) *The Application of Research in the Planning and Evaluation of Road Safety Publicity*, Proceedings of the European Society for Opinion in Marketing (Budapest) Conference, pp. 197–227.
100. Gemming, M. G., Runyan, C. W. and Campbell, B. J. (1984) A community health education approach to occupant protection. *Health Education Quarterly*, **11**, 147–58.
101. Tones, B. K. (1986) Preventing drug misuse: the case for breadth, balance and coherence, *Health Education Journal*, **45**, 223–30.
102. Kinder, B. N. (1975) Attitudes toward alcohol and drug abuse: experimental

data, mass media research and methodological considerations. *International Journal of Addictions*, **10**, 1035–54.

103. Blane, H. T. and Hewitt, L. E. (1977) *Mass Media, Public Education and Alcohol: a State-of-the-Art Review*, National Institute on Alcohol Abuse and Alcoholism, Rockville, Maryland.

104. Blane, H. T. and Hewitt, L. E. (1980) Alcohol, public education and mass media: an overview, *Alcohol, Health and Research World*, **5**, 2–16.

105. Block, M. (1965) *Alcoholism: Its Facets and Phases*, University Press, Oxford.

106. Breed, W. and Defoe, J. R. (1978) Bringing alcohol into the open, *Columbia Journalism Review*, **18**, 18–19.

107. Breed, W. and Defoe, J. R. (1979) Drinking on television: a comparison of alcohol use to the use of coffee, tea, soft drinks, water and cigarettes. *The Bottom Line*, **2**, 28–9.

108. Breed, W. and Defoe, J. R. (1980) Mass media, alcohol and drugs: a new trend. *Journal of Drug Issues*, **9**, 511–22.

109. Breed, W. and Defoe, J. R. (1979) Themes in magazine alcohol advertisements: a critique. *Journal of Drug Issues*, **9**, 511–22.

110. Breed, W. and Defoe, J. R. (1980) The mass media and alcohol education: a new direction. *Journal of Alcohol and Drug Education*, **25**, 48–58.

111. Breed, W. and Defoe, J. R. (1981) The portrayal of the drinking process on prime-time television. *Journal of Communication*, **31**, 48–58.

112. Gerbner, G. *et al.* (1981) Health and medicine on television – special report. *New England Journal of Medicine*, **305**, 90–4.

113. King, R. (1979) Drinking and drunkenness in 'Crossroads' and 'Coronation Street', in: *Images of Alcoholism*, (eds J. Cook and M. Lewington) British Film Institute, London.

114. Finn, P. (1980) Attitudes toward drinking conveyed in studio greeting cards. *American Journal of Public Health*, **70**, 826–9.

115. Caudill, B. D. and Marlatt, C. (1975) Modelling influences in social drinking: an experimental analogue. *Journal of Consulting and Clinical Psychology*, **43**, 405–15.

116. Garlington, W. and Dericco, D. (1979) The effect of modeling on drinking rate. *Journal of Applied Behavior Analysis*, **10**, 207–11.

117. Dembo, R., Miran, M., Babst, D. V. and Schmeidler, J. (1977) The believability of the media as sources of information on drugs. *International Journal of Addictions*, **12**, 959–69.

118. Brown, R. A. (1978) Educating young people about alcohol use in New Zealand: whose side are we on? *British Journal of Alcohol and Alcoholism*, **13**, 199–201.

119. Ogbourne, A. C. and Smart, R. G. (1980) Will restrictions on alcohol advertising reduce alcohol consumption? *British Journal of Addictions*, **75**, 293–6.

120. Bourgeois, J. C. and Barnes, J. G. (1979) Does advertising increase alcohol consumption? *Journal of Advertising Research*, **19**, 19–29.

121. Maloney, S. K. and Hersey, J. C. (1984) Getting messages on the air: findings from the 1982 alcohol abuse prevention campaign. *Health Education Quarterly*, **11**, 273–92.

122. Health Education Council (1983) *The Tyne-Tees Alcohol Education Campaign*, Health Education Council, London.

123. Health Education Council (1982) *Report of a Meeting held on 29th April, 1982: The Tyne-Tees Alcohol Education Campaign*, Health Education Council, London.

124. Wallack, L. and Barrows, D. C. (1983) Evaluating primary prevention: the California 'Winners' alcohol program, *International Quarterly of Community Health Education*, **3**, 307–36.

125. Reid, D. (1985) National No Smoking Day, in: *Smoking Control* (eds J. Crofton and M. Wood) Health Education Council, London.

126. Raw, M. and De Plight, J. V. (1981) Can television help people stop smoking? in: *Health Education and the Media* (eds D. S. Leathar, G. B. Hastings and J. K. Davies), Pergamon, London.

127. Cuckle, H. S. and Vunakis, H. V. (1984) The effectiveness of a postal smoking cessation kit. *Community Medicine*, **6**, 210–15.

128. O'Byrne, D. J. and Crawley, H. D. (1981) Conquest smoking cessation campaign 1980 – an evaluation, in: *Health Education and the Media* (eds D. S. Leathar, G. B. Hastings and J. K. Davies), Pergamon, London.

129. Puska, P. *et al.* (1979) A comprehensive television smoking cessation programme in Finland. *International Journal of Health Education*, Supplement to Vol. **XXII**, No. 4.

130. Best, J. A. (1980) Mass media, self-management and smoking modification, in: *Behavioral Medicine: Changing Health Lifestyles*, (eds P. O. Davidson and S. M. Davidson) Brunner/Mazel, New York.

131. Engleman, S. R. (1983) *The impact of anti-smoking mass media publicity*, Health Education Council, London.

132. Russell, M. A. H., Wilson, C., Taylor, C. and Baker, C. D. (1979) Effect of General Practitioner's advice against smoking, *British Medical Journal*, **2**, 231–5.

7

HEALTH PROMOTION
IN THE WORKPLACE

The workplace provides an interesting challenge to health educators – a challenge which has been accepted rather more readily in North America than in Europe. Knobel [1] has estimated that it is possible to reach 85% of the US population via the worksite and, for this reason alone, delivering health education to the workforce is of great strategic importance within the grand overall design of health promotion. Apart from this intrinsic merit, workplace health promotion has been included in the book because it exemplifies rather well two main propositions. First it illustrates conflicting philosophies rooted in the often different needs of key participants – workers and bosses. For management, success will normally be judged by hard economic indicators while for many radical health promoters, wellbeing may actually be incompatible with the profit motive! The workers' perceived needs are likely to be located somewhere between these two extremes.

Secondly, the workplace offers a tangible example of the ways in which success – however defined – is dependent on the synergy of individual behaviour and structural–organizational factors. For instance, smoking cessation programmes will be facilitated by a comprehensive workplace smoking policy. Similarly, the teaching of stress management skills without prior examination of the inherent stress-generating nature of work itself is neither efficient nor ethical.

This chapter will, therefore, seek to address the following questions: why deliver health education in the workplace? It is clearly assumed to be worthwhile (at least in North America!) – but who is the real beneficiary? What can we expect from work-based health promotion? How successful is it? What is its potential for enhancing wellbeing and preventing disease? What are its limitations?

In seeking to answer these questions we will need to consider two key issues: (i) the relationship between health and work; and (ii) the ways in which the different motives of the various actors in the workplace situation (management, workers, trades unionists, health professionals and health educators) relate to criteria for programme success. Having done this, we will consider worksite programmes by category in order to illuminate some of the philosophical differences dividing health education workers and to provide a

212

basis for a selective review of the extent of programme provision and effectiveness.

WORK AND HEALTH

The relationship between work and health is paradoxical. It stimulates vigorous debate and strikes a sensitive political nerve. On the one hand those of a Marxist persuasion may view work as a capitalist device to exploit the proletariat. At the risk of cheapening this point of view we might pose an oft-quoted rhetorical question: if work is so good, why don't the very wealthy do more of it? Bosquet [2] has expressed the point with some force:

> So deep is the frustration engendered by work that the incidence of heart attacks among manual workers is higher than that in any other stratum of society. People 'die from work' not because it is noxious or dangerous ... but because it is intrinsically 'killing'.

A more common (and better documented) standpoint is that unemployment rather than work is health-damaging. Indeed the evidence has been so extensively and comprehensively assembled and presented that the relationship between unemployment and mental, physical and social disease will be taken as axiomatic for present purposes. However, in terms of the models of health education outlined in Chapter One, both the above perspectives would favour a radical approach which sought to raise consciousness and stimulate social and political change in order to remedy what are viewed as serious social problems. Measures of success would, therefore, relate to the extent to which such social and political change actually occurs.

Less common but no less radical in its way is a third approach to the issue of health and work. It is concerned with the nature of work in a 'post-industrial society' [3] which is characterized by chronic unemployment, reduction of the working week, job-sharing, early retirement, part-time employment, and an increase in discretionary time and leisure. Preparation for a post-industrial society requires the same skills and competences needed to handle 'Future Shock' [4]. In other words the task of health and social education is not merely to provide an extensive preparation for greater leisure but will also involve fundamental questioning of the work ethic and the new, or rather re-discovered, enterprise culture. Since the futurologists' predictions of the nature of work will require a variety of social and personal skills associated with flexibility, resilience and proactivity, the appropriate health education model is that which develops self-empowered decision-making.

In the context of the hard and pragmatic concerns which are typically associated with workplace health promotion, the above approach might seem somewhat fanciful. However, the importance of considering fundamental questions of this kind was acknowledged by a conference on Health Promotion in the Working World organized by WHO [5]. This postulated several futuristic scenarios:

1. Business as usual. Assumes full employment will once again be achieved and this will be the predominant form of work with the associated consumption of goods and services and the centrality of paid work to individual self-esteem.
2. Hyper-expansionist. Postulates chronic unemployment as described earlier. Society will consist of two groups – employed and unemployed. The former will consist of a cadre of elite professionals using capital-intensive technology.
3. Sane, humane, ecological. Again, assumes chronic unemployment but posits a radical change in values which allows other useful activities to receive appropriate recognition and payment in addition to traditional paid work. Paid and unpaid work will be equally divided between men and women. Households and neighbourhoods will be the workplaces and production centres in society.
4. Variations on some of these themes were also proposed including 'Eco-Utopia' (small decentralized, self-sufficient eco settlements) and 'Findhorn' (characterized by spirituality and inner growth). By contrast 'Chinatown' postulated a population explosion with multimillion metropolises; alternatively the 'Dallas' scenario predicted a Western-dominated competitive Darwinistic imperialism – in which, presumably, the North American rationale for worksite health promotion would be even more popular!

Returning to the present, the more conventional analysis of work and health sees the workplace as a source of pathogens of one kind or another ranging from general work-produced stress to specific industrial hazards such as accidents, cancers and the like. Stress is of particular interest because it illustrates so well the conflicting perspectives of more radical health educators and the employers whom they accuse of 'victim-blaming'. The number of identified work stressors is legion. The World Health Organization [5] lists poor physical working conditions, shift work, job over-load and job under-load, role conflict, role insecurity, promotion blockage, two-career families, lack of opportunity for participation in decision-making, etc.

A more recent study by Braun and Hollander [6] examined job stress among employees in the Federal Republic of Germany. They showed that high job demands and low job decision latitude were related to stress. The study implications could be either to teach stress management skills or to alter the structure of the work situation. Although not in principle incompatible, the choice of one or other of these alternatives is, as we shall see, likely to reveal ideological differences in approach to workplace health promotion. A successful 'victim-blaming' strategy would be revealed by the acquisition of, say, relaxation skills or a reduced level of stress on an appropriate scale; the success of a more radical approach would be measured by actual environmental changes or intermediate indicators of progress towards such change.

DIFFERENT PERSPECTIVES ON SUCCESS

As will have been apparent from the discussion of health and work, successful worksite health promotion will be interpreted differently by the various actors: academics, futurologists, community physicians, public health workers and social scientists will have different value systems from employers and workers – although doubtless common ground exists. The health educator's perspective may well be dominated by the prospect of gaining access to a substantial proportion of the adult population. The choice of strategies will in part be dictated by the two principles of access and availability of skilled and credible health educators. Access to a generally hard-to-reach population is an outstanding feature of the workplace. It has been estimated in the USA that some 85% of the population may be contacted in this way – a proportion which compares very favourably with the 75% contact which the practice population has with general practitioner every three years and the 15 000 hours spent by students in school. The question of credibility and competence is, however, a different matter. Logically we would look to the occupational health service to deliver health education but this, of course, depends on the existence of such a service! McEwan [7] noted that in 1977 about '... 85% of all firms (in the UK), employing about 34% of the workforce, had no occupational health service other than first-aiders employed less than ten hours a week ...'. Buck [8], after a small-scale survey of firms in a district health authority in northern England, was more optimistic. Occupational health staff reported that their two most frequent types of health work were first, treatment and second, environmental visiting. Fifty-five of the 59 respondents recognized the existence of opportunities for health education in the treatment situation and 29 commented that opportunities arose 'often' or 'sometimes' in their visits to the working environment. Clearly recognition of opportunity did not mean that they actually took advantage of the situation to provide health education. Moreover since the response rate was only 47% it would not be unreasonable to expect a distinct lack of commitment in the non-respondents!

A national survey in the USA by Vojtecky *et al.* [9] provides a useful indication of the involvement of occupational health services in health promotion. A sample of 1953 was drawn from a sampling frame of 11 000 occupational health professionals. Again there was a low response rate of 34% so observations should be treated with caution. Five categories of health professional were identified: industrial hygienists, doctors, nurses, health educators and others. The proportion of total work time which the groups claimed to spend on health education was respectively, 33%; 22%; 38%; 89% and 23%. Major programme categories were health promotion, accident prevention and hazard protection. The proportion of each professional group having involvement with broader health promotion work ranged from 31% (industrial hygienists) to 98% (nurses). A wide range of teaching methods were used with the health educators using the broadest spectrum (50% using 10 of 13 listed methods). Interestingly, when the groups were asked to say whether their objectives were primarily changes in knowledge, attitude or practice, it was the health educator group which seemed more determined to change behaviours (80%) whereas 50% of nurses were concerned only to provide knowledge. Whether this indicates a difference in philosophy or whether nurses tended to assume that knowledge would automatically lead to behaviour change is not clear. Notwithstanding the relatively small response rate, the situation appears distinctly more healthy than in Europe – although the researchers lament the fact that only 62% of the occupational health professionals delivering health education had had any specific training in doing so.

THE MANAGEMENT PERSPECTIVE

The motivation of managers in respect of workplace health promotion may be summarized in three words: economic self interest. This viewpoint is sharply illustrated by a comment attributed to Xerox top management that the loss of one executive from preventible illness would cost the organization $600 000 [10]. It should be noted that the received wisdom that health promotion in the worksite will in fact save money has not gone unchallenged. Walsh [11] cites three sceptics [12, 13, 14] in her own critique of workplace programmes. Nonetheless the general feeling appears to be that appropriate educational and promotion programmes will result in increased productivity and sales and generate a reduction in costs. The rationale for these programmes in terms of productivity and cost reduction is summarized in Table 7.1.

Clearly some of these arguments are peculiar to the US health care delivery system with its emphasis on private health insurance. We are reminded, however, of the significance of these costs by Alexander [16]:

> During the past decade, large corporations have become increasingly concerned that providing health care benefits no longer constitutes an incidental cost of doing business. In 1961, such benefits were 25.5% of payroll. By 1981, they were 41.2%. Between 1978 and 1980 corporate health insurance premiums escalated markedly from $43 billion to $63 billion. The most notable impact on the manufacturing sector was documented for General Motors, which in 1977 was believed to have

Table 7.1 A summary of the main benefits of worksite health promotion programmes in North America in relation to productivity and cost reduction

Increased productivity
1. Reduction in sickness absence
2. Reduced absenteeism
3. Increase in worker morale
4. Presentation of a good corporate image★
5. Attracting competent staff in a competitive market situation

Reduction in costs
1. Decrease in accidents and associated compensation claims
2. Decline in health insurance costs as a result of lower demand for in-patient care, reduced treatment costs and fewer disability and death benefits
3. Decline in staff replacement and training costs as a result of lower staff turnover

★ According to Conrad [15] this desirable image is acquired by 'capitalizing on cultural wellness'!

added $176 to the cost of every car and truck to offset the $825 million it spent during the same year for employee benefits. A recent survey of a sample of Fortune 500 companies and the largest 250 industrials suggested that health insurance costs will equal profits after taxes in about 8 years.

The attractiveness of an effective health promotion service – and the victim-blaming nature of the programmes become understandable in the light of these statistics. The economic motivation of managers is thus hardly surprising – and is supported by Davis *et al.*'s [17] investigation of worksite health promotion in Colorado. Companies surveyed which had established programmes were asked to provide reasons for having started health promotion activities; companies interested in starting were also asked to indicate their motivation for so doing. Survey results are shown in Table 7.2. The economic motivation underlying decisions is self-evident – particularly for those companies contemplating adoption.

THE WORKER PERSPECTIVE

The worker perspective has probably received less consideration than that of management – presumably because of an assumption that workers might welcome interventions designed to enhance their wellbeing whereas managers would have to be subjected to a 'sales pitch'. It is doubtless true that trades union will welcome moves which can be shown to be for their members' benefit and workers will respond to the same initiatives – particularly if these happen in 'management time'! Several studies in North America have sought to ascertain the reasons for worker participation. For example Conrad [18]

Table 7.2 Reasons given by companies for starting health promotion and disease prevention programmes (from Davis *et al.* [17])

Reason	Companies with existing programmes (%)	Companies interested in starting programmes (%)
To improve health and reduce health problems	82	68
To improve employee morale	59	52
To reduce health care costs	57	67
To reduce turnover and absenteeism	51	57
To improve productivity	50	64
Response to employee demand or interest	33	20
To be part of innovative trend	32	11
To improve public image	20	18

identified a major concern with fitness and weight control. Spilman [19] noted gender differences in motivation which were consistent with generally recognized views about women's health – for instance, a general high participation rate, concern with weight loss for cosmetic reasons, concern with their nurturant roles as unpaid family health care workers. Kotarba and Bentley [20] described motivation to participate in a workplace wellness programme in terms of either a '... commitment to wellness, or as a vehicle for experimenting with or establishing a new style of self, the identity of a 'well person' so highly valued in contemporary western culture.' This latter observation will serve as a cautionary note: worker motivation is clearly culture-bound and will reflect general health norms. There can be no guarantee that the UK workforce will identify with the North American healthist pursuit of 'high level wellness'! Indeed suspicion about management motives might well predominate. Moreover in the context of our earlier discussion of health and work, the workforce in Britain is more likely to be concerned about unemployment than even exposure to hazardous substances let alone participation in the pursuit of fitness in order to reduce management overheads!

TYPES OF WORKSITE PROGRAMME

Before commenting on the relative effectiveness of health promotion in the workplace, it is as well to consider the variety of activity incorporated under the general rubric and examine the main sources of controversy generated by certain of these activities. The definition of workplace health promotion is in no way esoteric. Parkinson [21] refers to a '... combination of educational, organizational and environmental activities designed to support behaviour conducive to the health of employees and their families.' (Cited by Conrad [15]). Davis *et al.* [17] provide an operational definition in their criteria for deciding whether or not a given firm had a health promotion programme. 'A company was considered to have a HPDP (health promotion and disease prevention) programme if it provided health screenings, classes or preventive health services on an ongoing basis.' The philosophical basis which determines evaluative criteria, however, is less readily handled.

Alexander [16] in an article on the 'ideological construction of risk' points out this philosophical underpinning. Not only is health promotion predicated on a need by '... the American state and almost all sectors of capital to curtail their share of the social wage ..', but '... corporate managers choose selectively from a body of theoretical knowledge regarding illness and disease etiology in a way that restores sanctity to the individual, eschews history and social complexity and legitimates existing social relations.' No apology is made for making a further reference to the inherent tendency for workplace health promotion to focus on the individual at the expense of general social structures and particular organizational influences on health and illness. McEwan [7] is also concerned to make this point and cites Navarro [22] who not only asserted the economic and political etiology of alienation of the individual in society, occupational diseases generally and cancer in particular, but also pointed out how the power balance in western industrialized society inevitably favours the individualistic approach of traditional health education.

> ... one of today's most active state policies at the central government level in most Western capitalist countries is to encourage and stimulate these health programs, such as health education, that are aimed at bringing about changes in the individual but not in the economic or political environment.
>
> It is interesting to note that while much of the disease affecting the working class in Engel's time was supposedly due to the poor moral fibre of the workmen and their families, today the poor health conditions of that class and the majority of the population are assumed to be due to the lack of concern for their own health and their poor health education. In both cases, the solution to our public lack of health is *individual* prevention and *individual* therapy.

Walsh [11] notes the 'healthist' aspect of the American fitness programmes. 'Could it be', she asks, 'that health promotion is a lifestyle enclave in the worksite and if so is it deflecting energy from collective efforts to improve the quality of worklife for all?' Gordon [23] also notes the victim-blaming tendency but in addition comments on the possibility of ethical difficulties relating to confidentiality and trust in work-based medical practitioners and, more importantly for our purpose here, the intrinsic tendency to exert explicit or implicit pressure on workers to participate in health promotion programmes. Such coercion – however benevolent – together with an associated 'top-down' approach, is not only inconsistent with WHO's principles of health promotion but militates against the spirit of the British Health and Safety at Work Act (1974) which emphasizes responsibility, self-regulation and participation – all of which processes are consistent with WHO's view of health promotion. However, let us turn now to a categorization of major kinds of work-related health promotion programmes.

Consistent with the earlier discussion of health and work, we might usefully identify a variety of programme which is concerned to educate about work. Perhaps the best recognized of these has a radical intent and is concerned to raise critical consciousness about working conditions either in a specific workplace or in a particular category of workplace – for example, chemical industries. Freudenberg's [24] description of attempts to activate the workforce and pressurize employers to provide a healthier environment and compensate workers for industrial diseases illustrates this approach nicely.

Education about work is also an integral part of personal and social education and includes vocational guidance and career choice. Many programmes would also seek to have students think critically about workplace conditions and the implications, say, of working on an assembly line for health and wellbeing. The underlying rationale is one of fostering self-empowerment choice.

Education designed to empower the workforce is relatively rare – for obvious reasons! It is, therefore, worth reporting on a Canadian mental health initiative [25]. The Mental Health and the Workplace Project is unusual in that it acknowledges the importance of environmental variables both within and without the workplace. The programme philosophy is fundamentally concerned with self-empowerment. Novick, chairperson of the project, describes a 'New Work Agenda into the Nineties' based on the following assumptions:

1. Employment is a form of work which is done for remuneration as well as for psychological and social benefits.
2. Persistently high levels of unemployment are detrimental to the health and well-being of Canadian citizens and are an unacceptable waste of human resources.
3. A lack of more secure, stable, quality employment opportunities is increasing the stress and anxiety of working Canadians.

It acknowledges the 'future shock scenario', noting that groups '... previously excluded or only marginally employed (e.g. women, youth, disabled people) are making their claim for fair access to the workplace'. Wide income disparities between high paid and low paid workers and the polarization between a low skilled underclass and a high skilled elite must be taken into account by a programme concerned to educate about work. The importance of balancing employment with family life, life in the community and personal development must be recognized.

Six propositions are finally made by Novick [25]:

1. Employment should be structured and organized in ways that are compatible with and reinforcing to the quality of Canadian family life.
2. Working life should include opportunities for continuing learning for job advancement, work skill development, retirement and general personal betterment.
3. There should be recognition of the importance of alternative forms of work, such as household, voluntarism, recreational and cultural activities as well as paid forms of work.
4. All Canadians should have access to a fair share of meaningful and dignifying employment during their adult lives.
5. People should have more worklife choices in terms of how they arrange their employment time weekly, monthly and yearly in order to complement other pursuits and interests which they have.
6. Real worklife choices must entail provisions for both income security and employment stability within a framework for economic renewal.

The approach of 'Worklife Education' is perhaps summarized in the view that, 'The workplace is a community. All of its members should be empowered to care better for themselves and for each other.' This self-empowerment approach is substantially different in emphasis from mainstream workplace programmes in which disease prevention and health protection provide the main justification for intervention (with or without the cost-benefit implication).

The next category for consideration is, then, that which embodies traditional health and safety goals. It is concerned to identify and educate those at high risk – either for personal health problems such as coronary heart disease (CHD) or in the context of a specific occupation. More recently, broader-based health promotion programmes have focused on general health and fitness. All three approaches are consistent with agreed goals of an occupational health service as McEwan [7] points out in these terms:

1. Protecting the workers against any health hazard which may arise out of their work or the conditions in which it is carried on;
2. Contributing towards the workers' physical and mental adjustment, in particular by the adaptation of the work to the worker and their assignment of jobs for which they are suited;
3. Contributing to the establishment and maintenance of the highest possible degree of physical and mental well-being of the workers.

Examples of these programmes are readily available. For instance Ippolito-Shepherd *et al.* [26] describe an agricultural occupational health education programme in Latin America; Schenk *et al.* [27] present results of research into rubber industry workers' beliefs and attitudes about safety which might be used to devise risk reduction health education interventions. In the UK a general health and fitness programme originally developed by the Health Education Council for adult learners has been translated into the workplace. This 'Look After Yourself' (LAY) programme involves teaching about exercise, relaxation, healthy eating and other lifestyle health factors [28]. It is made available to the workplace on request; its goal is to train tutors within the work situation so that the programme becomes routinized. Although not substantially different from worksite health promotion in general, there is one well recognized category of intervention which merits separate consideration.

Although there is considerable overlap between the two, health promotion programmes may be distinguished from one well recognized category of worksite intervention – particularly in North America. This category is usually referred to as an Employee Assistance Programme (EAP). Roman and Blum [29] provide a useful comparison between EAPs and Health Promotion Programmes (HPPs). They offer two definitions of EAPs:

> ... mechanisms to increase the chances for continued employment of individuals whose job performance and personal functioning are adversely impacted by problems of substance abuse, psychiatric illness, family difficulties or other personal problems.

> (Roman and Blum [30])

> ... job-based programs operating within a work organization for purposes of identifying 'troubled employees', motivating them to resolve their troubles, and providing access to counselling or treatment for those employees who need these services.

> (Sonnenstuhl and Trice [31])

It is immediately clear from these definitions that EAPs are concerned with secondary prevention whereas other health promotion programmes would tend to focus on primary prevention. Roman and Blum also observe that whereas trades unions (in the USA) are probably suspicious of HPPs, they almost unanimously support EAPs. They, additionally, note that both HPPs and EAPs are 'mission-driven' ('The zealotry that accompanies many HPPs is often matched by the zeal with which EAP practitioners view the urgency of recovery from alcoholism..')! A key difference between both types of programme centres on the potential stigma associated with EAPs compared with HPPs. Clearly EAPs require confidentiality and a conviction by workforce and unions that admitting to problems will not lead to job loss. This latter point is of especial importance for the implementation of alcohol policies in the workplace. Indeed the development of worksite policies may be considered a separate category of health promotion exercise – at least in the UK.

HEALTH POLICIES IN THE WORKPLACE

The notion of a health policy is of particular importance in any discussion of health promotion. Indeed, as has been noted on more than one occasion, health promotion is usefully defined as a combination of education and policy. A prerequisite for a maximally effective intervention is the existence of an appropriate environment, and the establishment of a policy centres on the creation of such an environment in conjunction with various kinds of health education. Typically policy development has centred on alcohol, smoking, fitness and nutrition (often in the context of preventing CHD) and, less often, stress reduction. The elements of a workplace smoking policy will be briefly adumbrated below prior to considering implications for indicators of effectiveness (for further details see Jenkins *et al.* [32]).

First, a smoking policy would have the following environmental goals: a ban on smoking in areas where special safety or health hazards exist; at least 50% of cafeteria areas would be designated non-smoking provided that smoke did not affect the non-smoking zone; all common areas would be non-smoking; smoking areas would be provided for smokers; smoking cessation facilities would also be made available. Appropriate signs would be displayed; information would be disseminated to the management and workforce; the policy would apply to all members of staff; there would be no discrimination against anyone exercising their rights under the policy.

Secondly, generally agreed steps are involved in implementing policy as follows:

1. Establishment of a working party;
2. Definition of objectives;
3. Survey of employee attitudes and request for suggestions for policy implementation;
4. Construction of draft policy;
5. Consultation exercise;
6. Adoption of agreed policy by senior management; and
7. Implementation
   (a) Creation of non-smoking environment
   (b) Provision of help for smokers
   (c) Institution of measures for policing and maintaining policy provisions.

IMPLICATIONS FOR EVALUATION MEASURES

Evaluation measures for policy development are simple to define. In terms of outcome, success would be determined by the extent to which the various environmental goals listed above had been achieved. In relation to process evaluation, the seven implementation steps would be monitored and the illumination thus gained would be used to enhance efficiency and ensure steady progress to the next stage.

In the more general context, success would be ultimately determined by the philosophical orientation. Cost containment goals would be measured by hard cash saved and productivity – or, in terms of intermediate indicators, by the extent to which appropriate lifestyle/behaviour change had occurred or there had been a change in underlying and associated knowledge, beliefs, attitudes, etc. Radical or self-empowerment goals would again be evaluated in the ways discussed in Chapters One and Two, e.g. in relation to worker participation in union activities, in enhanced consciousness, in the acquisition of self-efficacy beliefs and skills.

A recurrent theme in this book is the importance of ensuring that the philosophy is complemented by appropriate technology. Unless the conditions appropriate to the adoption of innovations are supplied, an effective workplace programme will not materialize. Unless approved educational methods are used, learning will not occur. A discussion of both of these requirements in relation to the worksite is beyong the scope of this chapter but it is clear that the workplace has its own special needs – not least of which is the adoption of teaching methods appropriate to the adult learner. An example of programme planning which seeks to meet adult learning requirements is provided by Manning [33].

Finally we will provide a selective review of studies of the effectiveness of health promotion in the workplace commencing with some observations about the extent of provision.

HEALTH PROMOTION IN THE WORKPLACE: A SELECTIVE REVIEW

In 1970, in the USA, an Occupational Safety and Health Act was enacted '... to assure so far as possible every working man and woman in the nation safe and healthful working conditions and to preserve our human resources ...'. The achievement of this goal was to be ensured by, *inter alia*, '... education and training programs in the recognition, avoidance, and prevention of unsafe or unhealthful working conditions ...' [9]. In Britain similar legislation in the form of the Health and Safety at Work Act was introduced in 1974. Symington, in a conference on *Health Promotion in the Workplace* [34], commented on this Act and the Employment Protection Act which followed it in 1975, and argued that while they were primarily concerned with health and safety issues, '... this new awareness... provides a climate and a platform from which health promotion activities of a general nature can thrive'. He went on to point out that while not required by the Acts, screening programmes, alcohol and smoking policies emerged as a useful by-product. While this is undoubtedly true, the fact is that developments in Britain have not kept pace with those in North America. Indeed it is interesting to note an assertion by Webb at the same conference that after 20 years of decline in work-related diseases and injuries, '... figures for recent years show an alarming rise from 70.4 per 100 000 employees in 1981 to 87.0 per 100 000 in 1984'. He goes on to speculate that '... some workers are paying in health terms for the economic changes of recent years'.

At the time of writing no comprehensive survey of UK workplace health promotion activities is available. However examples of good practice in Scotland were presented in the conference report referred to above: these included programmes operated by seven commercial organizations, various district councils on alcoholism, trade unions, health education departments, the employment medical advisory service and local health boards. Topic areas discussed were safety, alcohol, exercise, nutrition, smoking, mental health, women's health and heart disease.

It will by now be clear that the situation in North America is very different. Fuchs *et al.* [35] commented on the escalation of interest between 1975 and 1985. They provided a selective review of 11 key textbooks, referred to 30 journal articles on general health promotion at work and listed 101 topic-specific articles together with 25 exemplars of more popular magazine pieces. The distribution of topics by popularity is as listed in Table 7.3. If these figures are representative, it is clear that the impact of safety legislation has been less

Table 7.3 The most popular worksite health promotion programmes (after Fuchs *et al.* [35])

Rank order	Topic	Number of references
1	Exercise programmes	33
2	Hypertension and CHD	19
3	Drugs and alcohol	17
4	Stress management	12
5	Smoking	8
6	Weight reduction	5
7	Safety	4
8	Cancer screening	3

than the more general health promotion movement – with, of course, its implication for cost containment!

Davis *et al.* [17] recorded an even greater range of topics in their survey of Californian workplaces. Between 16% and 72% of companies provided a wide range of screening services. These were, in ascending order of popularity: cervical cancer, colon/rectal cancer; diabetes; pulmonary function; annual medical examination; work-related problems; height and weight; general risk appraisal; high blood pressure; pre-employment medical examination.

Between 30% and 78% offered a wide range of information programmes. Again in ascending order of popularity, these were: seat-belt use; cervical cancer; breast self-examination; cancer prevention; work-related injury; low back pain; high blood pressure; alcohol and drug abuse; nutrition; smoking; stress; exercise.

Various services (e.g. group instruction; individual counselling; referral to community resources) were on offer with provision ranging from 28% of firms to 80%. Services provided were: industrial alcoholism programme; employee assistance; self-defence for women; low back pain; smoking cessation; weight management; stress management; exercise.

Hollander *et al.* [36] carried out a systematic survey of Fortune 500 companies (i.e. 500 largest US firms) to determine the nature and extent of health promotion provision (in 1984). The response rate was approximately 50%. Of these, two-thirds had a worksite programme and two-thirds reported plans to expand these. One third of those not having programmes planned to initiate health promotion activities. In general, the larger firms were more likely to have programmes which also tended to be more extensive. The number of health promotion activities reported ranged from 5.7 to 8.9.

Walsh [11] cited an unpublished manuscript of the Office of Disease Prevention and Health Promotion which reported a 1985 national survey of private sector employers having 50 or more personnel. This recorded at least one health promotion activity at nearly 66% of establishments; larger establishments tended to have many more programmes.

It would seem unlikely from the survey data presented above that health and safety legislation alone would be responsible for the accelerating provision of health promotion programmes in the USA. A more realistic estimate would be based on the general cultural pressure towards fitness and wellness along with the belief in the cost-effectiveness of interventions. Doubtless further impetus has been provided by the particular reference to the Surgeon General's report, worksite health promotion in *Healthy People* [37], which comments on the worksite as a locus for health education and health promotion:

> The worksite may provide an appropriate setting for health promotion as well as health protection activities. A number of companies have already shown leadership in providing employee fitness programs and encouraging worker participation, but more can be done.

The report also urged advertisers to be aware of their key role in influencing consumer behaviour and noted that advertising, '... particularly for food products, over-the-counter drugs, tobacco, and alcohol – has generally not been supportive of health promotion objectives'.

The report was published in 1979 and aspects of worksite health promotion were subsequently incorporated into the influential 'Objectives for the Nation' [38] in 1980. Since then the appropriateness of the setting has indeed been increasingly recognized. But what of success? To what extent has the faith of employers been justified?

First, there is little doubt that if appropriate educational techniques are used, the impact of particular interventions can be positive – even in behavioural terms. For instance, Street [39] describes two safety education interventions [40, 41]. The first revealed a pre-post programme difference in knowledge, beliefs and attitudes towards wearing hearing protection. Moreover after the intervention, fewer people stated that they 'never used hearing protection'. However the familiar gap between attitude and practice was noticeable in the reported results: whereas some 80% of the group agreed that it was important to protect their hearing, only 65% stated that they actually wore protectors most of the time.

The second programme was concerned with eye protection. It employed relevant precursor 'educational diagnosis' of the target group and added a 'policy element' to the education in the form of threatened disciplinary action for non-compliance. Actual injuries fell over an eight week period from 72 to six.

However, rather more substantial and extensive justification for large-scale investments of money and effort in workplace programmes would be expected if programmes were to continue. Davis *et al.*'s study [17] indicates that those employers operating health promotion programmes think that they work. Perceptions of benefits accruing are reproduced in Table 7.4.

Of course employer perceptions may well have been biased by wishful thinking! However, their views on reduced absenteeism may well be justified if Blair *et al.*'s [42] study is generally applicable. After an intensive 10 week programme of fitness teaching, there were not only significant differences in physiological and clinical characteristics in the 3846 participants receiving the instruction but there were also, on average, 1.25 days less absenteeism in the group. The researchers calculate that the programme had therefore resulted in savings of $149 578!

Many other reviews have reported similar kinds of success. Knobel [1] reported a reduction in disability costs for each $1000 of total wage payments from $13.28 in 1976 to $9.43 in 1978 at Southern Bell. This cost saving was ascribed to a co-ordinated prevention and promotion programme.

Knobel also commented on the Campbell Soup company programme which resulted in the removal of approximately 20 polyps each year at a cost of $6500 with estimated annual reductions of $100 000 in direct insurance payments.

Table 7.4 Employers' perceptions of the benefits of worksite health promotion programmes (from Davis *et al.* (1984) [17])

Category health promotion	Perceived as benefit by (%)
Improved morale	81
Improved health	52
Improved productivity	46
Reduced illness and injury	46
Reduced turnover of staff and absenteeism	40
Reduced medical care utilization	30
Reduced health care costs	23
Attracted better calibre applicants	17

The company detects and treats between 60% and 90% of hypertensives thus avoiding over a ten year period an estimated $130 000 in hospitalization, rehabilitation and disability costs.

Northern Natural Gas reported reduced absenteeism by approximately five working days a year after a fitness programme. School administrators and teachers – according to Knobel – had 17% reduced absenteeism after a programme of exercise, stress management and nutrition teaching. A nine-component health promotion programme, which cost New York Telephone approximately $2.8 million in 1980, generated savings of $5.5 million from reduced absenteeism and treatment costs.

Blair *et al.* [43] described the programme at Johnson and Johnson whose 'Live for Life' scheme includes health risk appraisal, fitness, diet and nutrition, smoking cessation, hypertension control, stress management, weight control and general health education. Over a two year period 20% of women and 30% of men had adopted vigorous exercise compared with 7% and 19% of a control group of company employees. Overall fitness and sense of wellbeing had also apparently improved. And again the 'bottom line' calculation: there were fewer hospital admissions and in-patient days in Johnson and Johnson employees and an estimated annual in-patient cost increase of $43 compared with $76 for non-programme employees (Blair *et al.* [44]).

The Canada Life Assurance Company's Fitness and Lifestyle Project [45] provided similar evidence of success. A saving of more than 0.5 hospital days per employee was claimed which was associated with a financial saving of $84.5 per employee year.

Sloan [46], in reviewing several of the projects mentioned above, presents a critique of the prevailing paradigm in North America. He reminds us again that '... some obvious alternative and complementary approaches are overlooked'. In particular he mentions the psychological and organizational climate of work. It should, perhaps, also be noted that there are instances where the worksite does not appear to generate successful results! For instance smoking cessation programmes may well achieve worse results than alternative modes of delivery and Klesges *et al.* [47] reported only 17% mean success rate at six months. Jason *et al.* [48] reported that work-based support groups increased the effectiveness of a smoking cessation programme using television and self-help manuals but reported only 7% continuous abstinence at 12 months – admittedly utilizing stringent criteria.

It is worth reiterating at this point the general assertion that any given programme will be more effective when it is part of a general integrated programme of education and policy and when it is supported by a consistent and integrated approach within the wider community. Part at least of this requirement obtained in a reported campaign strategy for weight loss at worksites [49]. As part of the Pawtucket Heart Health Program, worksite volunteers implemented a weight control campaign with 512 employees from 22 companies. At the end of the programme, a total of 1818 pounds has been lost at an average of 3.55 pounds per person and a cost of $0.81 per pound lost.

Although Chen [50], after reviewing a sample of worksite programmes, concluded that proper experimental or quasi-experimental research designs were relatively rare, the general view in North America appears to be that worksite health promotion is successful. Impact evaluation of the kinds described above is virtually non-existent in Britain. However, where a company has initiated a comprehensive programme, there seems to be a view that it was worth the effort. For instance, the personnel manager of Polaroid UK argued that for an outlay of £16 000 there had been a significant effect on people's lifestyles [35] in relation to diet and exercise and a claimed reduction in absenteeism from 6.3% to 3.7% over a four year period.

One of the more thorough and comprehensive workplace endeavours is the Look After Yourself (LAY) programme developed by the Health Education Council. An evaluation of a pilot programme revealed evidence of effectiveness. First in relation to indirect indicators, 73% of the 60 initial recruits attended all eight sessions. Additionally various intermediate measures gave evidence of heightened awareness of stress together with a positive attitude towards, and competence in controlling, it. Outcome measures of changes in eating, exercise, alcohol consumption and smoking demonstrated lifestyle changes: between 26% and 89% of 85 participants recorded change in one or more of these behaviours. Changes were also observed in various physiological indicators, viz. aerobic capacity, body fat, blood pressure and lung efficiency. Programme participants also expressed satisfaction with and interest in the programme as a whole [41].

The research designs of these programmes would doubtless not impress those favouring 'proper' experimental techniques which might allow us, in Chen's [50] words, to '... be better able to prove that "health education indeed is worthwhile".' However, it is worth reiterating one of the main contentions of this book, namely that although rigorous research design is often eminently desirable in order to generate internal validity, in general, such designs are not essential. Indeed in the interests of external validity, process evaluation will often be more useful provided that it is based on sound theory and utilizes relevant intermediate and indirect indicators.

The bulk of the evidence discussed in this chapter leads us inexorably to the conclusion that workplace heath education can work in producing behaviour change, reducing risk and even reducing costs. Cost-benefit analysis although doubtless attractive to many decision-makers in UK, is clearly of much greater relevance to North America and its peculiar system of health care delivery and payment. Nonetheless the behaviour changes which generate cost savings and increased productivity are in most cases the same changes which will enhance wellbeing and can thus justify both the inclusion of health promotion in British workplaces and the use of less rigorous measures of programme effectiveness in evaluation.

The discussion of behaviour change and economic indicators of success has, in this chapter, perhaps appeared almost obsessive! This is due to the excess of data of an economic kind and the dearth of evidence of effectiveness in other domains of a more radical nature! We will, however, finish this chapter by reporting Freudenberg's [24] account of successful examples of consciousness raising and community action. He points out that:

> Work-related diseases afflict at least 4 million people a year; as many as 400 000 Americans die annually from these diseases. In addition, 9 million workers are injured on the job each year and 13 000 people die from these injuries. .. 20% of all cancers are related to work place exposure to carcinogens.

He cites examples of consciousness-raising health education designed to provide a radical response to the situation described above. The case of the Carolina Brown Lung Association was mentioned in Chapter One. This radical health promotion programme provided workers with understanding and skills to monitor health hazards and take action in the case of violations. It also incorporated the broader health promotion tactics of lobbying and advocacy – for instance in order to achieve fair compensation and ensure the availability of proper health care for the victims of industrial disease.

The New York Committee on Occupational Safety and Health is also cited as an exemplar of radical health promotion. This group has sponsored educational forums on health hazards and has lobbied vigorously in order to achieve 'Right-to-Know' legislation. It also provides technical assistance and advice for trade unions and sponsors lectures at union meetings in addition to producing educational materials.

Criteria for success are readily defined: outcome indicators might include the achievement of legislation which will improve safety standards. Intermediate indicators could document the increasing level of awareness in a community and different degrees of social action. In a later article Freudenberg [51] provides further instances of radical health promotion. Indicators of success have been extracted from these and categorized in Table 7.5.

Table 7.5 Indicators of 'radical' health education

Indicators of success	*Examples of process involved*
Outcome	
January 1981, City of Philadelphia enacted the nation's first municipal Right-to-Know law.	Results from several years of community and workplace education by Delaware Valley Toxics Coalition.
Intermediate	
United Automobile Workers produce a handbook *A Manual for Cancer Detectives on the Job* which '… teaches members across the country how to conduct an investigation, file an OSHA complaint and bargain for health and safety'.	Stimulus from an organized coalition of tenants' associations, environmental groups and Vietnam veterans.
Tenants' Associations develop a flair for creative use of media (skills acquisition).	Learning how to produce reports; hold demonstrations; organize public meetings.
A mortality study is produced by workers which identifies potential carcinogens. Improvements are made to ventilation.	Workers approach National Union for help.

These last examples of workplace health promotion are very different from many earlier examples: not only do they adopt a radical approach which is philosophically and ideologically distinct from the narrower individually-focused and frequently 'healthist' programmes, but they also have moved us outside the bounds of the worksite and into the community. The final strategic approach which will be discussed in this book also focuses on the community. At one level of analysis it will examine the notion of community-wide approaches and consider integrated programmes which would incorporate worksite health promotion as one element in a broader but, hopefully, coherent strategy. At another level it will concern itself with a much narrower and geographically more limited approach having a very particular philosophy. This strategy is termed community development: its rationale and ideology and the methods it employs to achieve its goals have much in common with the radical formula for workplace health promotion delineated by Freudenberg.

REFERENCES

1. Knobel, R. J. (1983) Health promotion and disease prevention: improving health while conserving resources. *Family and Community Health*, **1**, 16–27.
2. Bosquet, M. (1977) *Capitalism in Crisis and Everyday Life* (translated from the French by J. Howe), Harvester Press, Hassocks.
3. Hopson, B. and Scally, M. (1981) *Lifeskills Teaching*, McGraw-Hill, London.
4. Toffler, A. (1970) *Future Shock*, Bodley Head, London.
5. World Health Organization (1987) *Health Promotion in the Working World*: Report on a joint meeting organized by the Federal Centre for Health Education, Cologne, 7–9 October, 1985, WHO, Copenhagen.
6. Braun, S. and Hollander, R. (1987) A study of job stress among women and men in the Federal Republic of Germany, *Health Education Research*, **2**, 45–51.
7. McEwan, J. (1987) Health and work, in: *Health Education: Perspectives and Choices* (2nd ed), (ed. I. Sutherland), National Extension College, Cambridge.
8. Buck, A. (1982) *Promoting Health and Safety at Work*, University of Nottingham/ Nottingham Health Education Unit, Nottingham.
9. Vojtecky, M. A., Kar, S. B. and Cox, S. G. (1985) Workplace health education: results from a national survey. *International Quarterly of Community Health Education*, **5**, 171–85.
10. Cooper, C. L. (1985) The road to health in American firms. *New Society*, **73**, 335–6.
11. Walsh, D. C. (1988) Toward a sociology of worksite health promotion: a few reactions and reflections. *Social Science and Medicine*, **26**, 569–75.
12. Russell, L. (1986) *Is Prevention Better than Cure?* Brookings Institute, Washington, DC.
13. Warner, K. E. (1987) Selling health promotion to corporate America. *Health Education Quarterly*, **14**, 39–55.
14. Schelling, T. (1986) Economics and cigarettes. *Preventive Medicine*, **15**, 549–60.
15. Conrad, P. (1988) Worksite health promotion: the social context. *Social Science and Medicine*, **26**, 485–9.
16. Alexander, J. (1988) The ideological construction of risk: an analysis of corporate health promotion programs in the 1980s. *Social Science and Medicine*, **26**, 559–67.
17. Davis, M. F., Rosenberg, K., Iverson, D. C., Vernon, T. M. and Bauer, J. (1984) Worksite health promotion in Colorado. *Public Health Reports*, **99**, 538–43.
18. Conrad, P. (1988) Health and fitness at work: a participant's perspective. *Social Science and Medicine*, **26**, 545–50.
19. Spilman, M. A. (1988) Gender differences in worksite health promotion activities. *Social Science and Medicine*, **26**, 525–35.

20. Kotarba, J. A. and Bentley, P. (1988) Workplace wellness participation and the becoming of self. *Social Science and Medicine*, **26**, 551–8.
21. Parkinson, R. S. *et al.* (eds) (1982) *Managing Health Promotion in the Workplace*, Mayfield, Palo Alto, Ca.
22. Navarro, V. (1976) *Medicine Under Capitalism*, Croom Helm, London.
23. Gordon, J. (1987) Workplace health promotion: the right idea in the wrong place. *Health Education Research*, **2**, 69–71.
24. Freudenberg, N. (1981) Health education for social change: a strategy for public health in the US. *International Journal of Health Education*, **XXIV**, 1–8.
25. Novick, M. (1987) The new work agenda into the nineties, *Work and Well-Being Quarterly*, Fall 1987, 26–30.
26. Ippolito-Shepherd, J. I. *et al.* (1987) Agricultural occupational health and health education in Latin America and the Caribbean. *Health Education Research*, **2**, 53–9.
27. Schenck, A. P. *et al.* (1987) A labor and industry focus on education: using baseline survey data in program design. *Health Education Research*, **2**, 33–44.
28. Daines, J. *et al.* (1986) *'Look After Yourself' 1978–86: Innovation and Outcomes*, Dept. of Adult Education for Health Education Council, Nottingham.
29. Roman, P. M. and Blum, T. C. (1988) Formal intervention in employee health: comparisons of the nature and structure of employee assistance programs and health promotion programs, *Social Science and Medicine*, **26**, 503–14.
30. Roman, P. M. and Blum, T. C. (1987) The relation of employee assistance programs to corporate social responsibility attitudes: an empirical study, in: *Research in Corporate Social Performance and Policy*, (ed. L. E. Preston) **9**, 213–35, JAI Press, Greenwich, Conn.
31. Sonnenstuhl, W. and Trice, H. (1986) *Strategies for Employee Assistance Programs: The Crucial Balance*, IRL Press, Ithaca, NY.
32. Jenkins, M. *et al.* (1987) *Smoking Policies at Work*, Health Education Authority, London.
33. Manning, D. T. (1983/4), Suggested strategies for occupational health promotion. *Hygie*, **II**, 44–51.
34. Symington, I. (1987) Health promotion in the workplace: legislative aspects, in: *Health Promotion in the Workplace*, (ed. H. Matheson), Scottish Health Education Group, Edinburgh.
35. Fuchs, J. A., Price, J. E. and Marcotte, B. (1985) Worksetting health promotion – a comprehensive bibliography. *Health Education*, **16**, 29.
36. Hollander, R. B. and Lengermann, J. J. (1988) Corporate characteristics and worksite health promotion programs: survey findings from Fortune 500 companies. *Social Science and Medicine*, **26**, 491–501.
37. US Department of Health, Education and Welfare (1979) *Healthy People: The Surgeon General's Report on Health Promotion and Disease Prevention*, Washington DC.
38. US Department of Health and Human Services (1980) *Promoting Health/Preventing Disease: Objectives for the Nation*, Washington DC.
39. Street, C. G. (1987) Unpublished MSc Dissertation, Dept. of Community Medicine, Manchester.

40. Foster, A. (1983) Hearing protection and the role of health education. *Occupational Health*, **35**, 155–8.
41. Denyer, B. (1986) Reducing the incidence of eye injuries. *Occupational Health*, **38**, 112–14.
42. Blair, S. N. *et al.* (1986) Health promotion for educators: impact on absenteeism. *Preventive Medicine*, **15**, 166–75.
43. Blair, S. N. *et al.* (1986) A public health intervention model for work-site health promotion. *Journal of American Medical Association*, **255**, 921–6.
44. Bly, J. L., Jones, R. C. and Richardson, J. E. (1986) Impact of worksite health promotion on health care costs and utilization. *Journal of American Medical Association*, **256**, 3235–40.
45. Shephard, R. J. *et al.* (1982) The influence of an employee fitness and lifestyle modification program upon medical care costs. *Canadian Journal of Public Health*, **73**, 259–63.
46. Sloan, R. P. (1987) Workplace health promotion: the North American experience, in: *Health Promotion in the Workplace*, (ed. H. Matheson) Scottish Health Education Group, Edinburgh.
47. Klesges, R. C. *et al.* (1987) Competition and relapse prevention training in worksite smoking modification. *Health Education Research*, **2**, 5–14.
48. Jason, L. A. *et al.* (1987) A 12 month follow-up of a worksite smoking cessation intervention. *Health Education Research*, **2**, 185–94.
49. Nelson, D. J. *et al.* (1987) A campaign strategy for weight loss at worksites. *Health Education Research*, **2**, 27–31.
50. Chen, M. S. (1984) Proving the effects of health promotion in industry: an academician's perspective. *Health Education Quarterly*, **10**, 235–45.
51. Freudenberg, N. (1985) Training health educators for social change. *International Quarterly of Community Health Education*, **5**, 37–52.

8

COMMUNITY ORGANIZATION AND STRATEGIC INTEGRATION: PROMOTING COMMUNITY HEALTH

The purpose of this final chapter is to consider the evaluation implications of community organization. The whole of this book might be said to rest on the thesis that maximal success (however defined) will be achieved by strategic planning which is (i) based on the principles of sound learning theory, and (ii) seeks to combine in synergistic fashion the full range of delivery possibilities. The most important of these have received attention in previous chapters, viz.: schools, the health care context, mass media, workplace and, now, the community itself. At one level of analysis we might say that community health education was the sum total of these delivery strategies. However certain approaches within the community and which are characterized by informality, lay involvement and more or less deliberate dissociation from official institutions and organizations merit separate consideration, They are variously labelled 'community development', 'locality development', 'community organization' and the like. We will, therefore, be identifying the particular characteristics of this 'micro' community education movement while arguing that its potential for empowering disadvantaged or resistant groups renders it of central importance to an effective 'macro' intervention in the community at large.

THE MEANING OF COMMUNITY

Before attempting to provide some insight into the distinctions between various approaches designed to foster change in under–privileged communities, we should note that while the definition of various forms of community organization is difficult, there are also problems in deciding on the meaning of the term 'community' itself! For instance, Hubley [1] has commented on the imprecision of the concept and cited one reviewer who had unearthed some 94 definitions. For the purposes of the present discussion, a community is distinguished from any other social aggregation in respect of its relative size, geographical contiguity and the nature of the social network and norms prevailing within this circumscribed locality. The report of the Calouste

Gulbenkian Foundation [2] provides an apt description:

> 'Community' ... refers to a grouping of people who share a common purpose, interest or need, and who can express their relationship through communication face to face, as well as by other means, without difficulty. In other words, in the majority of cases we see a community as being related to some geographic locality where the propinquity of the inhabitants has relevance for those interests or needs which they share.

Henderson and Thomas [3] emphasize the focus on a relatively small geographical neighbourhood: they argue that the appropriate catchment area for community development should be between 6000 and 20 000 population. However, while the above definitions clearly apply to many varieties of community organization, the more extensive programmes such as the North Karelia Heart Disease Prevention Programme will have much larger geographical areas as their target for intervention. Again, although the potential for face-to-face communication and associated social networks are of major importance in planning 'typical' community projects, there is obviously no clear-cut distinction between a community and a geographical area of more than, say, Henderson and Thomas' upper limit of 20 000 people. In fact, MacCannell [4] has provided an interesting continuum based on three guiding principles of 'differentiation', 'centrality' and 'solidarity'. This helps him to categorize and record key features of different social aggregates – ranging from isolated settlements to highly differentiated city communities having their own television station and other commodities of relevance for health education interventions. Such a classification system would therefore be able to incorporate the separate study towns of the Stanford Heart Disease Prevention Project – to be discussed later. Classic definitions of community development would not, however, be able to accommodate this. Neither scheme would apply – except by exclusion – to the larger rural area of North Karelia.

It is worth noting in passing that for many programmes concerned primarily with mental and social health, the mere act of creating a community where none existed before might be considered a major triumph. That is to say, building a social network characterized by interpersonal interactions sometimes referred to as *Gemeinschaft* by comparison with its unhealthy antithesis, *Gesellschaft* – a state of impersonal interactions typical of many western urbanized societies. More usually, though, community development or organization would be concerned to move into a community in order to stimulate some healthy developments–which might well be facilitated by, or even contribute to, the Gemeinschaft goal.

COMMUNICATION OF INNOVATIONS THEORY

Both health promotion generally and community organization in particular are concerned with how communities (large or small) come to change and adopt new ideas or practices. It is, therefore, worth briefly re-visiting Communication of Innovations theory [5] which was first referred to in Chapter Three in the context of defining indicators of success. Apart from describing the rate of adoption of innovations by a community in relation to an S-shaped curve, Rogers and Shoemaker provided important insights into the principles governing the likelihood of adoption – principles which can be used by anyone seeking to foster change in communities. The theory is based on an appraisal of seven major research traditions after analysis of 1084 publications in ' ... anthropology, early sociology, rural sociology, education, medical sociology, communication and marketing.' A full discussion is inappropriate to present needs but four of Rogers and Shoemaker's major observations should provide useful background information for understanding evaluative issues. They refer to: (i) the characteristics of the community (or more accurately, the social system) in relation to their willingness or otherwise to adopt an innovation, (ii) the main factors determining whether or not the social system will 'own' the innovation, (iii) the role of leaders in the change process, and (iv) the peculiarities of the innovation itself.

Community Characteristics

With regard to the first of these, Rogers and Shoemaker have provided a five-category analysis of adopters within the community. This is reproduced in Table 8.1. In a **top-down** programme, the change agents would seek to coerce the community into adopting the healthy innovation. Attempts would therefore be made to prod the 'late majority' into taking action and 'get through to' the hard core of resistant laggards. On the other hand **bottom-up** community developers would posit socio-structural reasons for the laggards' lack of receptivity – such as learned helplessness or a disadvantaging environment. Ultimately they would acknowledge the rights of this group to reject the innovation if it did not meet their felt needs. Both varieties of community worker would be advised to note the evidence presented by Rogers and Shoemaker that change may take a very long time!

Ownership of Innovation

The second observation, which concerns the importance of a community 'owning' an innovation, is acknowledged by both bottom-up and top-down programmes. For community development it is an ideological requirement: change should only result from the identification and satisfaction of a community's felt needs. For top-down planners it is a technical rather than a

Table 8.1 The communication of innovations: major adopter categories. Adapted from Rogers and Shoemaker [5], pp. 183–5

Adopter category	Characteristics
Innovator	2.5% of population: eager but a 'deviant'; probably mistrusted by the safe majority
Early adopter	13.5% of population: respectable but amenable to change; good candidate for opinion leader or community aide
Early majority	34% of population: according to Rogers and Shoemaker their motto might be 'Be not the last to lay the old aside, nor the first by which the new is tried'!
Late majority	34% of population: the sceptics reluctant to change until benefits of innovation have been clearly proven
Laggards	16% of population: the diehard conservatives! Will doubtless incorporate a sub group who will never change and appear to be against everything most of the time

It will be noted that these adopter categories represent ideal types and their distribution is viewed by Rogers and Shoemaker as matching the normal or Gaussian curve.

philosophical matter: programmes will fail unless by chance the innovation is perceived to meet a pre-existing need. Many mainstream preventively oriented health educators strive desperately to persuade a community to increase the priority they give to various measures such as improved dental health or smoking cessation. Rogers and Shoemaker describe the likelihood of change in terms of the interaction of two dimensions: firstly, community perception of

Recognition of need for change	Origin of new idea	
	Internal to social system	*External to social system*
Internal: Recognition is by members of the social system	Imminent change	Selective contact change
External: Recognition may be by change agents outside the social system	Induced imminent change	Directed contact change

Figure 8.1 Paradigm of types of social change. From Rogers and Shoemaker [5, p. 8].

the originators of the proposed change, and secondly, the extent to which the community itself recognizes a need for the change. Their model is described in Figure 8.1. And so, where an external source – perhaps doctors, teachers or a government agency – seek to impose change on a community ('directed contact change') the chances of adoption are virtually non-existent. On the other hand where the community recognizes the need and discovers the remedy ('immanent change'), change is virtually inevitable: The notion of 'induced immanent change' is especially interesting. Observers examining a community from outside may note some objectively measurable health need which is unrecognized by the people. The critical consciousness raising function of community workers is then to facilitate recognition of need and provide the skills necessary to meet it. The informal leadership provided by the change agents is epitomized by the oft-quoted traditional Chinese poem [6] which might almost be termed an ode to immanent change!

> Go to the people
> Live among them
> Love them
> Start with what they know
> Build on what they have
> But of the best leaders
> When their task is accomplished
> Their work is done
> The people all remark
> We have done it ourselves.

Role of Leaders

The third series of observations by Rogers and Shoemaker extends the notion of leadership embodied in the poem cited above. Leadership is intimately related to the invaluable principle of homophily – an idea originated by Lazarsfeld and Merton [7] but extended by Rogers and Shoemaker who define it thus:

> Homophily is the degree to which pairs of individuals who interact are similar in certain attributes, such as beliefs, values, education, social status and the like.

Interpersonal communication and general influence processes are more effective when individuals are homophilous. Where homophily cannot apparently exist – e.g. because change agent and client are from different social backgrounds – a functionally equivalent state is possible provided that the change agent has acquired the art of empathy – or to be more precise the cluster of social interaction skills necessary to be empathic. The two fairly obvious implications of the homophily principle are the use of community aides in development work and the provision of appropriate social skills training for community workers.

Characteristics of the Innovation

Finally, Communication of Innovations Theory reminds us of the importance of taking account of the particular characteristics of the innovation. These may be summarized as: relative advantage; compatibility; complexity; trialability; and observability. For example, if a community perceives that a recommended dietary change has benefits for them by comparison with their existing diet; if the proposed change is compatible with lifestyle and culture; if it is not too complicated – e.g. to grow, collect and cook; if it is relatively easy to try out without fully committing oneself; if the community can readily and quickly observe the benefits – then the innovation stands a pretty good chance of being adopted!

Summary

This analysis and brief report of Communication of Innovations Theory has been presented not only because of its relevance for understanding the distinctions between different approaches to community health programmes but also because it provides clear performance indicators for monitoring programmes – e.g. whether or not community felt needs have been recorded; whether community aides have been appointed and opinion leaders identified; whether staff have been trained; and whether the characteristics of the innovation have been identified and pre-tested on the community. These intermediate and indirect indicators are of special importance in the present context since the experimental/clinical trials approach to evaluation is singularly inappropriate for community programmes – a point which will receive elaboration later in the chapter.

COMMUNITY ORGANIZATION: VARIATIONS ON A THEME

Bivins [8] has described community organization as 'an old and reliable grassroots approach to health education identified in the 1940s'. Kindervatter [9], in an influential book on nonformal education, commented that 'Community organization first appeared in US social work textbooks in the 1920s and 1930s' but goes on to say that, '... not until the War on Poverty in the sixties did the concept and its application receive much attention.' Kindervatter suggests that community organization developed as a response to '... the conditions of poor people in Western urban settings, but is now practised in a variety of forms in urban and rural locales.' She considers its overall purpose, '... is to enable communities to improve and change their socio-economic milieu and/or their position in that milieu.'

These observations provide a strong flavour of this variety of community work. However, before considering some of the implications for evaluation we should note that various terms have been used to describe this general kind of community intervention: sometimes they are used interchangeably but sometimes they suggest a distinctive approach. The most common of these terms are: community organization itself, community development, locality development, social action, and technical or social planning. Rothman [10] identified three separate approaches to community work: locality development, technical planning and social action. According to Nix [11], locality development is the same as community development, community organization and the 'process approach'. Kindervatter considers locality development to be similar to community development insofar as it involves a non-directive approach to community work. She, however, views locality development, social action and 'social planning and co-ordination of services' as three different community organization approaches. Dodds *et al.* [12], in providing a 'North American Typology' of community development/ community organization, identify eight approaches which include self-help groups and 'public advocacy/pressure group tactics'. They also translate some of these terms into a British context.

While there seems to be some confusion over several of these terms, there seems to be general agreement about the nature of 'social action' which is almost universally associated with the work of Saul Alinsky [13]. According to Kindervatter, locality (community) development '...essentially enables people to cooperatively and self-reliantly solve community problems.' On the other hand, '...social action strategies aim to enable people to jointly challenge and change existing community power relationships. In terms of the relationship between community members and outside authorities, locality development assumes collaboration and cooperation, whereas social action assumes either competition or conflict.'

According to Kirklin and Franzen [14]:

> Large numbers of people are organized to bring into being a new power aggregate ...to force the existing political/economic power structure to change public and private policies. The battle is classically seen to be between the 'power haves' and the 'power have nots'.

For the purpose of the present chapter, only two broad categories of community intervention will be considered. The first will be generally labelled **community organization** in accordance with Ross' definition [15]:

> Community organization ... is ... a process by which a community identifies its needs or objectives, orders (or ranks) these needs or objectives, develops the confidence and will to work at these needs or objectives, finds the resources (internal and/or external) to deal with

these needs and objectives, takes action in respect to them and in so doing extends and develops cooperation and collaborative attitudes and practices in the community.

The fundamental goal, then, is self-empowerment. This involves, in Kindervatter's words, '...people gaining an understanding of and control over social, economic, and/or political forces in order to improve their standing in society.'

Again, whether the formula is social action or community development, the goal is fundamentally political as is apparent from the following extract from the Gulbenkian Working Party Report [2]:

We see community development as a main strategy for the attainment of social policy goals. It is concerned with the worth and dignity of people and the promotion of equal opportunity ... Community work is most needed in communities where social skills and resources are at their weakest. Community work involves working with those most affected by poverty, unemployment, disability, inadequate housing and education, and with those who for reasons of class, income, race or sex are less likely than others to be, or to feel, involved and significant in local community life.

In the light of the discussion which follows, the reader should be able to spot three major outcome/intermediate indicators in this passage!

By comparison, what Nix [11] has referred to as 'technical planning' and seen as equivalent to Rothman's notion of 'social planning' tends toward a top down approach. Thus the second broad category is that of **social/technical planning**, and is concerned with task rather than process goals and seeks to implement change in the community (for the good of the community) but without being concerned with the empowerment of people living therein. The assumption, of course, is that planners know what is best for the community (as indeed they may do). However the difference between a sophisticated social planning approach and more naïve (top-down) programmes is that in the former case, planners are aware of the need to take account of the dynamics of change in the community. They will thus employ outreach strategies, seek to identify opinion leaders and generally apply the accumulated wisdom of studies based on communication of innovations research. They will often, therefore, look like community organization programmes – at least at first glance.

The comparison between social/technical planning interventions and community organization is indeed intriguing since it embodies the fundamentally distinct philosophies of, on the one side, a radical, self-empowerment model of health education and, on the other, the preventive medical model seeking to change behaviour and maximize the efficiency of health and illness services. It also mirrors the dilemma associated with the adoption of the

WHO's primary health care philosophy. For instance it is clear that community development/community organization provides both a practically appropriate and philosophically sound approach to implementing the tenets of primary health care in developing countries [16] as well as handling problems of inequalities in health in 'fourth world' situations. The self-empowerment goals of community organization exactly match the aims of health promotion which are concerned with maximizing public participation.

While the main philosophical and ideological conflict described above relates primarily to notions of power – both political and professional – and the different world view of the medical model, Green [17] has identified an administrative stumbling block which militates against community organization. He argues that large-scale programmes require a degree of centralization of authority and responsibility almost by definition. In his words:

> This policy question has stalemated the implementation of the World Health Organization's primary health care approach in many countries where centralized planning is deeply ingrained in their systems. It also has limited the degree to which the community-based cardiovascular risk reduction programs, such as those managed by the Stanford and University of Minnesota research teams, have achieved a truly community-based initiative and follow-through.

It could equally be argued that unless the communities in question had genuinely identified cardiovascular risk as a major need, a true community approach was, by definition, impossible under such circumstances! The different evaluation goals of projects based upon the philosophy of community organization, as opposed to those derived from social/technical planning, will be discussed later. For the present, we should note that there are certain difficulties inherent in evaluating community organization – or so it is said. These will be examined later, but for now we might note that this is just one of the problems inherent in community organization initiatives. As Moynihan (in Hubley [1]) has said, community work will, '... promise a lot; deliver a little. Lead people to believe that they will be better off but let there be no dramatic improvement. Try a variety of programmes, each interesting, but marginal in impact and severely underfinanced.'

Constantino-David [18] has provided a more detailed and thoughtful critique of community organization. First she cautions against the members of a community becoming dependent on the workers so that the project collapses once the workers withdraw. Second, she warns of the possibility of creating a new elite of community aides/indigenous workers. Third she notes the dilemma for workers whose major self-empowering goal is to facilitate self-empowered choice and promote long-term outcomes such as literacy, autonomy or healthy lifestyles and yet find they must concentrate on specific felt needs – issues which may catch the community's imagination but which may be relatively insignificant in the longer term. She also highlights the 'facilitation vs. manipulation' dilemma in which there is a temptation for the worker to manipulate the attitudes and behaviour of the community to conform to the values and political motivation of the worker rather than facilitate empowered choice in the community members. Constantino-David also emphasizes the political paradoxes and problems which are usually greater in community organization than in other health promotion programmes which are more likely to be congruent with the dominant power structure in society. Loney's [19] analysis of the British Community Development Projects makes a similar point. The potential for initiating radical action may be limited when funding comes from central government. As Loney says, 'It is rather like pacifists suddenly finding they have army funding.' He does however note in his reference to the Community Development Project report, *Gilding the Ghetto* [20], 'That such a document could emerge from a state sponsored programme and could be printed at government expense must itself encourage a more cautious approach to summary dismissals of the possibilities of working in the state apparatus.' This is doubtless cheering news for many workers faced with the issue of programme evaluation. They might, however, be excused for a degree of scepticism since community programmes are more likely than most to give rise to a significant gap between the aspirations of funders and those of the workers themselves – to say nothing of the aspirations of the community! As the next section shows, there are other difficulties with evaluating community organization programmes.

EVALUATING COMMUNITY ORGANIZATION

In keeping with the aims of this book, no attempt will be made here to provide specific guidelines for evaluating community organization. Good practical texts are readily available [21, 22]. It is, however, essential to acknowledge the major issues. Voth [23] suggests that there are five main problems associated with evaluating community work: (i) ambiguity goals, (ii) absence of a model of the community development process, (iii) inability of the researcher to control assignment to treatments, (iv) weak effects, crude measurement, and small samples, and (v) political problems.

Although there are, as we have seen, difficulties over definition, the absence of a theoretical model hardly seems a major problem. It is clear that several detailed sets of suggestions for achieving community organization have been provided by many of the authors cited above. It may be the case that workers are not aware of them or prefer to reject theory – but that is a different issue. The question of political difficulties has already been explored – both in general in Chapter Two and more specifically above. No further discussion is necessary here. On the other hand the remaining issues do need further consideration: they have to do fundamentally with goal-setting and the writing of objectives and with the matter of experimental design.

First, with regard to goal-setting, it is undoubtedly true that community organization suffers from a tendency to state vague and/or over-ambitious aims – or even to refuse to state any aims at all! There are probably two main reasons why there is frequently a reluctance to carry out the essential task of operationalizing general aims. First, it is often argued that because genuine community development must be based on community-defined goals, i.e. felt needs, it is neither possible nor desirable to state programme objectives other than as general statements of intent such as 'empowering the community' or 'producing a shift in power'. Second, there may be an ideological objection to evaluation derived from a misconception that evaluation is inevitably associated with a logical–positivist approach and the much maligned medical model. These reasons or rationalizations are patently false. As we have said, community organization has broad goals such as reducing disadvantage and enhancing empowerment, and these can readily be operationalized into a series of process measures. One of these is, of course, to produce a 'needs assessment' of the community. Now while it may not be possible or desirable to establish objectives before this step has been taken, it is perfectly possible, not to say essential, to develop objectives after establishing felt needs. Success may then be judged by the extent to which these needs are met or modified in the light of subsequent education and consciousness raising. With regard to the ideological objection to evaluation *per se*, this is either a counsel of despair, an attempt at obfuscation or a decline into anarchy! It is, however, reasonable to challenge certain paradigms of evaluation. Indeed, as indicated earlier, this chapter is asserting that the clinical trials paradigm is inappropriate and damaging – as is its educational equivalent. Voth's remaining issues are in fact related to this matter and will, therefore, be considered now.

It is interesting to observe that Voth's suggestion that community developers need to combat the problem of 'weak effects, crude measurement and small samples' derives from an assumption that an experimental or quasi-experimental design cannot be expected to work in non-formal community settings. There seems to be an assumption that this is rather unfortunate. The approach adopted here, however, is that the alternative qualitative research designs discussed in Chapter Two are not merely appropriate but much more productive than their more quantitative counterparts. The reasons for the inappropriateness of the latter paradigm may be summarized as follows (and considered in the light of general comments made in Chapter Two).

1. Classic research design requires both experimental intervention and comparison or control groups. It is often inappropriate to utilize controls because of both the difficulty of avoiding cross contamination in community interventions and the ethical issue of not depriving the community of a beneficial input.

2. More importantly, because of the great complexity of the intervention, evaluators will need to use equally complex factorial research designs. These in turn will result in an unacceptable sacrifice of external validity to internal validity.

   Parlett and Hamilton [24] make this point graphically: 'To attempt to simulate laboratory conditions by "manipulating educational personnel" is not only dubious ethically, but also leads to gross administrative and personal inconvenience. Even if a situation could be so unnervingly controlled, its artificiality would render the exercise irrelevant; rarely can "tidy" results be generalized to an "untidy" reality.'

3. Community programmes must take account of the different needs of various stakeholders: community, funders, workers, health professionals, etc., and utilize an evaluation design which can record these various goals.

4. Community development is above all concerned with action research: it is inappropriate for evaluators to maintain an Olympian detachment and merely report on whether or not certain programme objectives have been achieved. Innovatory programmes require a continual flow of information in order to better change course in pursuit of relevant goals and react to changing circumstances.

5. Participatory evaluation is also a key element in the empowering process.

In general, then, formative rather than summative evaluation is needed: with a complex community programme, merely to be told that objectives have or have not been achieved is likely to leave the worker bemused and wondering why (s)he has failed or, paradoxically, why (s)he has been successful. This is not of course to disparage the clinical trials model or what, in education, Parlett and Hamilton have referred to as the 'Agricultural–Botanical Paradigm'. They are both powerful tools when used in the right circumstances. Although clinical trials might be excellent for avoiding placebo effects in testing the efficacy of a drug or single clinical intervention, complex health promotion programmes require illumination rather than the double blind.

It should be noted that the use of formative and process evaluation is not only the method of choice for community development, it is also equally appropriate for medically oriented programmes of the social/technical planning variety. As Means and Smith [25] have argued, there needs to be a pluralistic approach to evaluation. They apply this to the complex requirements of a community alcohol education programme whose goal is fundamentally one of prevention.

The arguments ranged against the clinical trials model should, of course, not be used to justify sloppy thinking and a refusal to develop objectives. Although it is important, through process evaluation, to accumulate evidence which illuminates the reasons for success or failure and provides guidance for more effective action, it is equally important to examine whether or not objectives have been achieved. It is equally possible to utilize experimental design within a programme to check a hypothesis or to compare the relative effectiveness of alternative approaches to achieving a given objective. Typically the objectives in question would give rise to indirect or intermediate indicators of performance. As indicated above, the literature on community development provides ready-made indicators of this kind. For example, consider the seven stages outlined by Batten [26] which are reproduced in Figure 8.2. These describe the impact of effective community work on members of a given community group in relation to a process of development from passivity to self-empowered action.

Process evaluation would provide illumination about worker activities indicating the worker's success in producing change in the groups and documenting the factors which facilitated or inhibited achievement of the developmental objectives. Intermediate indicators could be provided which described the knowledge, beliefs, attitudes and skills needed and acquired by the members of the group.

HOW SUCCESSFUL ARE COMMUNITY PROJECTS?

Having discussed some of the issues and strategies involved in evaluating community projects, we might reasonably ask about the degree of success achieved by community development when appropriate indicators are used. While it is probably true to say that many community workers are more concerned with achieving success than with measuring it, there are several examples of project evaluation in the development literature. Kindervatter [9], for example, describes a series of youth and village development workshops in Thailand. Although at first glance these would not seem to have great relevance for planning and evaluating community health projects in Western inner city areas, the fundamental principles are identical and many parallels can be drawn. For instance, the goal of the organizers of the Thai workshops (which they acknowledged as deriving from them rather than from felt needs) was encapsulated in the concept of 'khit pen'*. This notion is directly

---

* 'Some people translate 'khit pen' as critical thinking, others as rational thinking, still others as problem-solving. It is, in fact, the combination of these processes and more. A man (or woman) who has mastered 'khit pen' will be able to approach problems in his life systematically ... If due to outside circumstances or lack of certain necessary knowledge or skills, the solution of his choice can not be implemented right away, a 'khit pen' man will not become frustrated. Instead, he will adopt a lesser solution while preparing to make the solution of his choice possible ... In other words, this philosophy encourages people to change, but not to destroy themselves physically and mentally doing so.' Dr Kowit Vorapipatana, Thai Adult Education Division, July 1975, pp. 7–8, cited by Kindervatter [9].

	Members of the group	The worker (by asking questions)
Stage One	Vaguely dissatisfied but passive	
	↓ ←	Stimulates people to think why they are dissatisfied and with what
Stage Two	Now aware of certain needs	
	↓ ←	Stimulates people to think about what specific changes would result in these needs being met
Stage Three	Now aware of wanting changes of some specific kinds	
	↓ ←	Stimulates people to consider what they might do to bring such changes about by taking action themselves
Stage Four	Decide for, or against, trying to meet some want for themselves	
	↓ ←	If necessary, stimulates people to consider how best they can organize themselves to do what they now want to do
Stage Five	Plan what to do and how they will do it	
	↓ ←	Stimulates people to consider and decide in detail just what to do, who will do it, and when and how they will do it
Stage Six	Act according to their planning	
	↓ ←	Stimulates people to think through any unforeseen difficulties or problems they may encounter in the course of what they do. (The worker may again need to help them work through each of the preceding five stages in deciding how to tackle each problem)
Stage Seven	Satisfied with the result of what they have achieved?	

Figure 8.2 Stages in the thinking process leading to action by a group. From Batten (1967) *The Non-Directive Approach in Group and Community Work* [26].

compatible with Freire's [27] pedagogical aims and is consonant with the aims of self-empowerment – as described in Chapter One. The methods adopted by the 'facilitators' are akin to those recommended for use in various UK schools' health and lifeskills teaching – e.g. analysis of felt needs, team building, goal setting, problem-solving, etc. The goals of the Thai project, however, proved to be more tangible and immediate and included the acquisition of occupational skills which might be used to help the community by, for example, putting into practice a village project such as building a water drainage system. In other words, we have a scheme which incorporates the two classic goals of community organization/development: first the 'ideological' and all-embracing aim of self-empowering individuals and community; second the more specific objectives which emerge from the 'felt needs' of the participants.

As for the evaluation, planners utilized a number of simple tools to determine (i) a process effect – participants and facilitators' responses to the programme, (ii) intermediate indicators of participants' learning – attitudes and behaviours, and (iii) longer term outcome indicators. The process evaluation indicated for instance that '... outside resource people tended to present boring lectures'! This fact was taken into account when revising the programme along with various positive recommendations – that the occupational skills sessions were effective as were the morning calisthenics. With regard to intermediate indicators, various changes in attitude were recorded such as a greater awareness of village problems and a recognition that the individuals' abilities could be used to improve their lives. At the same time ambivalent results were noted in respect of such items as 'I am confident of my abilities' and 'I think my life will be better five years from now'. Clearly self-empowerment had been tempered by a recognition of the real social and environmental contraints.

As for outcome indicators; participants were reported to have become more active in discussion and had acquired increased skills in working in small groups (again it is interesting to note the parallel with school-based lifeskills evaluation measures). More importantly perhaps for the good of the community and the experience of success by the participants, most of the planned projects had been completed by the end of three months (e.g. raising $300 for village development projects; establishing a day-care centre; preparing a village learning centre; construction of three roads and the repair of a public hall).

COMMUNITY HEALTH PROJECTS

Let us turn now to community health projects – i.e. projects which utilize the strategies of community organization in order to address recognizable health issues. Again, although there are innumerable community projects concerned with some aspect of health (for instance the London Health Action Network listed almost 200 such schemes in 1984 [28]), evaluation is a relative rarity or incomplete or unhelpfully anecdotal. However before providing an account of a project which does provide a full account of itself, it is worth observing that the mere fact of being a community health project concerned with health in some way detracts from the notion of a 'pure type' of community organization which has been suggested above. The 'pure type' referred to here would be a development project whose only preconception was that of self-empowerment and equity. In other words the innovators would be concerned to modify feelings of learned helplessness and provide the community with the wherewithal to bring to fruition its own felt needs. By definition a health project – which in many cases might better be described as a medical project – seeks to identify one or more needs over and above those of self-empowerment and if not exactly imposing them on the community, at least seeks to have the community include them prominently among its list of felt needs. However, we can do more than reiterate an earlier point – namely that there are two kinds of community project: those which are top-down (social/technical planning) and those which are bottom-up (true community organization). Indeed consideration of a variety of community schemes would suggest there is a spectrum of activities having pure community organization at one pole and heavily coercive (medical model) outreach programmes at the other. A typical community health project might be located mid-way on such a spectrum and is shown at point three in Figure 8.3.

Clearly the nature of the goals shift from Type 1 to Type 5 in parallel with the criteria for programme success. Whereas the priority for Type 1 programmes would be to achieve self-empowerment and an improvement in socio-economic status, the most pressing goals of Type 5 programmes would be the achievement of preventive medical targets and their associated epidemiological outcomes. Because of their failure to gain community involvement, Type 5 programmes would have a much lower chance of success than those characterized by Type 4 practices. This latter type would include the major CHD prevention programmes to be discussed below. The top-down aspect which distinguishes these from more genuine community development can be seen in Farquhar *et al.*'s [29] discussion of the field application of community organization with its three stages of 'development, implementation and maintenance'. This systematic process of programme planning is summarized from their work as follows:

1. Development
   (a) *Goal definition.* Review of literature and baseline data to determine people's needs for information, motivation, skills, etc. in order to determine target groups and kind of programme needed to reduce their risks of disease.
   (b) *Resources definition.* Choice of appropriate resources for each risk factor.
   (c) *Community recruiting.* Identifying community leaders and enlisting aid of organizations to achieve programme goals.

Type 1 Innovators' goal for the community is primarily self-empowerment and improvement in socio-economic status.
Self-empowerment = health.

Type 2 As above but during the process of developing a community profile and identifying felt needs, the community itself acknowledges needs which are consistent with standard preventive medical/health education goals - e.g. need for better primary care services, accident prevention, dealing with child health problems.

Type 3 Characterized by 'community health projects'. Innovators' goals are to enhance health and prevent disease. They aim to do this by raising the profile of health but are prepared to help the community work through other more pressing 'felt needs' prior to their acknowledging a need to improve cardiovascular health for example.

Type 4 Innovators' goals are primarily those of preventive medicine. This type is epitomized by the various CHD prevention programmes. It is more 'top-down' than Types 1-3 but it understands the importance of taking the community with it and utilizing existing leadership patterns, etc.

Type 5 More limited 'out-reach' programmes; limited community participation but uses mix of agencies, e.g. media plus schools, plus drop-in centres and delivery of services to housing estate or workplace.

Figure 8.3 A spectrum of community organization programmes.

 (d) *Programme definitions.* Gaining feedback '... to fit the community's and the initiators' needs ...'; formative evaluation and design of programme are planned.
2. *Implementation.*
 (a) *Materials and programme developoment.* e.g. training of leaders; pre-testing materials.
 (b) *Consulting with community groups.* e.g. '... helping advisory boards become functioning community units ...'.
 (c) *Programme field testing.* e.g. redesigning and refining the programme.
3. *Maintenance.* This involves 'programme monitoring; programme multiplication; programme continuation.' The final goal is institutionalization and community ownership.

Simmons [30], in 1976, edited a series of reports from a workshop which represented, '... the first effort to present an overall picture of how health education principles were applied in the past decade to health programmes serving low-income and minority groups.' The six projects presented and analysed demonstrate the importance of community participation and run almost the whole gamut of types of intervention described in Figure 8.3. The communities in question ranged from hospital patients and staff to isolated villages in Alaska. One study in particular, the 'Forty Family Pilot Study', epitomizes the broader community organization programme which is representative of Type 2 community inverventions. The importance of locating medical goals which a broader framework and subordinating them to more fundamental socio-economic targets is highlighted by the project's philosophy which is reproduced below:

> Poverty is more than a lack of economic resources. It also includes a set of values and states of existence which exclude the poor from the opportunities offered middle-class persons.
>
> Citizens in the low-income group must be brought from the periphery of social living into the structure of the community. Nothing that the community does for the poor can be durably effective until the poor are a functioning part of the community.
>
> There is a need not only for medical, educational and occupational assistance for low-income people, but especially for a system of touching the lives and attitudes of the poor so that they can take advantage of all resources available to them.

The impact of the Forty Family Pilot Study project which applied the community education principles discussed above was dramatic. The various indicators listed below reveal not only standard epidemiological/clinical measures but much broader (and arguably more important) testimony of success.

1. Eighty-five per cent of families received dental and physical examinations during the first year compared with less then 5% previously.
2. Mothers became aware of nutritional aspects of meal planning; there was an improvement in general health knowledge.
3. The number of adults receiving the General Education Diploma increased by 19% in one year.
4. All but 0.9% of children were in school compared with a previous drop-out rate of 19%.
5. Thirty two per cent of people were now buying their own homes compared with 20% the previous year.
6. Average family income increased from $3900 in July 1972 to $4960 in July 1973.

While it is clear that community participation and empowerment is more easy to achieve within a relatively small locality or neighbourhood, as was clearly the case with the Forty Family Pilot Study, it should not be assumed that all interventions in relatively small communities will have general empowering goals. Indeed, one effective intervention [31] in an under-developed village community has an overtly medical brief – to eradicate scabies. A seven person health team used Type 5 tactics with the 3000 inhabitants of the Western Galilee village and achieved its goal – the eradication of scabies which prior to the campaign had been prevalent in 66% of the families!

Again, provided that there is a sufficient level of motivation, very good success can be achieved without full community involvement. Indeed one of the most thorough and well evaluated programmes, by Sayegh and Green [32], was organized within the American University Medical Centre in Beirut. Its concern was to develop an efficient family planning programme and although it is perhaps more properly regarded as patient education, it is worth noting its success here by way of comparison with the much more complex and problematic endeavours of full-scale community programmes. In short, from an initial rate of acceptance of family planning of 4.2%, an experimental group receiving efficient health education eventually settle at a level of maintained contraceptive use of some 37%. Bearing in mind that the acceptance rate of an International Post-partum Programme was 17% (population base of 497 622), it was possible to demonstrate not merely success in terms of behaviour change but also cost-effectiveness: the programme was cheaper per success rate than alternative methods of family planning education.

However, as indicated before, single goal programmes such as family planning embody fewer costs of all kinds than, say, alcohol education. For such programmes a community-wide approach would seem to be essential. Various such programmes have been documented – for instance Hersey *et al.* [33] demonstrated that an '... intensive combination of community activities and media exposure ...' could achieve desirable mental health goals. Apart from increases in knowledge and changes in attitude, respondents exposed to both media and community activities indicated '... substantial likelihood of engaging in support enhancing behaviour' compared with population groups receiving less extensive interventions. Undoubtedly, however, the most intense and comprehensive efforts in health education in recent years have been directed at the reduction of coronary heart disease. An analysis of these CHD prevention programmes is particularly illuminating therefore – not only because of the amount of research and evaluation incorporated in programmes but because the substantive nature of the programmes is of great interest. In short, whereas the complex nature of the risk factors involved in CHD pose a major challenge to health educators, the prospects for success seem a priori rather better than those facing alcohol educators (on the evidence discussed in Chapter Six on mass media).

THE MAJOR CHD PREVENTION PROJECTS

Farquhar *et al.* [34] describe ten community-based multiple risk-factor health education interventions. Four of these will be considered here: the Stanford Heart Disease Prevention Projects, the Minnesota Heart Health Study, the Pawtucket Heart Health Study and the North Karelia Project. A detailed review of each is beyond the scope of this chapter which will, therefore, be limited to discussing the following main features of the projects and their evaluation. First the main characteristics of the programme itself will be described. This will be followed by comments on the nature of the evaluation and, finally, observations will be made on the results of the evaluation – where these are available.

As regards evaluation, it should be noted that all of the programmes reject the clinical trials model – with greater or lesser reluctance and do so for the reasons discussed earlier in this chapter. Some projects, however, make strenuous efforts to compensate for the lack of a true experimental design by the introduction of various techniques to enhance the internal validity of their quasi-experiments. All projects utilize process evaluation – both to gain illumination and, in its formative mode, to monitor and improve interventions. In some instances, a true experimental design might be incorporated within a subprogramme.

Blackburn [35] describes the main strategies which are used to mitigate the effects of what is inevitably an imperfect experiment. These are adopted by the Minnesota Project and are listed below:

1. Creation of a degree of control by matching communities for anticipated important variables such as population structure, service provision, CHD mortality, etc.
2. Staging community entry to the programme thus allowing repetition of the experimental input and the consequent strengthening of inference of cause and effect.
3. Sensitive trend measures (allowing time series analysis) by means of cross-sectional surveys of communities and repeated measures of individual change within cohorts.
4. Dose–effect measurement which looks for different degrees of response in those subjected to increasing levels of educational exposure and programme involvement.
5. Establishing links between responses to specific elements of the educational programme and subsequent changes, e.g. links between participation in a nutrition programme and subsequent change of diet/reduction in risk factors.
6. Pooling communities/groups of people exposed to education and comparing them with similar pools in control communities.

In relation to the kinds of evaluation employed, the four projects will be compared in respect of:

1. Measures of mortality/morbidity, i.e. disease-related outcomes.
2. Risk factor reduction.
3. Intermediate measures of programme outcome ranging from the acquisition of knowledge, attitudes and skills to the various behaviours underpinning risk factor scores.
4. Process evaluation.

THE STANFORD STUDIES

The Stanford Three Community Study began in 1972 and has been extensively documented and described. It sought to examine the impact of two levels of intervention on two Californian towns by comparison with a control community. The populations of the towns ranged from 13 000 to 15 000. The Stanford Heart Disease Prevention Project (SHDPP) established the pattern for later schemes by building the interventions on a firm foundation of learning theory. This seems unremarkable but it is worth noting that many preventive interventions prior to this date (and many since!) had been educationally naïve – often making the assumption that providing information was the same as providing education. The theoretical element included an amalgam of social learning theory, attitude and communication theory and social marketing. This produced an almost standard formula which Farquhar *et al.* [29] described as a Communication–behaviour Change Framework. Effectively this meant ensuring a chain of events starting with agenda setting, moving on to the provision of information, enhancement of motivation, offering models, providing training and skills, offering 'cues to action' – which allowed programme participants to acquire self-management competences – and finally ensuring the availability of social and environmental support for newly acquired risk-reducing behaviours.

There were several points of especial theoretical interest in the main interventions used by the SHDPP and these centre on the role of mass media. One community, Gilroy, received only a mass media programme while Watsonville was subjected to the identical media influences and also provided with supplementary intensive instruction. For these reasons, the SHDPP found itself a kind of test case in the debate about the capabilities of mass media – a point of some interest in the light of Chapter Six. Before examining the impact of these measures however we should note the extent of the mass media programming employed by the Stanford team.

It consisted of some 50 television public service advertisements broadcast by four stations; three hours of television programmes; more than 100 radio spots and several hours of radio broadcasting; weekly newspaper columns,

255

advertisements and stories; poster advertising; direct mail including calendars and cook books mailed to each household; and kits for schools. This programme was continued for nine months after pre-testing in 1973 and repeated in 1974 after a second survey.

The intensive instruction received by Watsonville was derived from social learning theory and employed a range of behaviour modification techniques. It was delivered to a group of individuals at high risk (two thirds of a random sample of individuals falling into the top risk quartile) and consisted of home counselling/group sessions for a ten week period and included spouses who were willing to be involved.

The evaluation strategy involved baseline surveys in the three towns followed by three further surveys of the same samples at one yearly intervals. Participants' knowledge and beliefs about CHD and its prevention were assessed along with relevant behaviours. They key aspect of the summative evaluation, however, was a measure of reduction in a risk score derived from an equation incorporating cardinal risk factors of age, sex, systolic blood pressure, relative weight, amount of cigarette smoking and plasma cholesterol. Process evaluation was mainly concerned with various mini surveys which monitored the impact of media – in addition to materials pre-testing and developmental testing of the intensive instruction programme. An additional interesting example of process evaluation was provided by the results of a diffusion survey using network analysis to determine the nature of interpersonal contacts stimulated by the programme. This revealed, for instance, that whereas on average an individual only receiving a mass media input might have an average number of two interpersonal contacts and a frequency of two conversations with other people about CHD, someone receiving the media programme together with screening and face-to-face education from a health educator would make contact with eight people and have 13 conversations.

The results of the Three Towns Project were convincing. After one year there was evidence of significant shifts on the baseline measures with Watsonville leading the field – presumably thus justifying the assumption of the superiority of interpersonal education. For instance an overall improvement in knowledge about triglycerides was recorded (an increase from 18% to 45%) and belief in the statement that eating eggs could be harmful had increased from 67% to 77% in Gilroy, from 65% to 86% in Watsonville but showed no change in Tracy, the control town. As for behaviour change, there had been a decline in smoking: in Watsonville a 20% reduction was noted (44% in high risk group) but only a 3% drop had been observed in Gilroy. Of the high risk group, 31% had quit smoking during the first year of the programme. Using egg consumption as a behavioural indicator, the superiority of Watsonville at the mid-point in the intervention was again in evidence: the number of eggs eaten had declined 17% in Tracy, the control; 27% in Gilroy and 40% in Watsonville [38].

However, what created most interest and debate was the end-of-programme summative evaluation which demonstrated not only a significant reduction in risk but also revealed that Gilroy, the town exposed only to mass media, had virtually caught up with Watsonville. The relative risk in the control town had increased by some 6% while it had decreased by some 18% in the two experimental towns, yielding a net difference between control and treatment of between 23% and 28%. Among high-risk participants, the intensive instruction group had a 5% lower risk than the media only group [37].

What are we to make of these results which suggest that mass media can in fact yield results virtually as good as interpersonal education? The first point to note is that the intensity and extensiveness of the media programme per head of population was very substantial. The second point is, of course, that it is impossible to know the extent to which the media campaign triggered interpersonal education by health professionals and educators. The third point to note is that the media design was based on good learning theory and approximated therefore to interpersonal communication. However, Maccoby and Solomon [36] themselves state the case very appositely:

> We tentatively attribute much of the success of the community education campaigns to the quality of the media campaign and to the *synergistic interaction of multiple educational inputs* and to interpersonal communication stimulated by application of these inputs in a community setting (author's emphasis).

Farquahar *et al.* [37] add:

> Intensive face-to-face instruction and counselling seem important for changing refractory behaviour such as cigarette smoking and for inducing rapid change of dietary behaviour. But we must learn how to use these methods to correct obesity, and to employ them effectively with limited resources (e.g. by training volunteer instructors). Mass media are potentially much more cost-effective than face-to-face education methods.

The Stanford Three Towns Study – despite its manifest success – has been criticized on several grounds [39]. These objections may be summarized as follows. Firstly, it was argued that the study was wrong to confuse behavioural and medical indicators (a point made in Chapter Three). For instance, health education might well produce a change in behaviour such as a reduction in dietary cholesterol, without necessarily leading to a reduction in physiological risk and community levels of CHD. This issue of the wisdom of latching on to epidemiological indicators will be mentioned again later when considering the North Karelia experience. The second objection centres on an accusation that the SHDPP was unduly wedded to a medical model and missed the opportunity of appraising a genuine community study. As Leventhal *et al.* [39] say, 'We believe ... that the Stanford study is better described as a quasi-experimental study of individuals in a community setting and that it retains many of the failings typically ascribed to laboratory investigations.' These critics also regret the lack of sufficient process measures to describe community activities and diffusion of information. The third objection related to problems of internal validity of the kind discussed earlier and which follow failure to employ a true experimental design.

Not surprisingly the Stanford team reacted somewhat tetchily to these criticisms – and with justification [40]. A detailed discussion of the case is not appropriate here – but we might with benefit note the impossibility of avoiding criticism on methodological grounds without the talisman of randomization! We should also note that the follow-up to the Three Towns Study sought to meet some of Leventhal *et al's* criticisms. This took the form of a five cities study. However, since final results have not been reported at the time of writing, full details of this extension to the Three Towns Study cannot be described here. A comprehensive account is provided elsewhere by Farquhar *et al.* [41] and this summarizes succinctly the differences between the three and five centre studies in the following way:

1. The two experimental cities receiving the health education intervention are much larger and more socially complex. The health education is aimed at the entire population.
2. Three moderate sized cities are used as controls; total population size is 350 000 compared with 43 000.
3. The project will run for nine years and annual rates of fatal and non-fatal cardiovascular events will be monitored.
4. The project will incorporate a community organization approach.
5. A wider age range will be used in surveys [12–74]. In contrast to the cohort design of the Three Centres Study, repeated independent samples will be used to monitor programme effects.

In the context of the present chapter, the inclusion of community organization within the Five City Project is of special significance. The rationale for doing so seems to have more to do with ensuring that the project continues after the expiry of its funding than with notions of self-empowerment and the like. Community organization is, moreover, a feature of the remaining cardio-vascular disease/coronary heart disease (CVD/CHD) prevention projects to be examined here. The structure of these programmes owes a good deal to the pioneering work of the SHDPP.

THE MINNESOTA HEART HEALTH PROGRAM

The major difference between the Minnesota Heart Health Program (MHHP) and the SHDPP is the community organization aspect and the ways in which a wide variety of agencies and lay people are orchestrated to achieve project goals. Clearly its medical goals are identical with SHDPP and it thus represents a prime example of a Type 4 community programme (Figure 8.3). The goals of the Project are succinctly stated by Jacobs *et al.* [42]. It is interesting to observe how these have taken account of the general downward trend in cardiovascular disease (CVD) risk in their reference to accelerating the change process.

> Major MHHP hypotheses are that a systematic and multiple-strategy community-wide health education program is feasible and will lead to a change in the way people think about heart disease and its prevention; in behaviours related to risk for heart disease; in physiologic risk factors; and ultimately in disease rates. Some of these changes are occurring naturally. The MHHP aims to accelerate this change, and hypothesizes that an intensive education program of five years duration in a community will inititate risk factor changes leading to decreased disease rates. A further MHHP hypothesis is that the program will be taken over by the community after the researchers leave.

Three pairs of education and reference/control communities have been chosen for study and were enrolled in a phased manner (to enhance evaluation power as indicated earlier). The communities are matched and represent three different types: Mankato paired with Winona represented small free-standing towns; Fargo, North Dakota paired with Sioux Falls, South Dakota represented large free-standing cities; Bloomington paired with Roseville, Maplewood and North St. Paul represented large suburban areas.

The comprehensive education programme involves three major thrusts: mass media, direct education and community organization. Education is delivered through health education centres, by means of short courses, lectures, workshops and seminars and, of course, via school programmes. Target groups are community organizations and community leaders, youth, adults and health professionals. An over-riding aim is to ensure there is at least one direct contact with the majority of individuals within the community [35].

The intensity of the programme may be judged from an account of the health centre operation. This contact is designed to provide screening and 'exposure to educational and motivational messages'. It involves an audio-visual presentation for the family group to introduce them to the programme; the family rotates through various screening stations and receives further audio-

259

visual inputs about risk factors; their physical activity level is ascertained at an interactive computer station; finally they receive a whole family counselling session.

The nature of the schools programme is well illustrated by recent articles by Perry *et al*. which describe a 'needs assessment' of young people's nutrition and exercise status [43] and the development of a 20-session heart healthy nutrition education curriculum for third and fourth grade students [44].

The model of community organization is described by Carlaw *et al*. [46]. It is defined as a partnership between community and the MHHP development team, and the WHO's [45] reference to participation is cited by way of philosophical justification:

> Participation – or more correctly involvement – is a process in which individuals and communities identify with a movement and take responsibility jointly with health professionals and others concerned, for making decisions and planning and carrying out activities.

The procedures described are somewhat different from the classic grassroots bottom-up approach in, for example, disadvantaged inner city communities. The first step involves 'Community Analysis' by the team which consists of identifying geographical and interest sector representatives to serve on heart health boards and provision of training. It is followed by the establishment of 'Task Forces' which identify strategies and seek to influence their communities. Ideally this leads to the third stage, development of 'Social System Support' which includes skill development sessions in churches, school districts, trade unions, health clubs, etc. This hopefully leads to a 'strengthening of community norms and values'. The final stage should result in 'Organizational commitment to an improved social environment' and lead to a shift in the balance of power from the initiating researchers to the community itself. However the impression created is that the main focus is on institutions and community leaders rather than the 'hard-to-reach' targets of traditional locality development initiatives. For instance, as part of the process of 'organizational commitment', i.e. what has been described above as the final stage in the programme, the main target group consists of employers and managers who are asked to take responsibility for the provision of gentle coercion to lead the population to a healthier lifestyle. Those in authority are asked to encourage and reinforce '... consistent heart healthy behaviour through financial and other incentive systems' and 'insurance companies, banks and related organizations providing favourable rates for heart healthy families and individuals.' These last quotes point up one further way in which MHHP differs from Stanford: it incorporates many of the 'healthy public policy' aspects of health promotion. As Carlaw *et al*. [46] state:

> A second aspect of Phase I was the development, in the community, of the opportunities to practice healthful behavior. In practical terms

this translated into choices available to the consumer through services such as grocery store labelling, indexing of heart healthy menus in restaurants, improved smoking cessation services and attractive opportunities for physical activity for all age groups. Food packaging and food preparation are directed by marketing factors having little or no relationship to the health of the consumer. Considerable community initiative is needed to modify these services so that heart healthy behavior is encouraged.

Programme evaluation incorporated a wide range of measures. It is interesting to note that although the possibility existed of random allocation of communities to experimental or reference situations, this tactic was deliberately rejected since the small number of units involved could not guarantee equality: matching was therefore a superior strategy. Intermediate and outcome measures comprised '... *net* changes in awareness, participation, cognitions, behaviours, risk factors and disease endpoints.' [42]. Process measures included 'linkage' between education components and behaviour change and 'coincidence' of community change with the staged entry of different communities to the programme.

The MHHP provides a nice illustration of three broad categories of measure representing final outcomes, intermediate indicators and indirect indicators. The final outcomes include the disease endpoints: mortality and morbidity data on CHD and cerebro-vascular accident (CVA). The intermediate indicators include risk factor measures of blood pressure, smoking, total serum cholesterol and high-density lipoprotein (HDL) level together with associated behaviours relating to blood pressure control, smoking cessation, physical activity in leisure time and diet. More indirect cognitive and attitudinal measures which are related to these variables are also measured.

Jacobs *et al*. [42] provide an excellent example of indicators occurring at an early stage on the proximal-distal/input-output chain in their 14-point list of ways in which the community might participate in the programme. These are listed in Table 8.2. The MHHP also provides a very apposite illustration of the way in which it is possible to utilize true experimental design in community studies. These do of course fall within the broader quasi-experimental framework. As Jacobs *et al*. point out, although '... it is not possible to randomly withold from some persons television campaigns, a community walk, or a grocery store labelling program...', it is possible '... to randomly delay invitation to the MHHP Heart and Health Center to a random group of persons.' Such sub-experiments serve to test and improve specific methods and interventions.

Process measures/formative evaluation include telephone surveys to check on particular education programmes and the use of focus groups to evaluate media messages. Blake *et al*. [47] also describe in full detail a process evaluation of a physical activity campaign which illustrates the value of such research for

Table 8.2 Intermediate indicators of programme participation: Minnesota Heart Health Program (MHHP)

---

1. General awareness of the existence of the programme and/or its goals

2. CHD risk factor screening in the MHHP Heart Health Center

3. Exposure to general MHHP messages in the media

4. Exposure to specific MHHP messages in the media (such as television programme or a pamphlet or book)

5. Participation in the Shape-Up Challenge (a worksite physical activity programme)

6. Recognition/use of the restaurant menu labelling programme

7. Recognition/use of the grocery store labelling programme

8. Doing homework with children who participate in a MHHP school programme

9. Contact with a health professional whose practice has been influenced by MHHP

10. 'Quit and Win' smoking classes and contest

11. Participation on a MHHP task force

12. Participation in other MHHP sponsored classes

13. Social contact with the precepts and ideas of MHHP

14. Speaking at or hearing a speaker at a club or organization meeting

---

programme refinement. They considered community awareness of and participation in five specific kinds of exercise opportunity using telephone surveys and observation of participation. These indicated, *inter alia*, that participation was highest for activities organized within existing organizations but awareness was highest for heavily publicized general population events.

Final evaluation results obviously await the conclusion of the programme but several encouraging indications have already been noted. For instance, Mittelmark *et al.* [48] reported that initial objectives had been achieved. After two years, 190 community leaders were directly involved as programme volunteers; 14 103 residents (60% of adults) had attended a screening education centre; 2094 had attended health education classes; distribution of printed media averaged 12.2 pieces per household.

One of the salient features of MHHP was the provision of medical education and training for doctors and other health professionals who would act as role models and active educators. After two years, 42 of the 65 physicians in Mankato and 728 other health professionals had participated in continuing education programmes offered by MHHP.

As regards young people's programmes, all third, fifth, sixth and eleventh grade students were involved in the MHHP heart health education teaching, and 1665 young people visited the heart health centre with their parents.

Population surveys also revealed higher levels of awareness of the various heart-related risk behaviours in Mankato compared with the reference community. A telephone evaluation revealed that about one sixth of smokers watched at least one segment of a local television's five day series of cessation hints and one per cent stopped smoking. A smoking cessation short course called 'Quit and Win' resulted in 5% of all smokers in the community committing themselves to give up smoking. Over 50% of those who signed up stopped for one month and 34% had not relapsed after two months [49].

Reference was made above to the inclusion of true experiments within the overall framework. One of these [50] compared the level of risk of an experimental group who had received the personalized risk factor screening programme with a control group. After one year, the former group had significantly lower risk factor scores in respect of: blood cholesterol, diastolic blood pressure, reduced fat and salt consumption and increased regular exercise.

In short, Minnesota's multi-intervention community programme appears to be having a substantial impact. The next project for analysis is that of Pawtucket. Its special interest lies in its peculiar interpretation of community participation.

THE PAWTUCKET HEART HEALTH PROGRAM

The special interest of the Pawtucket Heart Health Program (PHHP) in the present context is its approach to community organization and the theoretical rationale which underpins this approach. In short, this project seeks to get closer to the grass roots.

The PHHP study community is located in Rhode Island, New England. Its residents are described as predominantly blue collar. The City of Pawtucket has some 72 000 inhabitants and the population is described as very stable. For evaluation purposes it is matched with a control community of some 98 000 people. The project is planned to run from 1980 to 1991; professional guidance is to be provided for the first four years and thereafter the management is to be in the hands of a community volunteer system.

The observations made below are derived from reports by Lefebvre *et al.* [51] and Elder *et al.*[52]. The authors, in discussing the community-level approach of PHHP, make a distinction between locality development and social planning – as discussed earlier in this chapter. Their definition of the former makes reference to the involvement of the people in goal determination and action, democratic procedures, training of indigenous leaders and educational self-help methods. Social planning is seen as an alternative view of community organization in which social change is planned by designated experts. 'Citizens are seen as being passive recipients of services ... the practitioner role of 'expert' in social planning strategies contrasts markedly with the 'enabler' posture of locality developers.' [51]. The PHHP is, in practice, considered to offer a blend of both of these theoretically discrete approaches together with Rothman's [53] model of social action in which experts ... 'seek to organize coalitions of concerned interests to attack the problem.' Within the framework of PHHP Lefebvre *et al.* see these social action tactics as involving, '... campaign tactics; employment of facts; and persuasion within the context of voluntary association, mass media, and legislative bodies to change institutional and community policies and norms ... citizens can be either recipients or agents of action, while the practitioner role is defined more as that of a coalition builder, fact gatherer, and policy analyst.' The researchers consider that PHHP's use of churches as heart health delivery systems illustrates this social action approach within Pawtucket.

Elder *et al.* identify four principles operating within the general approach. These are: (i) the importance of local ownership, (ii) the use of inexpensive resources and facilities (to make community ownership more feasible after external funding has ceased), (iii) the importance of interpersonal education – with media being used as awareness-raising devices, and (iv) the use of multilevel programming,i.e. reciprocal contributions of community, organizational, small group and individual programmes.

Elder *et al.* also record the change in emphasis during the first 26 months of PHHP from organizations to community. During the first 11 months the focus was on worksites, churches, schools and other organizations. Progress however was slow and this produced a strategic shift after 11 months when an attempt was made to accelerate progress by directing the programme to the community at large in association with media publicity. By the end of this stage perhaps the most singular feature of PHHP had emerged – the 'volunteer delivery system'. Lefebvre *et al.* have argued that there are at least eight reasons for using volunteers in preventive heart health programmes: they serve as peer models (cf. the principle of homophily); they provide a support network for others who have made changes in lifestyle; their own healthy behaviour is reinforced; they promote diffusion through social networks; effective volunteers can be deliberately 'networked' to help change norms; a volunteer system helps promote community ownership; it is cost effective; it has a multiplier effect.

The goals of PHHP are similar to those of the other major cardiovascular disease prevention programmes and they are similarly 'theory-driven'. Lefebvre *et al.* summarize this aspect of the project as an 'Intervention Cube' where the risk factor and disease endpoints of fitness, weight reduction, fat and cholesterol control, management of blood pressure and reduction of smoking are to be attained via four programme phases. These latter involve motivating the community; providing skills training for risk factor reduction; developing support networks, and finally ensuring the maintenance of ensuing change. The programmes are seen as having an impact at four levels: the individual, group, organization and the community at large.

Evaluation results to date are largely concerned with process. The general situation [51] is described thus:

> Children are involved in Heart Health Clubs, smoking prevention programs, and classroom heart health education;
> parents learn to raise heart healthy children;
> people shop at grocery stores where shelf labels identify foods low in salt, fat, and calories, and eat in Four-Heart restaurants offering good-tasting menu items that are low in fat, sodium, and cholesterol;
> senior citizens are active in Walk Jog Clubs and exercise programs; and
> all residents attend community events such as Octoberfest or 'Meet us in the Park' weekends where the PHHP Heart Check trailer and van are prominently located.

Fourteen Pawtucket companies sent 23 co-ordinators to training sessions; 3604 of 5700 eligible employees were screened.

Twenty one churches have been involved in social action and devoted some 2105 volunteer hours.

Trained volunteers have been accepted by both the lay community and the medical professionals. Between 600 and 1000 blood pressure readings are taken monthly at 14 Walk-In Blood Pressure Stations. In its first three years more than 30 000 hours have been invested by volunteers in the programme and the PHHP has had over 30 000 contacts with people seeking to improve their heart health.

It is, of course, too soon to look for the impact of these activities on disease endpoints. Some intermediate outcome measures have, however, been recorded. For instance people participating in the worksite screening programme succeeded in reducing their blood pressure: prevalence of readings greater than 180/100 dropped from 34 out of 409 screened to zero.

Again, after a 'Community Weigh-In', 138 residents recorded a joint loss of 1061 lbs after ten weeks. Six months later, a follow-up interview of 70% of the 211 original participants revealed that 80% had lost weight and 75% were continuing to do so.

In conclusion, we can reasonably say that the PHHP has again demonstrated that a community-wide programme can achieve substantial changes. In the case of PHHP the suggestion has been made that by using a more informal community effort centering on lay workers and volunteers, changes can be produced in a lower socio-economic status community. The methods used, however, still fall short of the 'true' community development approaches (presumably being somewhere between Types 3 and 4 in Figure 8.3) and whether these strategies would be effective within deprived and under-privileged inner city ghettos must remain a matter of conjecture. Again, whether the same degree of success would be achieved in a national context where healthist norms are less evident must also be a matter for speculation. Two important questions would, therefore, still seem to require answers. Firstly, whether the undoubtedly successful North American experience will generalize to disadvantaged neighbourhoods and to different national populations where health has a lower profile. Secondly, the question which sceptical clinicians and epidemiologists are constantly posing: will the lifestyle changes recorded by the CVD prevention projects result in a demonstrable decline in mortality and morbidity which can unequivocally be attributed to the health promotion? The final example, that of the North Karelia Project, demonstrates clear success in fostering lifestyle change in a European setting. It has also claimed to have an impact on mortality and morbidity but not without challenge!

THE NORTH KARELIA PROJECT

One of the principle features of the North Karelia Project (NKP) is its community focus and the circumstances which led to the establishment of the project are of particular significance. Indeed one of the most noteworthy features of NKP was the frequently cited popular petition to the Finnish government to deal with the problem of premature death from coronary heart disease (CHD) which had apparently forced itself on the consciousness of the population. In fact, following the Seven Countries Study of CHD mortality [68], it became apparent that Eastern Finland held the unenviable record of heading the league table of deaths. However, it apparently took three public reports before community leaders – at the end of the 1960s – began to demand action. This coincided with Karvonen, who was leading the Finnish investigation, having a WHO advisory role and being president of the Finnish Medical Association. It is also reported that the awareness-raising effect of epidemiological data was vigorously supplemented by lobbying by the Finnish Heart Association and its volunteer task force. These somewhat serendipitous circumstances are of importance because it would be wrong to assume that the NKP was the result of some popular upsurge of opinion. Indeed if the petition to government by community leaders had been a fundamentally grassroots eruption, the generalizability of NKP to other European countries would have been in considerable doubt. On the other had it would be wrong to ignore the importance of community awareness: the personal exposure of community members to CHD deaths in friends and relations doubtless concentrates the mind and creates a level of perceived susceptibility which the Health Belief Model requires as an antecedent to preventive action.

At all events the petition which was signed on 12 January 1971 by the Governor, all members of parliament and representatives of official and voluntary bodies signalled the start of a ten year programme which has continued to have repercussions and has influenced the development of health promotion nationally and internationally. Again, somewhat fortuitously, the start of the project was accompanied by the establishment of a medical school at the University of Kuopio and a new public health act which reorganized primary health care. The World Health Organization provided its support and documented the first stages of the project [54] and the thinking underlying the Stanford Project was incorporated.

A full description of NKP is beyond the scope of this book. Suffice to say that its theoretical foundation – the learning theory principles – was similar to the projects discussed above and included social learning theory; communication and attitude theory; Communication of Innovations Theory; and community organization principles. It is, however, worth noting one particular point of emphasis which distinguishes NKP from the North American schemes – and which, perhaps, reflects the different political climates of those countries. Unlike the American projects there is a more overt concern with the socio-economic and physical environment and its effect on the individual's health choices. This is seen in item six [55] in the '... seven key steps to help individuals to modify their behaviour':

1. Improved preventive services to help people to identify their risk factors and to provide appropriate attention and services.
2. Information to educate people about the relationship between behaviours and their health.
3. Persuasion to motivate people and to promote the intentions to adopt the healthy action.
4. Training to increase the skills of self-management, environmental control, and necessary action.
5. Social support to help people to maintain the initial action.
6. Environmental change to create the opportunities for healthy actions and improve unfavourable conditions.
7. Community organization to mobilize the community for broad-ranged changes (through increased social support and environmental modification) to support the adoption of the new lifestyles in the community.

The organization of the NKP was truly community-wide involving the national health service – and especially the new primary health care centres and the public health nurses – together with mass media, doctors, social workers, business leaders, voluntary organizations, administrators, trade unions, sports organizations and local political leaders. A special school and youth programme was developed [56] and in addition to the kinds of environmental change mentioned in, for example, the MMHP, local industry was prevailed upon to make available low-fat dairy products and a new sausage product. This latter move was apparently helped by the fact that two managers had recently experienced heart attacks [57]! Only one aspect of the many interventions described above will receive further comment: the use of voluntary groups and lay leaders.

From the start NKP sought to gain community involvement. As with PHHP, it utilized volunteers extensively. Local 'lay leaders' were identified by informally interviewing shopkeepers and other knowledgeable people in the community. These opinion leaders were then trained to act as models and educators. Over a four year period more than 1000 of 'the most influential members of the local communities were involved ...'. The work of these lay opinion leaders was extensively documented [58, 59] in the general context of diffusion theory. Measures were obtained of: participation in training; perception of relative ease of discussing the various risk factors with people; attitude to these changes; extent to which these leaders had discussed risk factors with three or more people during the preceding week; difference modes of action taken (e.g. direct requests to change behaviour, provision of advice, reference to own example, etc.); frequency of discussion with different target groups; frequency of contact with health centre; perception of their effectiveness in influencing smoking, dietary behaviours and hypertension problems; involvement in the project's television programmes and involvement in general health education. The picture emerging from this evaluation is one of considerable activity with evidence of genuine influence.

In addition to the lay leader tactics, the involvement of the MARTTA Organization proved to have been successful. This voluntary local housewives' association introduced, *inter alia*, 'Parties for a Long Life' in which women were taught how to cook heart-healthy meals and as a result of the experience came to believe that healthy cooking could be tasty! Three hundred and forty four of these sessions were recorded with 15 000 participants. At the 1976 follow-up, 9% of men and 18% of women in Karelia had been involved at least once [57].

Final observations on NKP will be concerned with outcome measures. Before considering the customary risk factors it is worth noting an interesting finding on CHD-related knowledge [60]. Repeated tests of total CHD health knowledge during the early phase of NKP revealed only minimal changes (admittedly from a relatively high starting point). The net change in North Karelia (NK score minus the reference area score) was 4% for men and 2% for women. The researchers comment on interventions which have produced knowledge change but no behaviour change and others which, like SHDPP, recorded an increase in knowledge and a reduction in risk. They rightfully remark on the dubious relationship between knowledge and behaviour change by comparing the minimal shift in knowledge in North Karelia with the 17% and 12% respective decrease in risk factor levels during the same period.

In relation to behaviour change, changes in self-reported dietary behaviours were recorded which indicated a decline in fat consumption. The influence of the programme on smoking was also extensively analysed [61]. Puska *et al.* [55] report a net change in North Karelia of 28% in amount of reported daily smoking by men and 14% for women over the period 1972–82. Elsewhere, in a comparative report of the results of various community projects [49], the decline in male smokers in North Karelia is recorded as a shift from 44% to 31% compared with 39% to 35% in the rest of the country. By the fifth year, the net percentage decline in prevalence was 2.5% for men and 6.1% for women (bearing in mind that a general decline was also occurring in the reference area and in the country as a whole).

With regard to risk factors generally, a decline was noted in mean serum cholesterol. This decline occurred in both the study and the reference areas but was greater in North Karelia. The net decline was 3% in men and 1% in women for the period 1972–1982. Again, a significant net decline in both systolic and diastolic blood pressure was observed in the experimental area. The net change between 1972 and 1982 was 3% in systolic blood pressure (SBP) and 1% diastolic blood pressure (DBP) for men and 5% and 2% respectively for women. As with other measures an overall decline was also occurring in the reference county and the net decline was greater during the first five years of the programme – suggesting a general diffusion effect.

The NKP also evaluated its programme in terms of late primary and secondary prevention. For instance, Salonen *et al.* [62] state that a higher proportion of men recovering from heart attacks in North Karelia did not resume smoking compared with a similar sample from the reference area. McAlister *et al.* [57] noted an increase in the proportion of hypertensives receiving medication from a level of 13% in both Karelia and the reference area to 45% in the study area and 33% in the reference county. The proportion of hypertensives was also alleged to be lower in the intervention area.

Before reporting on disease end-point measures, we should consider an outcome measure which did not figure in the North American CHD prevention projects described above and which serves to illustrate the comprehensiveness and thoroughness of the NKP. The survey questionnaires included questions which attempted to assess the psycho–social consequences of the programme. In addition to items checking perceptions of health status, questions were also asked about stress, psychosomatic symptoms and the like with a view to checking the possibility that the interventions might have generated hypochondria or other negative side-effects. There was in fact no evidence of this, and a statistically significant shift for both men and women in the direction of improved subjective health status was reported. The increase was greater in North Karelia than in the reference area while a greater decline in the 20-variable survey of 'complaints' about stress, etc. was noted in the experimental area. It seems then that subjective wellbeing was enhanced without creating negative effects – all of which was taken to indicate a greater degree of satisfaction with health enhancement in the intervention county.

MORTALITY AND MORBIDITY: THE LAST FRONTIER?

The North Karelia Project, along with the other interventions discussed in this chapter, has demonstrated unequivocally that it is possible to mobilize community resources – both professional and lay – and generate changes in knowledge, beliefs and attitudes. Skills can be provided and lifestyle can be influenced such that the risk of premature death and morbidity from contemporary diseases can be reduced. And yet the most important question remains to be answered. Is it possible to demonstrate that the changes wrought in a community like North Karelia will actually reduce the numbers of deaths and the amount of illness caused by the factors which the programme is designed to prevent? The NKP certainly has something to say on the matter and, as the longest running project which has recorded mortality and morbidity events, it would seem to be in a good position to comment. Unfortunately the issue remains clouded – a situation which is due to the quasi-experimental status of the intervention and the fact that a general decline in CVD is occurring in the country as a whole.

It has been quite clear that there has been a decline in mortality from CHD in Finland as a whole and, as Salonen *et al.* [63] have shown, the decline in North Karelia was greater still. This reduction, between 1969 and 1979, was 24% in men and 51% in women compared with a decline of 12% and 24% respectively in other counties of Finland. McAlister [57], writing in 1982, commented on the implications of this relative reduction when he observed that there had been a comparable reduction in cardiovascular disease pension payments in North Karelia. As he put it, 'Estimates from pension disability data already suggest that payment of over $4 million dollars in disability payments may have been avoided by the less than $1 million expended on the project's intervention activities.'

Tuomilehto *et al.* [64], writing in 1986, described the mortality trends in Finland from 1969 to 1982. They remarked that the annual decline in CHD mortality in men was 2.9% in Karelia whereas in the rest of Finland it was 2.0%. For women the respective annual declines were 4.9% and 3.0%. The net decline in North Karelia was 100 deaths per 100 000 men. On the face of it it seems reasonable to ascribe the substantial progress in North Karelia to the NKP. Indeed Tuomilehto *et al.* were moved to comment 'As we cannot think of any reason for the greater decline of mortality from ischaemic heart disease in North Karelia other than the prevention programme it is reasonable to argue that it was a consequence of the project.' Others, however, could think of alternative explanations and Salonen in 1987 [65], one of the principal investigators, felt obliged to produce a disclaimer which acknowledged four potential sources of bias ranging from differential rates of decline in different regions of Finland to the possible effect of general unspecified changes in Finnish society.

Needless to say, this retraction was greeted with barely disguised pleasure by more conservative clinicians [66] who could not see the logic of changing risk factors unless they have an aetiological role in disease reduction. However, in the last analysis – and given the undesirability/impracticability of using randomized controlled trials for community studies – the implementation of such programmes involves an act of faith. The act of faith is however based on a mass of supportive if not conclusive evidence – not least of which is the Oslo study [67] which was a randomized controlled trial and demonstrated a 47% reduction in incidence of first major CHD event after health education about diet and smoking in a group of 1232 high risk middle-aged men. Perhaps the single most important piece of advice which could be offered to those seeking to measure the success of health education programmes is to avoid 'premature evaluation', i.e. taking the risk of measuring educational success by using clinical outcome measures when the links between educational outcomes and disease end-points are by no means clear-cut.

CONCLUDING REMARKS

As indicated earlier, this final chapter might be said to encapsulate certain key features of the book as a whole. First, the focus on a community-wide interventions reiterates the notion that success will be more readily attained when all delivery systems operate in a co-ordinated way and within a context of healthy public policy. In the absence of evidence of what might be achieved by an all embracing, fully integrated health promotion programme, we can only speculate about the degree of success which might be expected in ideal circumstances. However, the recent CHD prevention projects discussed in this chapter foreshadow what might be possible. They also indicate the complexities involved in co-ordinating a programme directed at only one health topic and, thus, highlight the importance of a specialist health promotion service which would take on the more demanding task of integrating a wide range of programmes at regional or district level.

The chapter, however, does more than urge the cause of integrated and co-ordinated health promotion programming; it also makes reference to the wide variety of research designs and indicators of performance from which the health educator is expected to make a judicious choice. Examples have been presented of evaluations at both the qualitative and quantitative ends of the spectrum and case studies have demonstrated the need to adopt a sophisticated and non-partisan approach to choice of strategy. Furthermore, while acknowledging the fact that medically approved tactics such as the randomized controlled trial (or its educational equivalent) may often be entirely inappropriate in certain programmes, we have questioned the reluctance of some workers to adopt any kind of systematic evaluation. We have also noted the impact of ideology on evaluation – particularly in the review of different understandings of community organization. Perhaps the most powerful lesson to emerge is that, once removed from epistemological debate, the pragmatic reality of evaluation leads to a reconciliation of approach. Both qualitative and quantitative methods will usually be needed to satisfy the research and evaluation requirements of any given programme.

Hopefully, this final chapter has also reminded us of the importance of theoretical considerations. The various international CHD prevention programmes not only provide an impressive display of evaluation techniques, they also ground their programmes firmly in theory which seeks to explain how best to promote the adoption of health innovations based on an awareness of the psycho–social and environmental factors which govern decision-making and the maintenance of behaviour change. It is encouraging, in the face of demands that we demonstrate that health education really works, to note the extent of our understanding of the theoretical principles which provide a foundation for effective practice.

Our final point takes us back to the very first chapter. The importance of philosophy is epitomized by the conflict between the diametrically opposed aims of what might superficially appear to be similar community education programmes. While all community education ventures need the theoretical grounding provided, for example, by Communication of Innovations Theory, the success of pure community organization with its radical empowering philosophy must be judged according to very different criteria from the top-down outreach strategies described in this chapter as social/technical planning. In the last and first analysis, the definition of success must be based on a critical consideration of the fundamental purposes of health education.

REFERENCES

1. Hubley, J. H. (1985) *Papers on Community Development* (mimeo), Leeds Polytechnic.
2. Calouste Gulbenkian Foundation (1984) *A National Centre for Community Development: Report of a Working Party,* Gulbenkian Foundation, London.
3. Henderson, P. and Thomas, D. N. (1980) *Skills in Neighbourhood Work*, Allen and Unwin, London.
4. MacCannell, D. (1979) The elementary structures of community: macrostructural accounting as a methodology for theory building and policy formulation, in:

References

Community Development Research, (ed. E. J. Blakely) Human Sciences Press, New York.

5. Rogers, E. M. and Shoemaker, F. F. (1971) *Communication of Innovations*, Free Press, New York.

6. Chabot, J. H. T. (1976) The Chinese system of health care. *Tropical Geographical Medicine*, **28**, 87–134.

7. Lazarsfeld, P. and Merton, R. K. (1964) Friendship as social process: a substantive and methodological analysis, in: *Freedon and Control in Modern Society* (eds M. Berger *et al.*), Octagon, New York.

8. Cited in Lazes, P. M. (ed.) (1979) *Handbook of Health Education*, Aspen Systems Corp., Maryland.

9. Kindervatter, S. (1979) *Nonformal Education as an Empowering Process*, Center for International Education, Amherst, Mass.

10. Rothman, J. (1970) Three models of community organization practice, in: *Strategies of Community Organization* (eds F. Cox *et al.*), F. E. Peacock, Itasca, Ill.

11. Nix, H. L. (1970) *The Community and Its Involvement in the Study Planning Action Process*, US Dept of Health, Education and Welfare, Atlanta, Georgia.

12. Dodds, J. *et al.* (1986) *Community Development Approaches to Health Promotion in North America: Comparative Underinvestment and Untapped Potential in the United Kingdom?* Health Education Council, London.

13. Alinsky, S. D. (1946) *Reveille for Radicals*, Vintage Books, New York.

14. Kirklin, M. J. and Franzen, L. E. (1974) *Community Organization Bibliography*. Institute on the Church in Urban Industrial Society, Chicago, Ill.

15. Ross, M. G. and Lappin, B. W. (1967) *Community Organization: Theory Principles and Practice*. Harper and Row, New York.

16. Feuerstein, M. T. and Lovel, H. (1983) Introduction: community development and the emergence of primary health care. *Community Development Journal*, **18**, 98–103.

17. Green, L. W. and McAlister, A. L. (1984) Macro-intervention to support health behavior: some theoretical perspectives and practical reflections. *Health Education Quarterly*, **11**, 322–39.

18. Constantino-David, K. (1982) Issues in community organization. *Community Development Journal*, **17**, 190–201.

19. Loney, M. (1981) The British Community Development Projects: questioning the state. *Community Development Journal*, **16**, 55–67.

20. Community Development Project (1977) *Gilding the Ghetto*, CDP Inter-Project Editorial Team, Mary Ward House, 5 Tavistock Place, London WC1H 9SS.

21. Feuerstein, M-T. (1986) *Partners in Evaluation*. MacMillan, London.

22. Hedley, R. (1985) *Measuring Success*. ADVANCE, 14 Bloomsbury Square, London, WC1.

23. Voth, D. E. (1979) Problems in the evaluation of community development efforts, in: *Community Development Research: Concepts, Issues and Strategies*, (ed. E. J. Blakeley), Human Sciences Press, New York.

24. Parlett, M. and Hamilton, D. (1972) *Evaluation as Illumination: a New Approach to the Study of Innovatory Programmes*, Occasional Paper 9, Centre for Research in the Educational Sciences, University of Edinburgh.

25. Means, R. and Smith, R. (1988) *Implementing a pluralistic approach to evaluation in health education policy and politics*, **16**, 17–28.

26. Batten, T. R. (1967) *The Non-Directive Approach in Group and Community Work*. University Press, Oxford.
27. Freire, P. (1972) *Pedagogy of the Oppressed*. Penguin, Harmondsworth.
28. London Community Health Resource (1984) *London Health Action Network* (3rd edn), LVSC, 68 Chalton Street, London NW1.
29. Farquhar, J. W., Maccoby, N. and Solomon, D. S. (1984) Community applications of behavioural medicine, in: *Handbook of Behavioural Medicine*, (ed. W. D. Gentry). Guilford Press, New York.
30. Simmons, J. (ed.) (1976) *Making Health Education Work*. American Public Health Association, Washington, DC.
31. Kanaaneh, H. A. K., Rabi, S. A. and Badarneh, S. M. (1976) The eradication of a large scabies outbreak using community-wide health education. *American Journal of Public Health*, **66**, 564–7.
32. Sayegh, J. and Green, L. W. (1976) Family planning education: programme design, training component and cost effectiveness. *International Journal of Health Education*, **19**, (Supplement).
33. Hersey, J. C., Klibanoff, L. S., Lam, D. J. and Taylor, R. L. (1984) Promoting social support: The impact of California's 'Friends Can be Good Medicine' campaign. *Health Education Quarterly*, **11**, 293–311.
34. Farquhar, J. W., Fortmann, S. P., Wood, P. D. and Haskell, W. L. (1983) Community studies of cardiovascular disease prevention, in: *Prevention of Coronary Heart Disease: Practical Management of Risk Factors* (eds N. M. Kaplan *et al.*) W. B. Saunders, Philadelphia.
35. Blackburn, H. (1983) Research and demonstration projects in community cardiovascular disease prevention. *Journal of Public Health Policy*, **4**, 398–421.
36. Maccoby, N. and Solomon, D. (1981) Experiments in risk reduction through community health education, in: *Health Education by Television and Radio* (ed. M. Meyer). K. G. Saur, München.
37. Farquhar, J. W. *et al.* (1977) Community education for cardiovascular health. *Lancet*, i, 1192–5.
38. Maccoby, N. and Farquhar, J. W. (1975) Communication for health–unselling heart disease. *Journal of Communication*, **25**, 114–26.
39. Leventhal, H., Cleary, P. D., Safer, M. A. and Gutmann, M. (1980) Cardiovascular risk modification by community-based programs for lifestyle change: comments on the Stanford study. *Journal of Consulting and Clinical Psychology*, **48**, 150–8.
40. Meyer, A. J., Maccoby, N. and Farquhar, J. W. (1980) Reply to Kasl and Leventhal *et al. Journal of Consulting and Clinical Psychology*, **48**, 159–63.
41. Farquhar, J. W. *et al.* (1984) The Stanford Five City Project: an overview, in: *Behavioural Health: A Handbook of Health Enhancement and Disease Prevention*, (eds J. D. Matarazzo *et al.*). John Wiley, New York.
42. Jacobs, D. R. *et al.* (1985) *Community-Wide Prevention Strategies: Evaluation Design of the Minnesota Heart Health Program*, Mimeo. University of Minnesota, Minneapolis.
43. Perry, C. L., Griffin, G. and Murray, D. M. (1985) Assessing needs for youth health promotion. *Preventive Medicine*, **14**, 379–93.
44. Perry, C. L., Mullis, R. M. and Maile, M. C. (1985) Modifying the eating behavior of young children. *Journal of School Health*, **55**, 399–402.

References

45. World Health Organization (1983) *New Approaches to Health Education in Primary Health Care, Technical Report Series 690.* WHO, Geneva.
46. Carlaw, R. W., Mittlemark, M. B., Bracht, N. and Luepker, R. (1984) Organization for a community cardiovascular health program: experiences from the Minnesota Heart Health Program. *Health Education Quarterly*, **11**, 243–52.
47. Blake, S. M. *et al.* (1987) Process evaluation of a community-based physical activity campaign: the Minnesota Heart Health Program Experience. *Health Education Research*, **2**, 115–21.
48. Mittelmark, M. B. *et al.* (1986) Community-wide prevention of cardiovascular disease: education strategies of the Minnesota Heart Health Program. *Preventive Medicine*, **15**, 1–17.
49. Schwartz, J. L. (1987) *Smoking Cessation Methods: The United States and Canada, 1978–1985*, US Dept of Health and Human Services, Washington, pp. 62–71.
50. Murray, D. M. *et al.* (1985) *CHD Risk Factor Screening and Education: A Community Approach to Prevention of Coronary Heart Disease*, Mimeo. University of Minnesota, Minneapolis.
51. Lefebvre, R. C., Lasater, R. M., Carleton, R. A. and Peterson, G. (1987) Theory and delivery of health programming in the community: the Pawtucket Heart Health Program. *Preventive Medicine*, **16**, 80–95.
52. Elder, J. P. *et al.* (1986) Organizational and community approaches to community-wide prevention of heart disease: the first two years of the Pawtucket Heart Health Program. *Preventive Medicine*, **15**, 107–17.
53. Rothman, J. (1979) Three models of community organization in practice, in: *Strategies of Community Organization*, (eds F. M. Cox *et al.*). Peacock, Chicago.
54. World Health Organization (1981) *Community Control of Cardiovascular Diseases: The North Karelia Project.* WHO, Copenhagen.
55. Puska, P. *et al.* (1985) The community-based strategy to prevent coronary heart disease: conclusions from the ten years of the North Karelia Project. *Annual Review of Public Health*, **6**, 147–93.
56. Vartiainen, E. *et al.* (1983) Effect of two years of educational intervention on adolescent smoking (the North Karelia Youth Project). *Bulletin of the World Health Organization*, **61**, 529–32.
57. McAlister, A. *et al.* (1982) Theory and action for health promotion: illustrations from the North Karelia Project. *American Journal of Public Health*, **72**, 43–55.
58. Neittaanmaki, L., Koskela, K., Puska, P. and McAlister, A. L. (1980) The role of lay workers in community health education: experiences of the North Karelia Project. *Scandinavian Journal of Social Medicine*, **8**, 1–7.
59. Puska, P. *et al.* (1986) Use of lay opinion leaders to promote diffusion of health innovations in a community programme: lessons learned from the North Karelia Project. *Bullein of the World Health Organization*, **64**, 437–46.
60. Puska, P. *et al.* (1981) Health knowledge and community prevention of coronary heart disease. *International Journal of Health Education*, **XXIV**, (Supplement).
61. Koskela, K. (1981) *A Community-Based Antismoking Programme as a Part of a Comprehensive Cardiovascular Programme (The North Karelia Project)*, University of Kuopio, Finland.
62. Salonen, J. T., Hamynen, H. and Heinonen, O. P. (undated) *Impact of a Health Education Programme and Other Factors on Stopping Smoking after Heart Attack*, mimeo. University of Kuopio, Finland.

63. Salonen, J. T. *et al.* (1983) Decline in mortality from coronary heart disease in Finland from 1969 to 1979. *British Medical Journal*, **286**, 1857–60.
64. Tuomilehto, J. *et al.* (1986) Decline in cardiovascular mortality in North Karelia and other parts of Finland. *British Medical Journal*, **293**, 1068–71.
65. Salonen, J. T. (1987) Did the North Karelia Project reduce coronary mortality? Letter to the Editor. *Lancet*, **ii**, 269.
66. Oliver, M. F. (1987) Letter to the Editor. *Lancet*, **ii**, 518.
67. Holme, I., Hermann, M. D., Helgeland, A. and Leren, P. (1985) The Oslo Study: diet and antismoking advice. *Preventive Medicine*, **14**, 279–92.
68. World Health Organization Collaborative Group (1970) Multifactorial trial in the prevention of coronary heart disease. *European Heart Journal*, **1**, 73–9.

INDEX